Differential Therapeutics in Psychiatry:

The Art and Science of Treatment Selection

Differential Therapeutics in Psychiatry:

The Art and Science of Treatment Selection

By

Allen Frances, M.D.
John Clarkin, Ph.D.
Samuel Perry, M.D.

BRUNNER/MAZEL, *Publishers* • New York

Library of Congress Cataloging in Publication Data

Frances, Allen, 1942–
  Differential therapeutics in psychiatry.

  Bibliography: p.
  Includes index.
  1. Psychotherapy – Decision making. 2. Psychiatry –
Case Studies. I. Clarkin, John F., 1938–
II. Perry, Samuel. III. Title. [DNLM: 1. Mental dis-
orders – Therapy   WM 400 F815d]
  RC480.5.F675 1984   616.89   84-5883
  ISBN 0-87630-360-2

Published by
BRUNNER/MAZEL, INC.
19 Union Square West
New York, New York 10003

To
Vera, Audrey, and Anna
and to
Craig and Bobby,
Kevin and Brian, and
Maren, Kimberly and Daniel

Contents

About the Authors

Allen Frances, M.D., did his psychiatric training at the Columbia Presbyterian Medical Center and the New York State Psychiatric Institute. He completed his psychoanalytic training at the Columbia University Psychoanalytic Center for Training and Research and is now on its Faculty. Dr. Frances is also Associate Professor of Psychiatry at the Cornell University Medical College and Director of the Outpatient Department at the Payne Whitney Clinic of New York Hospital. He is Vice-Chairman of the Program Committee of the American Psychiatric Association and was a member of the DSM-III Personality Disorders Advisory Committee. Dr. Frances' major research interests have been in the areas of personality disorder and depression. He has also written widely on differential treatment selection and contributes a regular column on this topic for the journal, *Hospital and Community Psychiatry*.

John Clarkin earned his Ph.D. in Clinical Psychology from Fordham University. He completed his clinical psychology internship training at the New York State Psychiatric Institute and advanced training in family intervention at the Nathan W. Ackerman Family Institute. Formerly the director of the Outpatient Department of the Payne Whitney Clinic of New York Hospital, he is currently Director of Psychology, the New York Hospital-Westchester Division, and Associate Professor of Clinical Psychology at the Cornell University Medical College. Dr. Clarkin has edited a volume on behavioral treatments for depression and written on topics including the symptomatology of depression and borderline personality disorders, brief therapy, family therapy and differential treatment planning. He is currently co-investigator on an NIMH-supported research project on the efficacy of family therapy in an inpatient setting.

Samuel Perry, M.D., is Associate Professor of Clinical Psychiatry at Cornell University Medical College, Associate Director of the Consultation-Liaison Division at The New York Hospital, and Collaborating Psychoanalyst at The Columbia Psychoanalytic Center for Training and Research. His articles have addressed issues of medical student and psychiatric residency education, the management of acute psychotic states and the assaultive patient, selection criteria for the different psychotherapies, the pharmacological and psychological treatment of pain, and the psychodynamics of play. He is presently completing a five-year NIH-supported investigation of analgesia for burn patients and is launching a study of psychobiological responses to stress and loss by documenting psychological and physiological changes in parents of burned children.

Acknowledgments

This book is founded on a lesson we were taught by two very different groups of informants — our patients and our children. The lesson is that one never has much success in arranging plans for another unless the other person genuinely feels included in the decision-making process. Over the years, our patients have also taught us about treatment planning in other ways: They have told us what did or did not work in their past treatments and have offered explanations about why this was so; they have suggested new plans that at times to us made no sense; and they have refused to go along with our plans even when they seemed well conceived. In short, they have worked and argued and negotiated with us to settle on plans we could share; in so doing, they have allowed us the opportunity to watch how each treatment did or did not prove wise. These and many other shared experiences have enriched our lives in ways that are familiar to all psychotherapists.

We are also grateful to the Payne Whitney Clinic. Our colleagues have shown an unusual tolerance for diversity and uncertainty, while maintaining a scientific curiosity about how decisions are and should be made. By virtue of its location and reputation, Payne Whitney draws a patient population that is remarkably varied. The many case illustrations that we hope will bring life to these pages could only come from a clinic that is confronted daily with a wide range of presenting problems, diagnoses and treatment needs for those with very different social, family, ethnic, and economic backgrounds.

We cannot possibly mention the many teachers and colleagues who have in one way or another had an important impact on this book. Though the list may appear quite long, in our minds we have mentioned only a few: Nathan Ackerman, Anne Anastasi, Gordon Ball, Harvey Barten, Richard Brown, Arthur Carr, Arnold Cooper, Leonard Diamond, Richard Druss, Richard Frances, Shervert Frazier, William Frosch, Robert Glick, Howard Hunt, Helen Singer Kaplan, James Kocsis, Lawrence Kolb, Donald Kornfeld, Aaron Lazare, Robert Liebert, Roger MacKinnon, John Mann, Robert Michels, Mary Mylenki, Ethel Person, Arthur Phillips, Richard Rabkin, Phyllis Rubinton, Michael Sacks, Richard Sallick, Leon Salzman, Harold Searles, Kathy Shear, Robert Spitzer, Sanford Stevens, John Talbott, Milton Viederman, John Weber, and, of course, our parents.

The difficulties of a three-authored book were far outweighed by the education and support each of us received from the others. Most of the time we were pretty good-natured about disagreements and the book represents our collective wisdom, such as it is.

Carelyn Kane, Nancy Shepherd, and Lillian Conklin were remarkably clever, patient, and forgiving in deciphering scribbles that have bemused and bewildered our teachers ever since third grade. Finally, we are grateful to our editors, Ann Alhadeff and Susan Barrows, for their many helpful suggestions and gentle proddings.

A.F.
J.C.
S.P.

Foreword

The easiest way to practice psychiatry is to view all patients and problems as basically the same, and to apply one standard therapy or mix of therapies for their treatment. Although some may still employ this model, everything we have learned in recent decades tells us that it is wrong — wrong for our patients in that it deprives them of the most effective treatment, and wrong for everyone else in that it wastes scarce resources. We have progressed to the point where we can recognize and describe differences among patients, their disorders, and the problems that they bring to us; and we have developed an array of treatments along with different modes and settings for delivering them. We can help most of our patients, and most of our treatments are effective. Indeed, recent research suggests that we are easily on a par with other areas of medicine in this regard. However, not all treatments are equally effective for all patients. Our success brings with it the happy problem of developing a strategy for selecting the right treatment for each patient. The emerging field of differential therapeutics in psychiatry is the subject of this book.

The authors are experienced clinicians who are familiar with a wide array of patients, clinical settings, treatment philosophies, and the practical problems of integrating these. They have worked in inpatient, outpatient, and general hospital settings, in clinics and private practice, and are trained in psychoanalysis, various psychotherapies, family therapy, psychopharmacology, and psychodiagnostic testing. They have also conducted research on treatment evaluation, and know the strengths, the limitations, and the potential for knowledge from this source. Finally, they are master teachers and have a special skill in communicating what they know to others who are new to the field.

They discuss what kind of information is helpful for selecting a treatment plan – diagnostic, characterologic, historic, social, and situational – and how to collect and organize it. Their book then guides us through the complex matrix of relationships between goals, systems amenable to intervention, and capacities on the one hand and settings, formats, and processes of treatment on the other. It provides a modern approach to consideration of multiple treatments and treatment combinations, a welcome relief to a field cluttered by contradictory clinical maxims that reflect years of experience in making the same errors over and over again. In doing all of this, the authors draw on both clinical experience and research data, summarizing and critiquing what is known from each and particularly what is relevant to the practical problems that the consultant faces today.

Experienced clinicians will see this book as an opportunity to test their judgment against others, and to extend their knowledge with a critical, forced review of the research literature. Researchers will have a summary of the critical issues that make a difference in clinical practice. Students will have an introduction to strategies of clinical thinking, current professional practice, and new research findings, along with a wealth of clinical material to illustrate the issues.

This is the first textbook of differential therapeutics in psychiatry; it will certainly not be the last. I cannot imagine a more promising beginning. Future works will be measured against it. We are indebted to them for setting so high a standard.

Robert Michels, M.D.
Professor and Chairman, Department of Psychiatry
Cornell University Medical College;
Psychiatrist-in-Chief, New York Hospital

Introduction

Mrs. D. is a 45-year-old woman who begins her initial consultation by revealing that recently she has become seriously depressed for the first time in her life. The therapist soon learns that her youngest child has just left for college, that Mrs. D. suspects her husband is having an extramarital affair, and that her mother has had a series of depressions, each of which required hospitalization. Although she describes her problems in an entirely coherent manner, Mrs. D. looks distraught and complains of feeling preoccupied; she has been unable to sleep for more than a few hours at a time. She wonders if someone so helpless and worthless as she deserves to go on living.

Mrs. D.'s clinical presentation is familiar enough and, after a more thorough examination, the consultant readily arrives at an Axis I diagnosis of unipolar major depressive disorder with melancholia. In fact, with the recent availability of the Diagnostic and Statistical Manual, Third Edition, psychiatric diagnosis has become for many patients the most straightforward and reliable of the consultant's decisions. Far more difficult, unreliable, and controversial will be the decision about how best to treat Mrs. D. This really involves a series of related decisions. What is the optimal *setting* for treatment – a hospital? a day hospital? a crisis intervention program? Or can she make do with a regularly scheduled appointment to a therapist's office? What *format* or formats of treatment would be most helpful – individual therapy? group therapy? and/or family therapy? What theoretical approach or combination of approaches would be most applicable in understanding Mrs. D.'s problems and in planning interventions – a psychobiological model? a psychodynamic model? a behavioral model? a cognitive model? and/or a systems theory model? What should be the *intensity* and *duration* of treatment – every day for three weeks? once a week for three months?

four times a week for five years? Should medication be prescribed? What particular *combination of treatments* might be most advantageous — crisis intervention and pharmacotherapy? individual and marital therapy? marital therapy and environmental manipulation? Or perhaps the risks of treatment outweigh its potential benefits and no treatment at all is the prescription of choice. The consultant will judge what makes the most sense for this patient based on his own clinical experience, on what the patient wants, and also on the research evidence about treatment outcome for her particular problems.

We are well aware that the present knowledge about differential therapeutics is woefully incomplete and the topic remains highly controversial. Our motivation for writing this book emerged from the discovery that no reference source is available that discusses comprehensively the many issues that arise when choosing a method of treatment. We began working together at the Payne Whitney Clinic of The New York Hospital some seven years ago and assumed responsibility for all of the treatment assignments for the 100 or so new psychiatric patients who presented for evaluation each week at the outpatient clinic, emergency room, and consultation liaison service. We resolved to resist the temptation to refer patients to a particular treatment merely because it happened to be the one currently most available in our system. A policy that allows referrals to group or individual or other kinds of therapy *only* because the modality has "open slots" may be necessary in some settings, but is shoddy on clinical grounds and provides a poor model for trainees. Instead, we wanted the treatment programs offered by our hospital to be a dependent variable that would be molded gradually by the independent variable of patient need. We realized that this ideal would be limited, to some degree at least, by our available resources and perhaps to an even greater degree by our limited ability to devise what works best for particular patient problems.

The resolution to consider carefully our assignment of cases left us with the task of reviewing all new patients seen by our staff and trainees, discussing with them the various possible treatment options, and deciding upon an optimal, or at least acceptable, intervention. Of course, we had notions of our own — often very strong ones — based upon our interests, training, and clinical experiences, and were concerned about the possible influence of our own personal biases and limitations. One author (AF) is a psychiatrist and psychoanalyst who works primarily with outpatients; another author (JC) is a more behaviorally oriented psychologist and family therapist; and the third (SP) is a psychoanalytically trained psychiatrist whose main clinical area is in a general hospital working with physically ill patients. In an attempt to avoid imposing our own (perhaps too narrow) outlook upon our clinical services and patients, we began to search and study the literature on treatment outcome. Unfortunately, our plan to gather and integrate the opinions of leading commentators and to integrate these with the available scientific research yielded a surprisingly sparse and often bewildering yield. We had not expected there to be such a paucity of substantial and relevant discussions about why one treatment should be selected as opposed to another.

Upon reflecting upon our own training and teaching, we realized some of the reasons for the lack of attention in the literature to questions regarding differential therapeutics. Mental health trainees typically receive little education in the principles and practice of choosing a treatment modality. Too often treatment assignments are made routinely, based on customary practices, and with little discussion. Trainees are frequently asked to recommend a treatment choice from among a variety of treatment alternatives that they themselves have never had occasion to perform. Moreover, the assumptions behind recommendations may remain unclear, unspecified, and of uncertain validity. In our experience, the trainee and supervisor are likely to spend the bulk of their time together discussing phenomenology or psychodynamics. The discussion about the choice of treatment, if it comes up at all, is often tagged on to the waning moments and is dealt with as a practical necessity rather than an important part of the teaching.

As therapists interested in understanding our own behavior and that of others, we should try to explain the reluctance of the mental health profession to become more involved in the process of establishing guidelines for treatment selection. The importance of the topic is hard to deny. Most people present to a psychiatric clinic for help at what is likely to be their worst moment. They are in the midst of some crisis, have tried all sorts of solutions and advice without benefit, and are more or less at their wits' end. In the more desperate situations the particulars of treatment selection may mean the difference between life or death, sanity or madness, happiness or misery. Even the more commonplace decisions probably count in some way or other. If the middle-aged, unhappy housewife described above is referred to individual as opposed to family or group therapy, and receives or does not receive medication, these decisions could strongly shape the ultimate outcome of her treatment and her life. Different treatment experiences may provide radically different models of problem-solving and of human interaction and may shape attitudes in radically different ways (Bond and Lieberman, 1978). Why, then, has the field resisted investigating in more detail the process of differential treatment selection?

One reason for this reluctance is that, in some settings, the effort may appear to be an impractical, academic exercise. Those who administer an overworked and understaffed mental health clinic know that the facility can survive only if the hordes of new patients are assigned quickly enough to make room for the next wave of arrivals. In these circumstances, the assumptions that influence the choice of treatment are often not articulated or explored – in part because there is little time, in part because there is little choice. Treatment decisions then become a function of habit or availability; if group therapy is the clinic's specialty or is more available than other alternatives that particular week, everyone becomes a good candidate for a group. The excuse of having little time and limited facilities is an understandable, but we believe unacceptable, reason to avoid discussion about how various treatment decisions are made. Even if, as is often and perhaps always the case, the final treatment decision must be a compromise with resource availability, the selection of treatment should not be made expeditiously, unobtrusively, or as a matter of routine. When compromises are necessary, it should be recognized why and how they have been forged.

A second type of resistance to examining differential therapeutics is less administrative and more personal. Therapists are understandably unlikely to consider treatment modalities that they are not trained or inclined to do. Mental health clinicians have worked hard to become experts, but in most instances they are expert in only a few of the expanding variety of available treatment techniques. They are naturally committed to what they know and do best and are likely to formulate the problems of their patients within the context of their own training, interest, and skills. Therapists tend to recommend preferentially the treatment they have to offer rather than to consider systematically each of the alternative possibilities. As a result, the final choice of treatment is often determined more by the particular referral patterns that bring a patient to one or another consultant than by anything inherent in the patient's symptoms or character. The patient who presents himself to a psychoanalyst, a group therapist, and a family therapist may well receive three reasonable, but mutually contradictory, recommendations based more on the outlook of the consultant than on the specifics of the patient's problems or an appraisal of the literature concerned with treatment outcome.

A third resistance to considering differential therapeutics stems from the belief that any attempt to establish criteria for treatment selection is potentially dangerous. It is feared that guidelines for treatment selection are liable to encourage premature closure despite the fact that available research data do not yet warrant anything approaching firm conclusions. Many practitioners worry that criteria will be carved in stone (on the basis of scanty evidence) and that clinical judgment will be overruled by bureaucratic procedure sanctified by pseudoscience. Third-party payers will take advantage of any further treatment selection criteria in order to fund only the least expensive acceptable modality. Before long, a clinical and intellectual issue will have become primarily a financial one. Because this apprehension is understandably pervasive within the mental health professions, each aspect of the argument – the paucity of research, the premature closure, and third-party restrictions – is worth discussing in more detail.

What about these possible objections to a thorough discussion of different treatment selections? Regarding the existing shortage of outcome research, we do not believe that we or our patients can wait indefinitely for results to accumulate before attempting to summarize the current state of knowledge and art. The complexities of psychotherapy outcome research (to be discussed in Chapter 8) ensure that definitive findings will be extremely long in coming and will probably always be to some extent inconclusive. Research investigations generally measure the characteristics of whole populations and generate results that cannot be applied to any given individual without consideration of that patient's uniqueness. Furthermore, while the history of medicine reminds us that accepted clinical judgment is often very wide of the mark, an informed clinical decision is undoubtedly superior to blind chance as a guide to treatment. While we wait for more substantial data, decisions about treatment must be made – and, of course, are being made every day. It has become a necessary part of the therapist's task to follow in a critical manner the latest in research findings and to apply them as best he can to day-to-day clinical work. We hope that this book will help to foster an empirical orientation and motivate clinicians to study this inherently interesting topic. In sum, we think that the limitations of current research provide a reason to discuss treatment selection rather than a reason to avoid it.

Regarding the objection that our efforts may result in premature closure and rigidity, our intention is quite the opposite. The book is not designed in such a way that the current ignorance about differential therapeutics can be disguised under an elaborate and cumbersome system of criteria indicating who should have what treatment. On the contrary, by relying heavily on illustrative cases and discussing the various competing considerations in choosing a treatment plan, we hope to encourage debate and emphasize areas of controversy and ignorance rather than to sanctify simple (and therefore silly) rules of conduct that do not do justice to the complexity of the clinical situation.

Regarding the objection that the examination of differential therapeutics is liable to have a detrimental effect on the support rendered by third-party payers and governmental funding agencies, the concern that this book might incite new trouble is naive. The interest of outside agencies in regulating psychotherapy is already present and growing rapidly. The U.S. Senate has entertained numerous discussions and proposals intending in some way or other to guarantee that patients receive what is documented to be an effective psychiatric treatment at manageable cost. The U.S. Office of Technology Assessment (1980) has prepared a statement summarizing the difficulties involved in evaluating the effectiveness and cost benefit ratios of various forms of psychotherapy. The American Psychiatric Association has established a Commission on Psychotherapies charged with pursuing these questions, hopes to publish a monograph on treatment planning, and has already published one on psychotherapy research (APA, 1982). The National Institute of Mental Health is actively engaged in supporting research on the outcome of psychotherapy and in determining how best to apply the data being gathered to national health policy issues. Differential therapeutics has received increasing attention on all fronts during the past decade and simply cannot be avoided. The question is no longer *whether* to discuss and investigate treatment selection, but *how*.

Finally, a more interesting resistance to examining differential therapeutics stems from the profound, but rarely expressed, belief that the choice of particular treatment does not really matter all that much — that what really matters is the match between the therapist and patient. Thirty years ago, Nolan D.C. Lewis said that the right technique with the wrong therapist will do less good than the wrong technique with the right therapist. This statement is supported by many studies in the psychotherapy outcome literature that have failed to document specific effects of specific treatment techniques. Although we agree that the referring clinician is wise to use intuition when deciding who should treat whom, we must not assume that the match of personalities is all that is important. This is an unsubstantiated notion that can lead to idiosyncratic and thoughtless technique with the rationalization that therapy is all art and chemistry and no science.

A corollary to the position that all that matters is "a good relationship" is the argument that the healing properties of the different treatments are much the same; that is, no matter what the theoretical orientation and no matter what the therapists claim they are doing, the essential techniques and results are barely distinguishable. Jerome Frank (1978) has for many years insisted that basic healing properties are shared by all psychotherapeutic situations; i.e., in a state of high tension a client visits a wise authority who is rich with experiences, perhaps has overcome similar problems, and has acquired special powers; the client's problem is explained within the context of an ideology accepted by both; and a healing ceremony leads to relief.

There is much experimental data in support of Frank's views. One study (Sloane, Staples, Cristol, Yorkston, and Whipple, 1975) demonstrated that, although behavior therapists and brief dynamic therapists are very different in their approaches, the two types of therapy achieve similar results. Even more interesting, the patients in the two study groups perceived their therapists and treatments as being similar and rated as effective aspects of therapy that were common to both. Of note, the two modes of treatment were far apart in their origin (academic psychology vs. psychiatry), in their theoretical orientation (learning theory vs. psychodynamics), in their conception of a person and what cures him or her, and probably in the temperament of the therapists attracted to each field. Nonetheless, even though therapists of each school might argue adamantly about technical issues, this study suggested that the fine points of technique may not be the crucial factors in determining treatment outcome. The argument that treatments are more alike than different is also supported by the finding that more experienced therapists, despite their theoretical differences, resemble each other more in practice than do the neophytes in each school, who are more likely to maintain a caricature of technical purity.

If the crucial healing ingredients are more or less present in all treatments, is it worthwhile to pursue differential therapeutics and to attempt to specify the indications for one or another form of therapy? Obviously, we have forged ahead and think the effort has merit. Without ignoring the evidence that many treatments share the same therapeutic qualities, we believe each particular approach is likely to have its own advantages and disadvantages, benefits and risks, and to require different things from the patient. Some studies have already demonstrated the importance of choosing one approach instead of another, and we will cite these references throughout the text. As research designs become more sophisticated and specific studies demonstrate more specific treatment effects, it seems likely that an increasing awareness of the differential effectiveness of specific methods of treatment for particular problems will gradually come to inform clinical practice.

We do not deny the cogency of the reasons for caution in any discussion of the topic of treatment selection – that it is sometimes an impractical academic exercise, may constitute a threat to what the therapist can and wants to do, is potentially conducive to premature closure and rigid regulation, and may perhaps be unnecessary since a good relationship or nonspecific factors are so influential in determining treatment outcome. However, we also believe that, despite the obstacles, complexity, and insufficient available data, responsible clinical decision-making requires a careful consideration of the process of treatment selection. We hope that this book will enrich and inform such considerations.

ORGANIZATION

We have chosen an organization for this book that departs radically from the one routinely adopted by peer review manuals meant to be used in evaluating psychiatric treatment selection (APA, 1976). Peer review manuals list the possible treatment options considered to be appropriate for each diagnosis. Because so many psychiatric treatments are potentially appropriate for almost every DSM-III diagnosis, virtually the same lineup of recommendations is repeated over and over again. We believe that it is more useful to base the organization of our discussion on the treatments themselves and to outline the situations in which they are likely to be most useful.

This choice reflects the limited role of psychiatric diagnosis in treatment planning. As a medical specialty advances understanding of etiology, pathogenesis, and treatment effects, its nosology provides an increasingly clear call to specific interventions. In other medical specialties, diagnosis often leads directly to a specific plan of action: antibiotics for a strep throat, digitalis for congestive heart failure, surgery for a nonruptured but inflamed appendix, and so on. In psychiatry, few treatments are so closely linked to a particular diagnosis. Even though lithium may be the standard treatment for bipolar affective illness, phenothiazines for schizophrenia with hallucinations, sex therapy for premature ejaculation, and behavioral therapy for an isolated fear of flying, more often the psychiatric diagnosis by itself does not provide enough information to be comprehensive. Even these well established indications do not preclude alternative choices or include all possible necessary interventions.

In most instances, psychiatric treatment cannot be directed simply at the disorder; it must be tailored for the person and circumstances and also for the multiply interacting factors that influence how the patient is reacting to pathological processes and stressors. Close attention to the person beyond the diagnosis is well in line with the actual process of decision-making followed by most clinicians. When a patient presents with panic attacks and a fear of leaving home, the consultant goes beyond the psychiatric diagnosis to ask a number of questions about treatment: Does this patient require imipramine to alleviate the panic attacks? diazepam for the expectant anxiety? Does the patient have the psychological mindedness and clarity of conflict suitable for a dynamically oriented treatment? Will the patient expose himself to anxiety in a behavioral therapy? And other questions follow. In matching the patient's personal history, beliefs, values, and interpersonal style with the techniques, demands, and goals of the various treatments, the therapist considers aspects of the patient not included even within the five axes for DSM-III diagnosis.

The limitations of psychiatric diagnosis in predicting treatment are also a function of the relative lack of available knowledge about the syndromes that have thus far been described and differentiated from one another. The psychiatric syndromes of DSM-III are for the most part no more than collections of isolated symptoms that have been observed, clinically or in research studies, to correlate with one another and to occur together in the same patients. Although there is some hope that patients classed within each syndrome are relatively homogeneous in their etiology, course, prognosis, and treatment needs, little documentation supports this for most DSM-III diagnoses. It is often wise to focus attention primarily on the target symptoms included within the diagnostic label rather than to attach too much importance to the label itself. This is especially true for the many atypical patients who do not fall neatly into any of the existing categories. They should not be shoehorned to make for a tidy but unreliable and inaccurate fit. Treatment selection should be more closely addressed to target symptoms and not to a diagnostic label, especially when none of the labels fits very well. Whenever there is a heated argument about whether a patient is "schizophrenic" or "affective," it is wise to assume that neither categorization will be very helpful in this case and instead to treat the target symptoms in the context of the patient's overall circumstances. The insistence in arriving at a diagnosis of "schizophrenic" or "affective" or "schizoaffective" disorder for the atypical patient will add little of value to the process of treatment selection and reflects rather than resolves our confusion about such patients.

Although we have not used psychiatric diagnosis as a means of organizing this book, we do not underestimate its importance or support the past neglect that led to idiosyncratic decisions with negligible reliability among various centers across the country and abroad. We are enthusiastic about DSM-III, have worked on its development, and believe that often it does provide an important first step in treatment planning. It must be realized, however, that although DSM-III has achieved remarkably increased reliability, it cannot include many variables that are crucial in deciding about the choice of treatment. It is more efficient to consider the differential advantages of the various treatments than to attempt definitive treatment plans for each psychiatric diagnosis.

This book also differs in organization and intent from peer review manuals in another important way. These manuals are designed to eliminate treatment methods that are so far wide of the mark as to be deemed inappropriate. The goal of this book is quite different. By reviewing the literature and different current practices, our aim is to go beyond discussing what modalities seem appropriate and to determine what kind of treatment is potentially the best. By analogy, we want to find out not only what kinds of treatment might hit the target, but also, on the basis of available evidence and thoughtful reflection, what treatments have the best chance of hitting the bull's-eye. As we consider various clinical situations and wrestle with the distinction between what method of treatment is suitable and what method is most desirable, we hope to remind others and ourselves that the least expensive acceptable treatment is by no means necessarily the treatment of choice.

The book contains one chapter for each step in the decision tree that leads to a complete treatment plan, i.e., chapters on the choice of treatment setting, format, orientation, intensity and duration and medication, as well as one that discusses ways in which these treatment components are combined. One chapter is devoted to a discussion of no treatment as the prescription of choice. Another discusses how research informs differential therapeutics. There are chapters outlining the ways in which the clinical evaluation and psychological testing contribute to the data base upon which treatment decisions can be made. There is a chapter on methods of teaching differential therapeutics. Case presentations have been sprinkled liberally throughout the book because we believe that they constitute the second best way of improving and learning treatment selection skills. (The best way, of course, is actual clinical experience.)

The book presents suggestions for treatment selection that are based upon our reading of the research literature, the opinions of leading practitioners, and our own clinical experience. We will outline what we regard to be the most useful indications, patient enabling factors, and relative contraindications for each of the settings, formats, orientations, and durations that are discussed. By and large, the suggested guidelines are tentative and unproven. They need to be refined and superseded as evidence accumulates from increasingly specific treatment outcome studies. But for now, we have found that the process of writing this book has made an important contribution to our clinical decisions. We will be satisfied if this experience is also shared by our readers.

Differential Therapeutics in Psychiatry:

The Art and Science of Treatment Selection

CHAPTER 1

The Setting

The first step in planning a psychiatric treatment involves choosing the setting in which that treatment will occur. Although decisions about therapeutic setting are also pertinent in medical and surgical treatment planning (Should a patient be transferred to the intensive care unit? Should the minor surgery be performed in the operating room or in the doctor's office? etc.), the setting plays a particularly important part in the delivery of psychiatric treatments. In many instances, the setting chosen will itself provide an important element in the treatment (e.g., the structure and organization that only a total environment like an inpatient service or day hospital can confer on a patient's life). Moreover, the setting will always be, to a greater or lesser extent, a limiting factor in deciding what combinations of formats, orientations, and duration of treatment are possible.

Not infrequently, the urgency of a clinical situation demands that the decision about setting be made promptly and with relatively limited information available. The unavoidable uncertainty occasioned by such situations is all the more troubling because this choice may well have the most profound influence on the patient's treatment and prognosis. Whether or not a suicidal patient is hospitalized can literally be a matter of life or death. Conversely, if unnecessary hospitalization is recommended in preference to outpatient treatment, the iatrogenic social, legal, and financial repercussions may have serious and enduring adverse effects. Psychiatric hospitalization still carries certain prejudices, may predispose future consultants to suggest repeated hospitalizations, and may perpetuate the regressive process of making the individual a "career patient"—or, on the contrary, may incline the patient to avoid future help even when he or she desperately needs it. Cost is also an important and often neglected factor. The difference between

1

repeated hospitalizations for an acute illness and monthly visits to a clinic for maintenance medication can total $30,000 or more per year, a cost that is borne in one or another way (insurance rates, taxes, out-of-pocket) by the consumer.

Treatment selection is always based on many interacting variables, including age, diagnosis, severity and urgency of problems, motivation, level of prior functioning, available support and structure, response to previous treatments, and many others. With so much data to gather and weigh in a clinical situation that is pressing for timely response, we have found it useful to emphasize the following question in deciding upon the choice of therapeutic setting: *"What is to be the primary goal of this treatment at this time?"* Accordingly, we have subdivided this chapter into three sections; each considers a different primary treatment goal and the setting most appropriate to it. The first section discusses those settings in which the goal is to protect the decompensating patient and/or to resolve his/her urgent and severe problems so that he/she can return as quickly as possible to the previous level of functioning. Such *acute care* settings include: 1) intensive care psychiatric hospitals; 2) intensive care partial hospitals ("day hospitals"); 3) outpatient crisis intervention or homecare facilities. The second section discusses those settings, usually longer term and less intensive, in which the goal is helping the patient to function at a level higher than was previously obtained. Such settings for *rehabilitation* (loosely defined here) include: 1) longer term inpatient reconstructive hospitals; 2) longer term day or partial hospital rehabilitation programs; and 3) most traditional outpatient psychotherapy. The third section discusses those settings in which the goal is to maintain the severely impaired and chronic patient at the current level of functioning and thereby prevent either acute exacerbations or further insidious deterioration. The settings for *maintenance* include: 1) chronic care psychiatric hospitals; 2) chronic care partial hospitals; and 3) maintenance outpatient psychotherapy and pharmacotherapy. (See Table 1-1.)

Naturally, in actual practice these categories overlap considerably and the specific goals for any given patient often do not fall neatly into any one of the types described. For instance, the goal with an acutely delusional patient might be both to resolve the acute psychosis *and* to facilitate rehabilitation by helping to improve his marriage and job skills. Also, goals change over time. After a patient has been admitted repeatedly to inpatient facilities for acute psychotic disorganizations, the main goal of the next treatment episode should shift toward a rehabilitative model or even a maintenance model that attempts to alter

TABLE 1-1
Selection of Therapeutic Setting

Acute Care	Rehabilitation	Maintenance
1) intensive care inpatient hospital	1) longer term inpatient hospital	1) chronic care inpatient hospital
2) intensive care partial hospital	2) rehabilitation partial hospital	2) chronic care partial hospital
3) outpatient crisis intervention	3) outpatient psychotherapy	3) outpatient maintenance therapy

the patient's longitudinal course, rather than focusing on the repetitive, fruitless resolution of the acute episode.

Despite its limitations, the above scheme provides a necessary framework during the evaluation that helps to organize the data upon which to base decisions. It also makes clear that the choice of setting depends, at least in part, on the therapeutic aim and not only on the patient's psychopathology. There are many times when the sickest of psychiatric patients should not be admitted to an inpatient facility – e.g., a nonfunctioning patient with constant hallucinations and suicidal ideas whose symptoms have been present for years, have been refractory to treatment, and for whom an outpatient or partial hospital program might provide a more suitable setting. On the other hand, a successful corporate executive who is not nearly so impaired might require admission if his acute hypomanic episode is likely to lead to irreparable financial and personal damage before therapy can be effective. (See Table 1-2 for differential criteria for acute, rehabilitative, and maintenance care.)

After deciding if the primary goal of treatment is acute care, rehabilitation or maintenance, the consultant must next decide upon which of the particular available settings within the category has the best chance of meeting the goal. In order to illustrate how different variables might be balanced, we will begin each of the following sections with a case presentation describing a patient who characterizes some of the typical complex and conflicting issues that arise in deciding upon a therapeutic setting. Next, we will provide a brief description of the various settings most likely to be appropriate and the rationale for choosing among them for that particular patient. We will conclude each section by discussing how the available psychiatric research would or would not have been helpful in guiding the choice of therapeutic setting.

TABLE 1-2
Differential Criteria for Acute, Rehabilitative and Maintenance Care

Acute Care	Rehabilitation	Maintenance Care

Relative Indications
1) Patient requires attention for symptoms such as:
  (a) homicidal or suicidal behavior
  (b) acute psychotic state
  (c) unable to care for self
  (d) bizarre behavior that would ruin reputation
2) Need for supervised diagnostic tests, observations, or supervised administration of medication.
 	
Enabling Factors
1) Patient has a history or current indications of a rapid response to medications.
2) Family supports rapid, intense treatment.
	Relative Indications
	1) Chronic symptoms and long-standing character problems.
	2) Severe impairments in vocational or social performance of recent onset or extended duration.
	
	Enabling Factors
	1) Patient can gradually assume increasing vocational and social responsibility under supervision.
	2) Patient has sufficient frustration tolerance for the repetitive drilling necessary to acquire or reacquire social and vocational skills.
		Relative Indications
		1) Patient has a chronic mental illness that would require custodial care or result in patient's isolation and deterioration in the community.
		2) Patient requires a professionally organized and supervised social network.
		3) Patient requires regular treatment but would deteriorate in a more active treatment program.
		
		Enabling Factors
		1) Patient must be able to attend and form an alliance to the program, and ensure that his or her financial and living arrangements will not interfere with the program.

SETTINGS FOR ACUTE CARE

The following case illustrates the challenge and uncertainty in choosing a therapeutic setting for a despondent and bitter woman who requires prompt intensive attention for her acute problems.

THE CASE OF THE MELANCHOLIC MOTHER

Late one afternoon Mrs. A., a 52-year-old married mother of three, is brought to the hospital emergency room by her sister and husband. Wearing a wrinkled housecoat, loafers, and a make-do scarf over unbrushed hair, she paces up and down the waiting area wringing her hands and mumbling to herself. On occasion she stops, turns toward her husband, and demands boisterously to be taken home at once. When he refuses and softly tries to reassure her, she snaps irritably that "Everyone is a goddamned nuisance" and tearfully adds that she wants to be left alone to die. She greets the psychiatrist with the same disdain she has already expressed toward herself and her family. She complains that she is too young to understand her problems and that "I know for a fact that this hospital gives lousy care, but it's probably all I deserve."

The doctor ushers Mrs. A. into an adjacent room and evaluates her first alone and then with her husband and sister. Early in her marriage, Mrs. A. had experienced two severe bouts of depression, each of which required hospitalization for about two months. During the past few years, however, she has been doing very well as a conscientious mother for her adolescent children and as a part-time typist for a small business firm. Then, gradually and without apparent reason, Mrs. A. began to feel tired and listless and to skip work and dinner. For several months, she has found herself spending long periods of time in bed with severe headaches and back pain. She would cry herself to sleep only to awaken before dawn. Mrs. A. would then spend hours staring into the darkness, oppressed by the thought of another day.

When her husband tentatively suggested that she might have a recurrence of depression, Mrs. A. rejected this notion at once and refused any psychiatric treatment. Instead, she made appointments with a neurologist, a rheumatologist, an oncologist, and an endocrinologist. Although extensive medical tests revealed no physical cause for her ailments, she doubted the repeated reassurance of these specialists and became convinced that all the doctors were withholding the truth. She came to believe that she was suffering from an incurable cancer and would soon be dead. Mrs. A. had in fact dreaded cancer ever since she had watched helplessly as her mother died from cancer, slowly and in agony – "The cancer in her breast ate up her body and her mind."

Attempts by the family to comfort Mrs. A. seemed only to strengthen her conviction that they were conspiring with the doctors to deceive her. Preoccupied with trying to catch them in their lies and ruminating about her eventual fate, she became more and more distracted at work and made insignificant typographical errors which, to her, seemed of vital importance to the company. She imagined that everyone in the office was watching her every move and, indeed, her irritability, absenteeism, and withdrawal were causing concern among her coworkers. Mrs. A. took this concern to be a sign that she would and should eventually be fired. Rather than suffer this humiliation, Mrs. A. resigned abruptly. For the past six weeks, she has been at home in bed by day or pacing at night waiting impatiently for the tumor to consume her. She now wants no treatment whatsoever because she conceives her current misery as a just punishment for her sins. The thought – indeed, the pleasure – of killing herself is with her constantly but religious scruples make this escape unacceptable. Instead, she must burden her family just a while longer as she fills her remaining hours with a litany of prayers for their forgiveness.

From her husband and sister, the doctor learns that, when not depressed, Mrs. A. is a hardworking and affectionate, though somewhat fearful, person. Her previous hospitalizations occurred when she was 32 (just after the birth of her first child) and again when she was 37 (without any clear precipitant). Both times she responded well to antidepressants and the support of the hospital staff. If anything, Mrs. A. became too comfortable in the inpatient setting and was eventually frightened of returning home. Planning for discharge was stormy, as Mrs. A. developed a recurrence of symptoms and had to be virtually forced out of the hospital against her will. The reason why Mrs. A. finally was brought to the emergency room at the present moment, rather than at any time earlier during the weeks of her festering depression, became clear toward the end of the initial evaluation. The family was not particularly worried about suicide. Mrs. A. had never made an attempt and was not impulsive even when depressed. Instead, the reason for the visit was related to an unbearable tension developing within the home. Mr. A., a generally supportive husband, had lost many days of pay as a construction worker because his wife had refused to be left alone. He now felt forced to return to work and had asked the patient's sister to stay with Mrs. A. Her sister had more time, but was far less patient with Mrs. A.'s somatic complaints and constant criticism that no one was doing enough to help.

The children were also having increasing difficulty keeping their mother company, tolerating her gloom, and trying to cheer her up. On this particular day, the husband learned from his foreman that he must work overtime, the sister said she could take no more of this burden, and the children had all made plans to pursue their own interests. A visit to the hospital became the last resort.

This vignette, though brief and necessarily incomplete, helps to illustrate the issues one must consider when choosing a therapeutic setting for acutely disturbed patients. Mrs. A.'s five-axis DSM-III diagnosis was:

Axis I.   296.34 Major depression, recurrent with melancholia, with mood-congruent psychotic features
Axis II. 301.60 Dependent personality disorder with compulsive traits
Axis III. None
Axis IV. Moderate stress — "empty nest" — 4
Axis V.   Highest level of functioning past year — very good — 2

The psychiatric consultant realized very quickly that the major thrust of treatment needed to be directed at resolution of the acute problem with the goal of rapid symptom remission. The more difficult task was deciding which of the possible settings would likely be most therapeutic, least regressive, and most acceptable to Mrs. A. and her family. Each of the alternatives — inpatient care, day hospital, or crisis intervention — has advantages as well as disadvantages (see Table 1-3). We will first present a brief overview of these three possibilities before wrestling with what decision to make regarding Mrs. A.

Intensive Care Inpatient Hospital

For many years, psychiatric hospitals were considered the most obvious and safest setting in which to treat severe emotional problems. Only in the past two decades has this tradition been questioned and even those who suggest alternatives appreciate that some situations can best be managed within the confines of an intensive care hospital where medication management, seclusion, restraint, drug detoxification, and medical care are readily available. Here, a trained staff can provide maximum observation, protection, and support under the most structured and carefully monitored circumstances and, if the law permits and the occasion requires, treatment can be implemented — if absolutely

TABLE 1-3
Differential Criteria for Treatment Setting When the Goal is Acute Care

Outpatient Crisis Intervention	Intensive Care Partial Hospitalization	Intensive Inpatient

Relative Indications
1) Symptoms, distress, and risk factors severe enough to warrant urgent and intense attention—often to require hospitalization if crisis intervention is not offered. This degree of urgency could result from: suicidal threats or acts, acute psychotic symptoms, severe depression, anxiety or panic disorders, grief and/or grief reactions, excited states, somatic symptoms.
2) A major precipitating stress which provides a clear focus for the intervention. These may be:
	Relative Indications
	1) Patient would otherwise require hospitalization for:
	  (a) subacute homicidal or suicidal behavior
	  (b) acute psychotic state
	  (c) supervised diagnostic tests, observations, or supervised administration of medication
	2) Inpatient who would otherwise require a longer stay.
	
	Enabling Factors
	1) Patient is motivated to attend program.
	2) Patient is sufficiently organized to attend program or has social network intact enough to ensure treatment compliance and provide support on nights and weekends.
	3) Patient has a history or current indications of a
		Relative Indications
		1) Symptoms, distress, and risk factors severe enough to warrant urgent and intense attention, especially acute suicidal and/or homicidal behavior, violence, suicidal preoccupation, threats, attempts.
		2) Threats and/or attempts to hurt someone else physically.
		3) Severe impairments in functions such as reality testing, judgment, logical thinking and planning.
		4) Patient's condition deteriorating rapidly or failing to respond to active ambulatory intervention.
		5) Need for supervised diagnostic tests, observations, or supervised administration of medication.

(a) accidental – injury, illness, death, job loss, etc.
(b) interpersonal – an affair, bitter argument, etc.
(c) developmental – child born or goes to school, marriage, retirement, etc.
3) Relatively recent onset of symptoms.

Enabling Factors

1) Willingness to participate, keep appointments, be available for home visits, take medications, etc.
2) Social and family networks are adequate or can be mobilized.

Relative Contraindications

1) Active suicidal and/or homicidal behavior that cannot be handled on outpatient basis.

rapid response to medications.
4) Patient has a history of good outcome in partial hospitalization program.

Relative Contraindications

1) Significant organic mental syndrome.
2) Suicidal or homicidal behavior.
3) Medical illness requiring inpatient treatment.
4) Patient requires diagnostic tests and observation that can be performed only in a 24-hour hospital.
5) Patient's behavior is intolerable to or may permanently damage his social network.
6) Patient's behavior outside the program may permanently damage his reputation (for example, a manic physician who is calling all his patients).
7) Patient may require physical restraint.
8) Patient can be better managed in a less intensive treatment.

6) Pathological or noxious situation exists among family members such that initiation of treatment not possible without hospitalization.

Relative Contraindications

1) Possibility or history of regression in hospital settings.
2) Hospital addiction (e.g., patient with multiple hospitalizations who wants to check in at any crisis point).
3) Patient can be managed in less intensive treatment.
4) Stigma attached to hospitalization not worth the potential gain.
5) Financial limitations.

necessary – against the patient's will. Because these hospitals are based on a medical model (i.e., the staff treating "an illness"), the patient may be allowed and at times even encouraged to assume a sick role and to relinquish some day-to-day responsibility, while the critical situation can be decompressed and induction into a suitable treatment program in or outside the hospital can begin.

Intensive Care Partial Hospital

Although partial hospitals have been around since the 1930s, this setting of treatment emerged in the early 1960s as an important component of community-based psychiatric treatment. Partial hospitals have not met early expectations presaging the demise of the asylum (Klar, Frances, and Clarkin, 1982), but they have shown that for many patients "less can be more"; that is, less time during each day or night in the hospital is often more beneficial and less regressive than totally removing the patient from the home and work environment. The differences between intensive care inpatient and partial hospitals are to some extent differences only in degree; both offer a structured setting for evaluation, the induction into treatment, and the alleviation of acute symptoms while the crisis subsides. But the differences between the two settings are to some extent qualitative as well as quantitative. Partial hospitals are less accepting of the patient's assumption of the sick role and instead expect the patient and his family to take more responsibility in daily activities and to work toward recovery. This requirement is intended to short-circuit the propensity for regression that accompanies any illness and to mobilize the healthier aspects of the individual to deal with the problems at hand.

The partial hospital settings that serve as alternatives to acute care inpatient hospitalization are often located within the hospital setting, in some cases sharing the same physical space and staff as the inpatient ward. They tend to have a high ratio of staff to patients, to utilize the services of medical personnel, and to have relatively brief stays (Weldon and Frances, 1977). In these respects, the acute care partial hospital differs in its structure and functions from the rehabilitation and maintenance partial hospitals that are described below and resembles an inpatient unit that operates only part of the day.

Crisis Intervention

Crisis intervention is an intense, timely, brief (usually under one month), and goal-directed treatment intended to resolve a crisis of major and urgent proportions and recent onset. The treatment often requires frequent and prolonged sessions, 24-hour staff availability, rapidly increasing dosages of psychotropic medications, home visits, mobilization of family members and other community resources, environmental manipulations, and a multidisciplinary team. For severely disturbed patients, the most frequent differential treatment alternative to crisis intervention is inpatient or partial hospitalizations. Toward the other end of the severity spectrum, patients experiencing distress that is not urgent may be managed in the less intense formats of brief or longer term therapy. Urgency may result from suicidal or homicidal threats or acts, psychosis, severe depression, anxiety or panic disorders, grief, excited states, or somatic symptoms. Critical enabling factors include an adequate social and family network and a willingness to participate, keep appointments, be available for home visits, and take medication.

This brief review of the acute care inpatient, day hospital, and crisis intervention settings allows us to consider which option might be most suitable for Mrs. A. There are a number of very good reasons to hospitalize Mrs. A. First and foremost, her past depressions have responded well to hospitalizations. If this setting has worked before, the chances are good that it will work again. The best predictor of future treatment response is past performance. Furthermore, she has adamantly refused the psychiatric treatment or medication that has been suggested by her family. She is unlikely to cooperate with any form of outpatient therapy and is a high risk not to take her medicine as prescribed. Although Mrs. A. has not yet made any suicide attempt, this possibility cannot be discounted, since she is experiencing severe depression, agitation, and insomnia. The likelihood of suicide also increases as she continues to deteriorate at home. Mrs. A.'s despair is causing and is partly caused by increasing tension among family members, who are gradually diminishing their support. Hospitalization would provide better protection and observation, as well as an opportunity to free the family of a responsibility laden with guilt and ambivalence. Finally, if medication or ECT is to be used, the hospital setting can more easily provide the necessary close monitoring for side effects and adverse reactions.

There are also many good reasons not to hospitalize Mrs. A. She is reluctant to pursue any psychiatric treatment and she may become all the more resistant if this seemingly drastic recommendation is made. Moreover, the alliance between consultant and patient is already fragile and may strain beyond the breaking point if a battle develops over hospitalization. Mrs. A. is not at high enough risk to be eligible for involuntary commitment (at least in New York State), so any decision about inpatient care will require her acceptance and active participation. Moreover, because of Mrs. A.'s resignation from work and the subsequent financial strain, neither she nor her husband are currently carrying a health insurance policy to pay for hospitalization. To complicate matters even further, both husband and sister argue vehemently against and insist that they will not accept transfer to a less expensive municipal facility. Their attitude is fueled by the guilt they share for "betraying" and "abandoning" Mrs. A. by bringing her to the hospital for evaluation. A final and perhaps most telling reservation about hospitalizing Mrs. A. is that previously she became very dependent on the inpatient environment and had appreciable difficulty leaving it to return home.

A day hospital might avoid this regressive pull and Mrs. A. might accept this alternative as the lesser evil. She has a reliable family who agree to watch her carefully to insure that she gets to the program and takes any prescribed medication. The major disadvantage of the day hospital is the likelihood that her suspiciousness and resistance to treatment will prevail and prevent her participation or even attendance in the program. In spite of the family's efforts, she may not cooperate and appear for treatment each day. The family members might then become even more angry at Mrs. A. for staying sick and frustrating them, angry at themselves for being unable to make her better or even accomplish their assignment,and angry at the psychiatric consultant and the day hospital for suggesting a plan that could not really be implemented. Without further support for Mrs. A. or her family, the situation could deteriorate even further.

Crisis intervention as an option would be even more acceptable to Mrs. A., would require less from her and be less disruptive to her life, would make the family feel less guilty about relinquishing their responsibility, and would be the least expensive. And even if crisis intervention proved to be insufficient, it might facilitate Mrs. A.'s eventual acceptance of hospitalization. Crisis intervention is a flexible choice – Mrs. A. can always be hospitalized later if it becomes clear that this is necessary. On the other hand, crisis intervention would provide the least structure, observation, medical management, and protection from suicidal impulses, and it might stress rather than relieve a family already under great pressure as a result of Mrs. A.'s illness.

The difficulty in choosing among the three alternatives reveals that for Mrs. A. each might be reasonably suitable. If she were more acutely suicidal, more medically ill, less surrounded by a supportive family, or less likely to regress in hospital, then inpatient admission would be most indicated. Day hospital would be chosen over crisis intervention if there were very strong reasons to get her away from home and family for at least part of each day. Perhaps she has had too narrow a social network even when not acutely ill, or requires gradual separation from her children upon whom she has become too dependent, or needs prevocational evaluation and training. Crisis intervention is often the best first choice in situations that are not so dangerously emergent that more immediate structuring is clearly required. In addition to its therapeutic impact, crisis intervention provides a means of gathering the information necessary for making more informed decisions.

A partial hospital was chosen as the therapeutic setting most indicated for the treatment of Mrs. A. This decision was made jointly by the evaluating psychiatrist and the family (and with the passive acceptance of Mrs. A.). She had refused to take a more active part, claiming, "It makes no difference anyway," and "I'm too sick to make decisions." The psychiatrist believed that Mrs. A. was too enmeshed with her family to accept complete hospitalization, could not be committed, and did not have any pressing medical or psychiatric risks requiring the expense of around-the-clock observation and care. The husband and sister convinced him, however, that they were stressed beyond their limits, had no reserve left to participate in a crisis intervention program, and needed more relief and time for themselves than such a regimen could provide. In addition, despite her withdrawal and suspiciousness, Mrs. A. was willing to cooperate throughout the interview and to reveal her preoccupations and despair. This relatedness suggested a capacity to establish at least the beginnings of a working alliance with the staff and to comply with the daily program of a partial hospital. Accordingly, before going home, Mrs. A. briefly visited the day hospital, met some of the staff members and patients, and took her first dose of medication. She was brought back early the next morning by her husband on his way to work and picked up that afternoon by her sister.

As it turned out, Mrs. A. did remarkably well. In the day hospital, she was assigned to a young female therapist, to whom she immediately developed a strong attachment. The therapist, while investigating the stimulus for this instant positive transference, uncovered the circumstances that might have been important precipitants of Mrs. A.'s profound depression. Four months prior to admission Mrs. A.'s teenage daughter had taken a part-time job after school. For Mrs. A. this event represented the eventual loss of her only daughter, a loss that symbolically recapitulated the loss of Mrs. A.'s mother. Mrs. A.'s conviction that she had cancer was in part a sympathetic identification that continued her attachment to her mother. Interestingly, Mrs. A.'s first depression had occurred after the birth of this same daughter (who was named after Mrs. A.'s mother) and her second depression occurred shortly after this daughter started grade school. In short, the symbolic loss of Mrs. A.'s growing daughter replayed the painful and unresolved loss of Mrs. A.'s mother.

The combination of this dynamic understanding, therapeutic levels of imipramine, and the setting of the partial hospital helped Mrs. A. deal with her problems of separation and loss and recover from her depression. By spending time both at home and away from home Mrs. A. was able to experience the pain of separation concretely and discuss these difficulties with the staff. The family sessions helped to both reunite the family members and at the same time confront the issues about inevitable separation of children from parents. Mr. and Mrs. A. participated together in a couples group therapy which included other parents who were struggling with similar problems. In so doing, they tightened the bond of their marriage, which in turn gave Mrs. A. the support she needed to weather her daughter's eventual leaving. Mrs. A.'s depressed mood improved and her vegetative symptoms disappeared. Finally, and seemingly serendipitously, Mrs. A. befriended an elderly woman whose depression had begun with the unexpected death of her daughter. The combination of having an older woman as friend and a younger woman as therapist probably helped Mrs. A. to emerge from her depression over the ensuing weeks. To reinforce her growing autonomy, Mrs. A. was not discharged from the partial hospital until she had resumed working. Ten weeks after admission she was "back to her old self" – and perhaps even a bit wiser than before the experience.

Whether crisis intervention or inpatient care would have ultimately produced the same or better or worse outcome for Mrs. A. is, of course, not knowable. It is also possible that the chosen setting, whatever it is, provides no more than a holding environment necessary during the interim while the imipramine takes effect. Indeed, it is at least conceivable that Mrs. A. simply lived through an illness that might have resolved spontaneously. Such uncertainty is inevitable.

Research Review

While clinical judgment remains our best tool, a thorough knowledge of the literature does provide a helpful scaffolding on which to base decisions for an individual patient. Let us review research findings that pertain to the choice of settings for the resolution of acute psychiatric problems.

Three prospective studies would support the generalizability of Mrs. A.'s favorable outcome in an intensive care partial hospital. After comparing patients assigned to a day hospital with a control group assigned to an inpatient setting, Herz, Endicott, Spitzer, and Mesnikoff (1971) concluded, "On virtually every measure used to evaluate outcome, there was clear evidence of the superiority of day treatment" (p. 1379). Summarizing the findings of a similarly designed study, Wilder, Levin, and Zwerling (1966) stated, "The day hospital was a feasible treatment modality and was generally as effective as the inpatient service in the treatment of acutely disturbed patients for most or all phases of their hospitalization." Washburn, Vannicelli, Longabaugh, and Scheff (1976) also conducted a similar study and found the same result: In terms of subjective distress, functioning in the community, and family burden, day hospital patients fared better. Moreover, differences favoring partial over inpatient hospitalization held up during the first 18 months after discharge. Although 22% to 40% of patients assigned to partial hospitalization in various studies have eventually required admission to an inpatient service, these hospitalizations tend to be briefer than readmissions for those who were initially assigned to an inpatient setting (Fenton, Tessier, and Struening, 1979; Herz et al., 1971; Wilder et al., 1966). Further, studies show that patients' families view partial hospitalization more favorably (Herz, Endicott, and Spitzer, 1976, 1977; Wilder et al., 1966). Another advantage derives from the fact that the cost of partial hospital care is obviously far less than the enormous expense occasioned by even brief inpatient treatment.

Although these comparative studies have documented the efficacy of partial hospitalization, they have also reconfirmed almost inadvertently that for some individuals inpatient care is still and will likely always remain necessary. In each study, only a certain percentage of patients met the inclusionary criteria necessary to participate in both inpatient and partial hospital treatments. Some patients were simply too disruptive, confused, violent, suicidal, medically ill, or unsupported at home to be suitable for partial hospitalization in the judgment of the investigators and had to be hospitalized rather than assigned to treatment randomly. It is of great interest that the willingness to place an acutely disturbed patient in a day hospital varied from one setting to another, in spite of the fact that each study had about the same explicit criteria of suitability for randomization to either inpatient or partial hospitalization. One group (Herz et al., 1971) assigned only 22% of possible inpatient admissions to randomization, whereas other groups judged that 59% (Washburn et al., 1976) or 66% (Wilder et al., 1966) of potential admissions could be managed in either setting.

The reasons for the different evaluations of suitability for day hospital using similar criteria are not clear. Perhaps the patient samples differed. Another possibility relates to Hogarty's (1968) comment that "Preconceptions of who can or cannot be treated under outpatient or other community conditions lead the referring agent to choose the treatment of less risk, namely hospitalization." This speculation is supported by authors who have noted that consultants with experience in partial hospitals are more likely to admit patients to them (Platt, Knights, and Hirsch, 1980).

Those clinicians who have seen severely ill psychiatric patients successfully respond to partial hospital treatment will be less wary of admitting such patients to this setting. Furthermore, it is doubtful whether we will ever know for sure which and what percentage of severely disturbed patients definitely require inpatient admission rather than day hospital treatment. Such a determination would involve randomly assigning extremely suicidal or homicidal patients to either a partial or inpatient hospital, a study that is clinically and ethically untenable and will never be performed. From the available information, we can conclude that for a certain group of patients partial hospitalization is as good as, if not better than, inpatient care. We are unsure how large this group is likely to be in different settings and how to define the specific qualities of those patients who will do better in partial than in inpatient hospitalization.

The case of Mrs. A. also raises the question whether she would have done so well or better in a crisis intervention setting, which is even less disruptive and expensive. Psychiatric research does not provide a clear and satisfactory answer to this question. One problem is that studies often do not define precisely how many and which patients were excluded from the randomized group and admitted to a hospital from the start. As with the research comparing inpatient and partial hospitalization, many studies about crisis intervention are evaluating treatment outcome in a group that is highly preselected. Another problem in evaluating the literature in this area is that the services included under the label "crisis intervention" vary so much from one study to another to include such things as home visits by public health nurses (Pasamanick, Scarpitti, and Dinitz, 1967), family crisis therapy (Langsley and Kaplan, 1968; Rittenhouse, 1970), halfway house (Mosher and Menn, 1978), or a home run by private families (Polak and Kirby, 1976).

Despite the wide variations in the design of the studies and in the kinds of facilities labeled "crisis intervention," a common theme does emerge. For a certain group of disturbed patients requiring prompt resolution of their problems, crisis intervention does produce significant improvement. Butcher and Koss (1978) reached a similar conclusion in their review of brief and crisis therapy research. A pioneering study performed by Langsley and his colleagues (Langsley, Flomenhaft, and Machotka, 1969; Langsley, Pittman, Machotka, and Flomenhaft, 1968) is particularly applicable to Mrs. A. They randomly assigned patients who were judged by an independent clinical team to be in need of hospitalization either to inpatient care or to outpatient family crisis intervention. The results indicated that those patients who received family crisis intervention resumed functioning more quickly than did the inpatients and had fewer rehospitalizations. This study supports the clinical impression that for patients like Mrs. A. who are part of an integrated family, an acute hospitalization may not always be necessary or desirable.

Often the patient's family is very disturbed or inaccessible and cannot be used as an organizing structure for crisis intervention. A study by Polak and Kirby (1976) suggests that these patients can be treated in "crisis homes" run by private families. When such families provided assistance for several days or weeks, the majority of patients avoided hospitalization. This idea of a surrogate family was extended by Mosher and Menn (1978), who placed firstbreak schizophrenics in a relatively unstructured residential treatment setting so that they could be "looked after" by a paraprofessional staff. Patients stayed an average of 167 days and only two of the 30 needed to be hospitalized.

As intensive outpatient programs provide more and more support and structure, the boundary between crisis intervention and partial hospitalization becomes less distinct. For example, Stein and Test (1980) developed a community-based program called "Training in Community Living" (TCL). In this innovative program a mental health staff was transplanted into the community where they were available 24 hours a day. Patients were treated in their homes, neighborhoods, and places of work. Treatment included assistance in daily living, recreational programs, vocational guidance, and a variety of problem-solving methods. Unlike Mrs. A., the studied patients (50% of whom were schizophrenic) frequently had been in and out of hospitals, with an accumulated mean stay of 15 months. When these patients once again required intensive care for an acute problem, they were randomly assigned to the TCL program or to an inpatient service. The hospitalized control group had a mean stay of 17 days and were followed in more traditional aftercare services. After 14 months those patients assigned to TCL were functioning at a higher level and with less subjective distress; however, interestingly, after the study period was over and patients were put back into routine aftercare programs, many again began to deteriorate. The implications are that for a revolving door population a community-based program must be continuous and not simply crisis-oriented.

Although the above studies document the value of crisis intervention programs for some patients, one of the questions raised by Mrs. A. still remains: How do we decide who needs acute inpatient care?

Warner and associates (Warner, 1961; Warner, Fleming, and Bullock,

1962) developed a scale to help prevent community patients from being admitted against their will on the basis of inconsistent and unspecified criteria. This scale was divided into six weighted categories: 1) mental status, 2) ability for self-care, 3) availability of responsible parties, 4) patient's effect on the environment, 5) danger to self and others, and 6) treatment prognosis. By considering the degree of impairment in each category, the consultant could make the decision regarding hospitalization in a more systematic and less arbitrary manner. The efficacy of the weighted checklist approach was also shown by Whittington (1966). His list contained 12 weighted items regarding hospitalization, from which could be derived a total score. When he and his coworkers applied these criteria to a retrospective chart review, they found that the total score significantly separated hospitalized patients from outpatients, indicating that the criteria do have a correlation with actual decision-making in clinical practice.

Kirstein, Prusoff, Weissman, and Dressler (1975) were interested in studying systematic methods of deciding if a suicide attempter should be hospitalized. They first established nine guidelines derived from their review of the literature and charts. In a prospective study, they compared these guidelines to actual clinical practice and found that four of the nine guidelines were consonant with decisions made in the clinical setting. In a further study (Kirstein, Weissman, and Prusoff, 1975), the same research team found 15 cases who were hospitalized despite the fact that, according to the criteria, they should have been in outpatient treatment. A closer look at these aberrant patients revealed that they had significant depressive symptomatology. Accordingly, the initial criteria were modified so that the degree of depression would be given more weight. This study confirmed the value of establishing tentative guidelines. The empirical examination of their efficacy then served as a first step towards a more scientific differential therapeutics. However, the use of clinical decision-making as criterion is a serious methodological limitation unless one has great faith in the validity of the clinical decisions that serve as standards.

Before ending this section on therapeutic settings for the treatment of acute psychiatric problems, we would like to add one final note: Although evidence continues to accumulate from clinical experience and research studies that partial hospitals and crisis intervention facilities are at least as good as inpatient care for a certain group of patients, this finding has not yet had a significant impact on the delivery of mental health care. Inpatient hospitals remain by far the most frequently used setting for the treatment of acute, severe psychiatric problems. The reimbursement schedules established by third-party payers (both the government and private insurance companies) usually make admission to an inpatient hospital cheaper and easier for all concerned. The individual with full inpatient and no partial hospital coverage will find a $400 a day inpatient stay paradoxically much cheaper than a $75 a day partial hospital (Washburn, Vannicelli, and Scheff, 1976). This misallocation of resources has resulted in a shortage of partial hospital facilities and crisis intervention teams and encourages a probable excess of expensive inpatient psychiatric beds. In addition, training programs for future therapists generally do not emphasize day hospitals and crisis intervention and thus perpetuate the probably unjustified widespread preference for inpatient care.

Given the inordinate expense, the iatrogenic risks, and the potential personal and social repercussions of a psychiatric hospitalization, why have the other acute settings not been accepted more quickly and enthusiastically? No doubt one important reason is that the family and the therapist feel more secure when a disturbed and disturbing patient is hospitalized and becomes someone else's shared responsibility. The medical model of around-the-clock observation, the structured environment, and the access to emergency support all contribute to this (sometimes false) feeling of security. Less is immediately required of the patient, the family, and the outpatient therapist. Responsibility may be temporarily relinquished and placed in another's hands. Moreover, physicians are often instrumental in deciding which setting to recommend and doctors may be more inclined by training and prejudice to refer to a physician in a hospital rather than to the nonphysicians who are frequently prominent leaders and staff members in day hospitals and on crisis intervention teams.

It is perhaps more surprising that third-party payers have not been more eager to reduce their benefit expenditures by providing better reimbursement for the less expensive alternatives of partial hospitalizations and crisis intervention (Weiss and Dubin, 1982). This is probably due to some combination of custom, political pressure, and concern that utilization rates and overall costs of these alternatives are unpredictable. Insurance companies find it easier to pass on to clients the costs of easily predicted, very expensive inpatient stays than to risk losses should partial hospital utilization become very great once these services become covered and generally available.

SETTINGS FOR REHABILITATION

The following case illustrates some of the difficulties one faces in choosing a therapeutic setting for a bright young man who does not present a particular emergency but nonetheless appears destined ultimately for a terrible prognosis without effective psychiatric treatment.

THE CASE OF THE DESPONDENT DROPOUT

Mr. B. is 20 years old, but the whimsy in his eyes and his smooth, beardless face make him look no more than 16. He sits slumped in the therapist's office and mumbles laconic answers with the troubled yet appealing manner of the actor James Dean, whom he happens to admire greatly. He has come for the consultation reluctantly and claims to have agreed only because his parents threatened to kick him out of the house unless he kept the appointment; however, despite his seeming indifference to his parents' concern, Mr. B. responds to the therapist's interest by revealing painful aspects of how he views himself and his seemingly hopeless future prospects.

Early in the interview, Mr. B. announces that he plans to kill himself in one month on his 21st birthday because he feels bored to death already and because "maturity is undigestible." His intention is presented provocatively but engenders added concern because he has already made a serious suicide attempt by ingesting 10 Tuinals at age 18. Furthermore, in the past few months Mr. B. has increased his abuse of drugs in an attempt to self-medicate his boredom, loneliness, and despair. He is often too drunk or drugged by the time he gets home to remember how or when he got himself upstairs to bed.

Most of the time, with or without drugs, Mr. B. feels like "a Star Wars robot." He watches himself mechanically going through the motions of life and also views others as though they were "radar-controlled marionettes." He worries that his soft skin, slight build, and aesthetic interests are signs that he is a latent homosexual. Although he has had no sexual experiences of any kind with either sex, he considers the stares of other men as confirmation that he might be gay. Mr. B. also believes that he might have contracted venereal disease from a contaminated drinking cup and fears that he may have developed general paresis, a condition he learned about in a news magazine. When the consultant informs Mr. B. that these fears are based on a misunderstanding of the illness Mr B., instead of being reassured, becomes suspicious, wonders aloud if the consultant has a "dirty mind," and launches into a seemingly prepackaged sermon about the importance of personal hygiene and the dangers of sexual contact and exploitation. As his speech becomes more pressured and less interruptable, Mr. B.'s potential for idiosyncratic and referential thinking and formal thought disorder become apparent.

Later during the interview, Mr. B. reveals his anger and disappointment—toward his father, mother, and younger sister. His parents were divorced when he was 15 and his father remarried soon thereafter. Mr. B. claims he will not forgive any of them for their "vicious deed," but most of all he will never forgive his father, who is an "assman ruled by his cock." Mr. B. is no less vindictive toward his mother, who is still a youthful and extremely attractive woman, "a Star Wars starlet." She used Mr. B. as a confidant during the lonely period immediately after the divorce. At the time, Mr. B. hated the way his mother would cling to him and express her loneliness, but now he is equally resentful of her dating. He refuses to be in the same room with her current boyfriend, whom he considers a "jock strap." Mr. B.'s sister, three years younger, has sailed through the family storms unscathed, is now captain of the cheerleaders, popular with boys, and an honor student. She regards her brother with an open contempt that fuels his spiteful envy of her success and ease in life.

Mr. B. at first dealt with his turmoil over the divorce by frequently sneaking out of school and back into the house where he would spend listless hours in bed staring at the ceiling. He would try to imagine that each of his thoughts were being programmed into a computer which he would then imagine being short-circuited and destroyed. When he was forced to go to school, the computer imagery could not contain his distress—but marijuana did. He began to use the drug before, during, and after school. Although his IQ was over 140, his grades fell precipitously. A destructive cycle was now in motion: Ostracized by his peers, accused by his teachers, threatened by his parents, he used drugs for relief and to establish a new social network with older boys. He was subsequently caught several times and suspended from school for smoking pot on school grounds and once for selling. Each day brought a new crisis. His mother wanted him at school; the school wanted him out; his former friends wanted nothing to do with him. Finally, at age 16, just one year after the divorce, he dropped out of school and spent his days, evenings, and many nights wandering the streets, high on drugs or wishing he were dead.

Several previous trials of outpatient psychotherapy had been unsuccessful. In each instance, after pleas and threats from his parents, Mr. B. would keep a few appointments, become bored, have nothing to say, and eventually stop going. His parents reacted at first with anger, but then with helpless resignation and despair. They were not sure which was worse: forcing him out of the house to find a job and living with the fear that he would accidentally or intentionally overdose on drugs, or keeping him in the home and living daily with his disruptive, unpredictable, and self-destructive behavior. As for Mr. B., no place was tolerable, but it did not matter all that much because in just another month he was certain he would be dead. Mr. B.'s DSM-III multiaxial diagnosis was:

Axis I.   296.32 Major depression, recurrent without melancholia, with mood-congruent psychotic features
305.91 Mixed substance abuse – possible substance-induced delusional disorder
Axis II.   301.22 Schizotypal personality disorder
Axis III. None
Axis IV.   Moderate stress – reaching age 21 and having to support oneself – 4
Axis V.   Poor functioning in the past year – 5

Unless dramatic changes interfere with the pattern of Mr. B.'s life, he is clearly headed for disaster. The consultant must determine which of the alternative possible therapeutic settings has the best chance of facilitating these necessary changes. A short-term inpatient hospital might be a suitable environment for the acute treatment of Mr. B.'s depression and to protect him from suicidal impulses and the ready availability of drugs. In this acute setting, a therapeutic alliance might be forged that would serve as an induction into a more successful outpatient psychotherapy than has occurred in the past. Other possible settings place greater emphasis from the start on treating Mr. B.'s longstanding difficulties rather than focusing primarily on the resolution of the immediate problem. These settings would include: a longer term reconstructive inpatient hospital, a rehabilitation partial hospital, and outpatient psychotherapy (see Table 1-4). We will provide a brief overview description of these possibilities before indicating which setting was chosen for Mr. B. and what in fact happened regarding his care.

Reconstructive Hospital

These inpatient units have a length of stay that extends from several months to a year or more and the goal of radically intervening in the patient's life to change longstanding patterns and not merely alleviating symptoms. The national trend toward utilization review and reducing lengths of stay has profoundly reduced the number of beds available for this purpose. In the presence of high cost and little data on efficacy, opponents question the value of hospitalizing a patient for three months to a year or more. They challenge the argument that prolonged involvement with the staff, patient community, occupational therapists, recreational therapists, and especially the intense psychological involvement with the individual therapist will facilitate a fundamental change in the patient's psychopathology, character, and way of dealing with his emotional illness that would not be possible in other less expensive settings. There is also considerable risk in this setting of promoting regression and "sick role" behavior.

Advocates of specialized reconstructive hospitals maintain that for a highly selective group of patients, who have severe pathology, but also many assets, the investment is worthwhile and may enable the individual not simply to endure his problems, but actually to attain a much higher vocational and interpersonal level than would otherwise be possible. They point out that such patients require a secure and structured treatment environment available over a period of time in order to break or prevent a lifelong pattern of drifting from one in- or outpatient modality to another with gradually increasing deterioration. In a more structured and supportive inpatient setting, these same patients might come to form an intimate attachment to others, develop insight, work through their problems, and develop social and vocational skills which will thereafter allow them to be happier and function adequately in the community. A structured and stable long-term inpatient setting also allows for psychotherapeutic confrontations and a careful monitoring of psychotropic drugs; both are more difficult to perform in other settings.

Day Hospital Rehabilitation Programs

Like reconstructive hospitals, day hospital rehabilitation programs are based on the principle that a structured setting can help organize a severely disturbed patient and change him in a substantial and enduring way. The kind and degree of structure will vary from one program to another and ideally will be tailored to fit the needs of the individual patient. Some day hospitals are very intense brief therapy environments (Frances, Clarkin, and Weldon, 1979). Some rigidly structured programs for disorganized patients simulate a psychiatric inpatient environment; patients arrive early each morning and attend community, group, occupational, recreational, family, and individual meetings throughout the day on a tight schedule. Moderately structured rehabilitation programs often simulate a work rather than hospital community. These sheltered workshop rehabilitation facilities are usually geographically and theoretically removed from the general or psychiatric hospital. During the four to eight months in the program, the patient is viewed more as an on-the-job trainee than as a patient and is expected to attend five days per week, six hours per day, in order to approximate the work environment. Sessions for individual, family, group, or medication therapy are viewed as adjuncts and not as the central focus of the program. Less structured rehabilitation programs would include halfway houses in which patients live for several months as they make the transition from an inpatient environment to more normal and unsupervised community living. In some halfway houses, a professional or paraprofessional

TABLE 1-4

Differential Criteria for Treatment Setting When the Goal is Rehabilitation

Outpatient	Partial Hospitalization	Hospitalization
Relative Indications 1) Most psychiatric outpatients will fall into this category. Those who are more impaired will progress to either partial hospitalization or hospitalization. 2) Chronic problem with sufficient functional impairment to require psychiatric treatment.	*Relative Indications* 1) Patient has not been previously treated in a rehabilitation program but has severe impairments in vocational or social performance of recent onset or extended duration (for example, patient is unemployed with marked social withdrawal).	*Relative Indications* 1) Patient with repeated brief hospitalizations requires a major overhaul. 2) Environment is so noxious that treatment can be done only in a controlled setting. 3) Patient who requires repeated confrontations and/or structured reinforcements in a structured setting.
Enabling Factors 1) Patient capable of sustaining life in the community.	*Enabling Factors* 1) Patient must be able to attend and form an allegiance to the program, and ensure that his financial and living arrangements will not interfere with treatment. 2) Can gradually assume increasing vocational and social responsibility under supervision.	*Enabling Factors* 1) Motivation for extended inpatient stay. 2) Capacity to adhere to rules of the hospital system.
Relative Contraindications 1) Problem severity that requires more intense interventions (e.g., risk of suicide). 2) Treatment at this level in the past has		*Relative Contraindications* 1) Potential for or history of regression

been repeatedly ineffectual or harmful.
3) Patient addicted to multiple episodes of treatment at this level of care.

3) Has sufficient frustration tolerance for the repetitive drilling necessary to acquire or reacquire social and vocational skills.

Relative Contraindications
1) Patient can be handled in a less intensive treatment (for example, traditional psychotherapy, prevocational counseling, or group therapy).
2) Patient's symptoms are acute and require more intensive evaluation and treatment, such as intensive care partial hospitalization or inpatient treatment.
3) Patient has failed or become increasingly symptomatic in response to previous treatment in a rehabilitation program and requires less intensive treatment, such as chronic care partial hospitalization or a medication group.

in hospital settings.
2) Addiction to hospitalization with little gain.
3) Use of hospital to avoid painful but likely step outside the hospital environment.

staff provides supportive therapy; in other houses, the staff serve only as understanding "landlords" and the patient has major outside investments in school or work and receives outpatient therapy in another setting.

Outpatient Psychotherapy

Whatever the format or theoretical approach, outpatient psychotherapy differs markedly from both reconstructive hospitals and rehabilitation programs in that the patient's living environment is far less structured and influenced by the therapist. As opposed to altering the environment to change the patient, the intention of most outpatient psychotherapies is to change the patient, who then may or may not choose to alter his environment. The frequency and duration of outpatient therapy depend upon the goals and orientation of the therapist and patient, which we will discuss in detail in subsequent chapters.

This condensed description of reconstructive hospitals, partial hospital rehabilitation programs, and outpatient psychotherapy points out that, although the three settings have many differences, they share a common goal: They are all designed to increase the patient's previous level of functioning and not simply to resolve an acute problem. The consultant believed that in view of Mr. B.'s age, intelligence, and creative potential, as well as his quickly developing chronicity, the goal of treatment should be ambitious and address longstanding and not just immediate problems. The consultant was concerned that, although an admission to an acute inpatient hospital might temporarily decrease Mr. B.'s drug abuse, depression, and risk of suicide, it would not be enough of an intervention to alter his long-range prospects or to provide a meaningful induction into long-term outpatient therapy. The patient might "play the game," getting in and out of the hospital without ever becoming genuinely involved in treatment, and then return to his chaotic life with even less reason to hope that psychiatric treatment had anything substantial to offer. In choosing a more ambitious setting, the consultant realized that he was also influenced (and perhaps countertransferentially) by the appeal of Mr. B.'s looks, intelligence, charm, language, and manner.

One obvious setting to consider for Mr. B. was a long-term reconstructive hospital. This setting would remove him almost completely from the many noxious external influences in his life and from his conflicted family relationships and, in a sense, would give him a chance to start over in a new and different milieu. Old and well established interpersonal patterns would of course recur in the hospital in relation to his therapist, the staff, and other patients, but these would be less likely to be destructive because they would occur in an environment that fostered his capacity to better understand and change them. After receiving a thorough diagnostic evaluation and an assessment of his vocational skills, Mr. B. could also be started on medication and gradually encouraged to participate in new activities and develop a new social network. He could be involved in intense individual, family, and group treatment. His reactions to the ward setting and participation in it could be observed and discussed in a wider variety of therapeutic encounters and in greater depth than is possible in any other treatment setting. With relative protection against his drug abuse and suicidal impulses, the staff — especially the individual, family, and/or group therapists — would be relatively comfortable in more strongly and quickly confronting his maladaptive behavior and defenses than is ever possible in less structured settings.

However, with these advantages of a reconstructive hospital come certain serious risks and disadvantages. Instead of experiencing the hospital as a climate for change, Mr. B. might respond to being labeled a long-term psychiatric inpatient by allowing himself to go completely crazy (whatever that means to him) and, in a regressed state, to become even more symptomatic, delinquent, or unmanageable than he was out of the hospital. Even without such an extreme regression, Mr. B. might simply settle in to the environment and become comfortable with the relative lack of responsibility and demands. After a year or two or three, and after hundreds of thousands of dollars, he would then be discharged without significant improvement and be even less capable of autonomous functioning, having missed age-appropriate developmental experiences in the "real world." For the rest of his life in and out of acute care hospitals, Mr. B. might continue to yearn for the comfort and support of the expensive reconstructive facility, recalled by him as a kind of paradise lost.

The risk of a disabling regression might be reduced if Mr. B. were assigned instead to a rehabilitation day hospital. Forced to return home each night and encouraged to maintain a life separate from the treatment program, he would be less likely to become overly dependent upon the artificial community of the treatment setting and to retreat from "civilian" society. The day-to-day struggles with and transferences to his family and peers could be kept in view, immediately accessible to therapeutic intervention. This opportunity is lost in an inpatient setting. But partial hospitalization would also have risks and disadvantages of its own. Even a highly structured and observant rehabilitation program

cannot provide protection against drug abuse and suicide equivalent
to that afforded by an inpatient facility. Staff members and patients,
appreciating Mr. B.'s relative inability to tolerate uncomfortable feelings, would understandably approach him with more therapeutic and
interpersonal caution than is necessary on an inpatient setting. They
would fear that confrontation or intimate attachment might lead to Mr.
B.'s acting-out destructively when he left the day hospital at night. This
wariness might increase Mr. B.'s sense of alienation and reduce the opportunity for insight, learning new coping skills, and change. Moreover,
partial hospitalization reduces regression, but by no means eliminates
it, and so there may be great difficulty at the time of discharge.

At this point, outpatient psychotherapy would seem the least desirable alternative. Although Mr. B.'s intelligence and great need have
tempted some therapists to try a rescue operation in the past, they have
been unsuccessful and nothing has changed environmentally or intrapsychically in such a way as to suggest that outpatient treatment would
now have a different and more favorable result. The honeymoon period
might end abruptly the moment the therapist felt called upon to make
a necessary confrontation. Even if Mr. B. thereafter kept his appointments, the therapist would have to work tentatively with the fear that
at any instant the sword might fall and he would lose his patient.

After considering the advantages and disadvantages of each of these
settings, the consultant's choice for Mr. B. was a reconstructive inpatient hospitalization. A major factor in this decision was the concern
about Mr. B.'s drug abuse and suicidal impulses. In the consultant's
judgment, these destructive tendencies were by now so embedded in
Mr. B.'s character that they would not respond to treatment over a few
weeks in an acute care inpatient setting, while a day hospital could not
provide adequate protection, and these symptoms would make meaningful outpatient psychotherapy impossible. Furthermore, the consultant believed that, given Mr. B.'s hostility and disdain for both of his
parents and the absence of any reliable support from friends or employment, not much would be lost, and much was possibly to be gained, in
placing Mr. B in a completely new environment. A longer term, rehabilitation inpatient facility is often the best way station for youngsters
having great difficulty separating from their families and may serve as
the only setting in which they can negotiate the difficult steps toward
autonomy and adulthood. The family, although by no means wealthy,
had excellent medical coverage and was willing to make the additional
sacrifice necessary for longer term hospitalization. Mr. B. reacted to the
decision with a shrug of indifference, claiming "in one more month you
can find some other fruitcake to take my place."

During the first week in the hospital, Mr. B. drifted around the ward with a bemused smirk. He was aloof and seemed annoyed by the efforts of patients and staff to draw him out of his science fiction paperbacks and into conversation. The staff, appreciating that Mr. B.'s arrogant withdrawal was caused by anxiety, remained unintrusive and allowed Mr. B. time to become accustomed to the new community. He was given a complete battery of psychological tests, evaluated for vocational skills, and placed in occupational, recreational, and group treatment, but he was not forced to participate very actively in these activities at the start. Similarly, Mr. B.'s individual therapist, who by nature and by design was cautiously methodical, spent the first weeks of treatment once a day with Mr. B. for an hour in order to gather a painstakingly thorough psychiatric history. The rigor of these history-taking sessions proved helpful in organizing Mr. B.'s chaotic inner world and giving coherence to what had previously seemed a bewilderingly kaleidoscopic life. In addition, the therapist's methodical approach enhanced Mr. B.'s use of more adaptive intellectual defenses to control anxiety. This intellectualization also prevented what might have been experienced as intolerable intimacy. The doctor-patient relationship was allowed to evolve slowly in order to avoid the possible storm which might have led to acting-out or signing-out. Mr. B. was also begun on a regimen of the tricyclic antidepressant amitriptyline, with gradually increasing doses up to 250 mg/day. Family sessions were held once a week. The participants changed depending upon the needs of the moment and included at different times his mother, father, stepmother, and sister in varying compositions.

By the middle of the second month, Mr. B. admitted he actually felt comfortable in the presence of other people for the first time he could remember. The staff and patients gave him a surprise birthday party (on the day he had previously predicted would be his last on earth). Mr. B. at first devalued the gesture with snide remarks, but then became choked with tears as he cut the cake and handed out pieces. Three weeks later, he was elected president of the ward community and confided to his therapist, "With so many real sickies in this place I don't feel like such a weirdo."

Over the next three months the hospital milieu provided the necessary structure and support as individual sessions and the now occasional family sessions became increasingly intense and productive. Mr. B. wept longingly for his father and realized that his bitterness since the divorce was in part a defense against the loss of his father, whom he admired, loved, and missed. He also understood that his homosexual fears were in part related to his wish for a father to intervene between him and his mother, whom he experienced as doting and seductive. After five months of treatment, these longings for a rescuing father were transferred first to a kindly older ward attendant and then to the therapist himself. When plans for discharge to a halfway house were first discussed after six months of hospitalization, the trauma of his parents' divorce was in some sense replayed. Mr. B. once again felt he was losing his father and being "thrown to the mother hen." At one point during this difficult time, several patients at a ward meeting mentioned that they suspected that Mr. B. was again taking drugs during passes on the hospital grounds. The suspicion was never confirmed, but staff and patients got the message and provided additional support during Mr. B.'s transition out of the hospital, which was postponed for an additional month.

While at the halfway house for the next four months, Mr. B. continued to meet with the same individual therapist three times a week, worked at a bookstore, and completed his high school equivalency exam without difficulty. He then left the state for college. Two years later the admired ward attendant received a Christmas card from Mr. B., who said that he was currently doing reasonably well in a premedical program and living with a woman ten years older than himself.

A more complete follow-up is not available. At the time Mr. B. left treatment to attend college, his therapist felt that the risks of significant drug abuse or suicide were not serious and he believed that Mr. B.'s intelligence and wit would facilitate his academic and social adjustment. The therapist was more concerned about Mr. B.'s capacity to develop and sustain trusting relationships. For instance, during the final session, after nostalgically recalling all that the two of them had been through over the past year and a half, Mr. B. abruptly retreated from the closeness by glibly remarking, "Well, if nothing else, my checks kept you eating regularly." Mr. B. had already made it clear that he did not intend to contact his therapist again and wanted "nothing to do with further treatment with anyone . Once you wake up from a nightmare, you might as well get up. There's no sense going back to sleep."

Research Review

Even with these reservations about Mr. B.'s future, the referral to a reconstructive hospital would appear to have been a wise choice. Mr. B. was helped in that setting. The available psychiatric research, however, does not give much support to the consultant's recommendation that Mr. B. be admitted to a long-term inpatient facility. With few exceptions, the evidence reviewed below favors briefer hospitalization followed by treatment in a day hospital or outpatient setting.

However, there are many problems in interpreting the available studies that compare brief vs. longer hospitalization. None of them is designed to assess the more subtle and ambitious long-range goals of reconstructive, long-term hospitalization. Instead, they measure what are more easily measurable outcome parameters such as the incidence of rehospitalization or the recurrence of symptoms. The settings that were used for the available comparative studies were not specialized to serve as reconstructive hospitals, but were instead university or state hospitals that lacked the commitment to this kind of treatment and the necessary expertise and physical and staff resources. Moreover, the patients who have been studied were more severely and/or acutely ill and almost certainly lacked the assets and potential for change possessed by Mr. B. and other patients treated in longer term reconstructive hospitals.

In summary then, the available literature comparing brief vs. longer hospitalization does not really answer questions about the relative effectiveness of reconstructive hospitals because available studies test different settings, and possibly different patient populations, than those that are appropriate for reconstructive hospitalization.

The question of whether reconstructive hospitals are cost-effective is also unanswered. For those patients who become able to contribute to society and to avoid rehospitalization after one extended hospitalization, the cost/benefit ratio may prove to be quite favorable over the long haul, despite the enormous initial expense. However, it is possible that only a relatively select group of patients are differentially helped in so dramatic a fashion by such facilities. This raises the public health and ethical problem of whether the high cost for these few patients is warranted, as well as the clinical question of whether it is possible to predict in advance those who will do well in this setting and not in another less expensive form of treatment.

The early studies comparing short and longer term hospitalization are particularly hard to apply to patients like Mr. B. Many of these were conducted in the 1960s when the efficacy of the recently discovered psychotropic medications was being documented. Researchers wanted to establish that the previously customary prolonged inpatient care was no longer necessary. But as mentioned above, these early studies involved a sicker patient population than would be considered suitable for reconstructive hospitals. The focus of outcome measures was resolution of symptoms and reduction of rehospitalization rates — not the reconstructive rehabilitation of the patient. Even though these studies do not appear directly relevant to Mr. B., they are worth reviewing in some detail, particularly because they set a trend for progressively more and more abbreviated hospitalizations. This trend has continued and, according to some, has gone too far. Certainly, reconstructive hospitals must begin to prove their value and cost-effectiveness if they are to receive increased (or even continued) support in the future.

Caffey, Galbrecht, and Klett (1971) divided male schizophrenic inpatients into three groups: 1) A control group received the "standard" inpatient treatment of the time and stayed in the hospital for an average duration of 83 days before discharge to the usual variety of then existing aftercare facilities. 2) A second group received the same treatment in the hospital and stayed about the same length of time, but after discharge they were followed as outpatients by the same staff who had treated them as inpatients. 3) A third group had an accelerated hospital stay of only one month (mean 29 days) before being discharged and followed as outpatients by the inpatient staff. The results indicated essentially no difference in outcome among the three treatment regimens. The patients who were more rapidly discharged did just as well, and the reason did not seem related to the continuity of inpatient-outpatient staff.

In 1965, Dieter, Hanford, Hummel, and Lubach conducted a study of shortened hospitalization in which the control group was hospitalized for two months, while the experimental group was placed on a seven-day program of medication followed by a two-week program of preparation for readjustment to follow-up care in the community. Despite the difference in length of hospitalization (52 vs. 21 days), readmission rates during the subsequent year were equivalent for both groups.

These early studies showing no disadvantage of a briefer hospitalization were soon followed by studies which showed an actual advantage to a shorter inpatient stay. Burhan (1969) found that patients in an experimental group with a stay of two weeks (14.8 days) were four times less likely to be readmitted over the next two years than were patients in a control group whose hospitalization had been much longer (37.7 days). Mattes and his associates (Mattes, Rosen, and Klein, 1977; Mattes, Rosen, Klein, and Millan, 1977) assigned a diagnostically mixed group of patients to either a shorter or a longer term hospitalization. Three years after discharge, long-term patients were rated by relatives as having less pathology, but this one isolated positive finding was the only statistically significant indication that the longer stay was of value. No differences were found between groups in many other measures of pathology, and, in fact, the longer term patients required more frequent rehospitalization and these lasted for longer periods of time.

More recently, Endicott and colleagues (Endicott, Cohen, Nee, Fleiss, and Herz, 1979) have reconfirmed the value of brief hospitalization and by implication have questioned the value of longer stays. His research team studied three different groups of inpatients: those receiving standard inpatient care; those receiving brief hospitalization; and those receiving brief hospitalization followed by transitional day care. The standard group stayed 60 days, whereas the briefer groups stayed only 11 days. Long-term follow-up demonstrated little difference among the three groups. The authors concluded that for those severely ill patients who live with families, brief hospitalization with transitional day care is superior to long-term hospitalization on most measures of individual psychopathology, level of functioning, and family burden. The authors also emphasized that the cost/benefit ratio clearly favors brief hospitalization. Although the above studies confirm the value of brief hospitalization, the referring consultant must be cautious about generalizing these data beyond their field of applicability. It would be an error to assume that available research establishes that a patient like Mr. B. will fail to benefit from more extensive and ambitious inpatient care. As an example of how such information can be misinterpreted, we will discuss the methodological limitations of a study that was reported by Smith, Kaplan, and Siker (1974). They contrasted the outcome of first admissions to a regional community mental health center to the outcome of patients given traditional state hospital care. In a four-year follow-up period, the group admitted to a community center, even though they had a mean stay of 47 days, had done far better than the state hospital group who had been in the hospital three times longer, with a mean stay of 137 days. The community group had fewer days of rehospitalization and less disability at far less expense. But – and here is the important point – the two groups differed not only in length of hospitalization but also in the kind of treatment offered. Obviously, factors other than the shorter inpatient stay may have contributed to the favorable outcome of the community group. This sort of study does not tell us about the possible effectiveness of state-of-the-art reconstructive hospitals working with suitably selected patients.

Instead of comparing brief vs. longer hospitalization, a number of other studies have addressed a related issue relevant to Mr. B., namely: Is the addition of psychotherapy to the treatment regimen in an inpatient setting beneficial when compared to a regimen in which patients receive only psychopharmacotherapy, milieu, or custodial care? The conclusion of most such studies has been that psychotherapy given alone in the hospital is not very effective, but as an adjunct to pharmacotherapy can be helpful and cost-effective by reducing the subsequent amount of hospitalization. For example, McCaffree (1966) reviewed treatment in a state hospital system during two periods. In the first period, only custodial care was provided; in the second period, various forms of psychotherapy were provided as well. McCaffree assessed the cost for both types of treatment, including within his calculations both public costs, such as welfare subsistence, and private costs, such as loss of patient income. The overall cost for patients who received psychotherapy was about half the cost for those receiving custodial care. The largest saving came because patients who received psychotherapy had a briefer hospitalization (22 vs. 42 days). One must be cautious in interpreting these data because the study has many methodological limitations. It is possible that the group receiving psychotherapy may have been less disabled to begin with than the custodial care group. Furthermore, McCaffree did not evaluate improvement systematically and it is at least possible that the psychotherapy group may have been no better after receiving treatment. The only difference between groups may have been caused by changes in the criteria for patient discharge between the two data-gathering periods. Finally, since drug treatment was introduced during the second period, McCaffree may have been measuring the effects of pharmacotherapy and not psychotherapy.

May and Tuma (1964) performed a prospective and well controlled study that corrected many of these methodological problems. Schizophrenic patients were assigned during their hospitalization to five different kinds of treatment: 1) milieu therapy alone, 2) psychotherapy alone, 3) pharmacotherapy alone, 4) pharmacotherapy with psychotherapy, and 5) pharmacotherapy with milieu therapy. The use of drugs with psychotherapy was only slightly more effective than the use of drugs alone and both of these were significantly more effective than psychotherapy alone.

As research has become more advanced in differential therapeutics, increasingly sophisticated studies have been designed to address the complex and interacting variables that influence outcome and decision-making. For example, Endicott and her associates (Endicott, Cohen, Nee, Fleiss, and Herz, 1979) reported results of a data analysis designed to determine what specific patient characteristics indicated optimal response to either brief or longer term hospitalization. They found that for patients with no or few hospital admissions, the length of hospitalization made little difference in the outcome. However, as the number of previous admissions increased, longer term hospitalization was less helpful than brief hospitalization followed by either day or outpatient treatment. Their data also supported the clinical impression that extremely angry or violent patients do poorly with a brief hospital treatment followed by outpatient care. Angry patients have a better adjustment in the community and place less burden on the family if they are given a brief hospitalization followed by partial hospital treatment.

Glick, Hargreaves, Drues, and Showstack (1976) also went beyond examining the question of whether brief or long hospitalization was better in some general way in order to determine which patients should get which kind of treatment. Groups of patients hospitalized for three to four weeks were compared with groups hospitalized for three to six months. They found a slight advantage in favor of long-term inpatient care for schizophrenic patients. Perhaps ironically, the authors attributed the beneficial results not to the longer hospitalization per se, but rather to the posthospitalization treatment history of the longer term patients, who apparently were more likely to be successfully induced into and to remain in a suitable aftercare program. Three years later (Glick and Hargreaves, 1979), the authors used their accumulated data to further divide patients into subgroups with differential response to brief or longer term hospitalization. The data indicated that schizophrenic patients who function well prior to hospitalization tend to do better with longer term inpatient care, perhaps because these patients are more likely to continue in needed aftercare treatment than are shorter stay patients. On the other hand, for most patients who have a poor premorbid adjustment, brief hospitalization followed by maintenance community care is the disposition of choice.

With so many differently designed studies and so many variables, the accumulating data concerning the effectiveness of short vs. longer hospitalization will doubtlessly be interpreted in contradictory ways. Riessman, Rabkin, and Struening (1977), for example, concluded that every clinician must assume the burden of justifying the use of a hospital stay longer than 60 days. And Swartzburg and Schwartz (1976), after reviewing almost 2,000 patients, concluded that the entire issue about therapeutic setting and length of stay was missing the point; the key variable was not whether a patient was hospitalized or for how long, but rather whether certain crucial tasks were being accomplished during the hospital stay.

Things get even more confusing and uncertain when the consultant begins to consider the other two rehabilitation settings — the day hospital and outpatient psychotherapy. There are no available studies that compare all three of these treatment settings and only a few studies have compared rehabilitation day hospitals with more traditional outpatient care. Meltzoff and Blumenthal (1966) randomly assigned patients to outpatient and partial hospital treatment following discharge from an inpatient service. Eighteen months after discharge, partial hospital patients were more likely to be employed, less likely to be rehospitalized, and less symptomatic than those treated in the outpatient department. In a study with a similar design, Weldon, Clarkin, Hennessy, and Frances

(1979) randomly assigned 30 patients either to a rehabilitation partial hospital or to a conventional outpatient clinic. At three-month follow-up, they noted that partial hospitalization was significantly more effective than traditional outpatient treatment in returning recently discharged psychiatric inpatients to community functioning in work or training areas. However, the relatively short duration of the period that was studied precluded an evaluation of how this difference in response to the different therapeutic settings would hold up over the long haul.

Medicine has in general addressed itself first to the provision and study of acute care services before becoming interested in the treatment and rehabilitation of patients with more chronic conditions requiring longer term interventions. The indications for reconstructive inpatient and day hospital services are not at all clear, partly because these services have not yet been clearly described or systematically investigated. This will change with the realization that, although our acute treatments have become increasingly effective in reversing acute psychopathology, many patients are left in a relatively nonfunctioning limbo from which they can emerge only with the help of carefully structured, long-term, ambitious rehabilitative treatment environments.

SETTINGS FOR MAINTENANCE

The following vignette is about a man who has been severely incapacitated for most of his life. His case history illustrates the difficulties in finding a suitable therapeutic setting to help the chronically impaired patient to maintain a stable level of functioning and avoid further deterioration or acute exacerbations. The question here is not so much getting the patient better but rather holding the line at the highest possible level of functioning.

THE CASE OF THE MAN WITHOUT A HOME

It is midnight. Mr. P., a wrinkled man in his fifties, sits slumped alone on a bench in an emergency room of a metropolitan hospital. He has a wild flock of ghostly white hair going off in all directions and vaguely resembles a disheveled Albert Einstein. His unshaven and filthy face rests in gnarled hands as he mumbles to himself. Occasionally he flinches for no apparent reason and snarls against some imagined accusation. All that Mr. P. owns in the world is either on his back or in two large shopping bags by his side. Although it is summer, he is wearing an enormous wool coat that hangs over him like an old army blanket. The bags contain soiled underwear, a pungent sweater, a tin of cigar butts, a half-empty bottle of Southern Comfort, two potatoes, a dull kitchen knife, his grade school report cards, and several unknown items wrapped in newspaper. When approached by the psychiatrist on call, Mr. P. looks up and, with a surprisingly bright and responsive nod of recognition, shuffles toward the evaluating office. Introductions are not necessary. The entire staff knows Mr. P. well and he knows them. Hungry, dirty, tired, he has come yet one more time asking to be admitted.

In recent years Mr. P.'s thinking has been so illogical and idiosyncratic that no one is quite sure what has been going on in his head or in his life. His long and unhappy psychiatric history has been pieced together by reviewing old charts and talking to staff members who have known him over the years. As best as anyone can tell, Mr. P.'s severe problems became noticeable when in ninth grade he increasingly withdrew from peers, refused to take gym or go into the men's room, and began to giggle inappropriately in response to private thoughts. He began performing complex rituals, such as showering twice before each meal and laundering his entire wardrobe every Friday night. His chaotic and impoverished family, an assortment of cousins, stepparents and half-sisters, ignored his psychopathology and eventual truancy until they became frightened by his unprovoked screams – though he never actually struck out at anyone. At age 17, with the help of the family caseworker, Mr. P. was placed in a state hospital, where he was noted to have a variety of hallucinations and delusions. These symptoms did not improve and when he was sent home after three months, he was still unable to resume school or begin work. The family now viewed him as "a crazy," avoided him, and felt relieved when he was off by himself in his tiny room. Mr. P. spent hours each night pacing back and forth or writing obscenities on the wall, which he then spent the day scrubbing off with a steel brush. Primarily because of a rearrangement in the family and the arrival of a stepuncle and his wife to live in the home, at the age of 20 Mr. P. was again taken to a state hospital. This second admission lasted 17 years.

His cubicle on Ward F became more of a home than Mr. P. had ever had before. After a variety of medications in high dosages and an extended trial of ECT failed to diminish the symptoms of his schizophrenia, the staff resigned themselves to letting Mr. P. be – which was just fine with him. None of the hospital rules interfered with his daily rituals and after a while no one inquired what his bizarre sneers or gestures might mean. From time to time, especially in the fall, Mr. P. would become fanatically devoted to washing the cars of staff members. He would then hoard the small amount of money he had earned in this fashion and use it to buy cigarettes over the next year while he hibernated unobtrusively in his corner of the ward.

Mr. P.'s fate abruptly changed in the mid 1960s due to forces beyond his control. His hospital, following a national trend, sought to deinstitutionalize patients and return them to the community. After several months of meetings designed to prepare such patients for "reentry," Mr. P. was discharged with medication to a single-room occupancy (SRO) and given an appointment to an aftercare clinic in his new "catchment area." For Mr. P., with his lack of social or vocational skills, this was equivalent to being delivered into the 25th century. Thoroughly bewildered by the change, he promptly lost his medicine and by the second week could not find his way to his SRO. Soon he began to wander the streets and to live on doorsteps and out of garbage cans. After a month, Mr. P. was brought to an emergency room by the police after he had defecated in a phone booth. Although he begged to return to his cubicle in his old hospital, his new address was not part of its catchment area. Mr. P.'s old hospital (and home) would never again be available. Moreover, his family could not be found and there were no leads to track them down. The evaluating consultant was at a loss.

As a short-term solution, Mr. P. was admitted to his new district's city hospital, where he was medically and psychiatrically evaluated and placed back on maintenance medication. With some diminution in his hallucinations – or at least in his willingness to describe them – he was discharged after ten days to another SRO. He never kept his appointments at the aftercare clinic and was not seen again until three months later when he showed up in the emergency room, perhaps picking this night because it was the first bitterly cold spell of the fall. Thus began a cycle which was to recur every three to six months over the next 15 years. Typically, after losing a Welfare check or forgetting an aftercare appointment or hearing "new agents" telling him to avoid the day hospital or simply getting drunk (Mr. P. had developed a mild drinking problem), he would be found one night sitting in his customary spot on a bench in the emergency room. From time to time, an enthusiastic therapist would spend hours negotiating his transfer to a state hospital, but within a few days – in part because Mr. P. would make a suitable adjustment to the chronic care facility and appear so improved – he would be discharged ("deinstitutionalized" in the barbarous jargon of the time) against his wishes and sent back into the alien community, where his sad scenario would be replayed yet again.

Mr. P.'s DSM-III diagnosis is:

Axis I.   295.12 Schizophrenia, disorganized, chronic
Axis II.   None

Axis III. Essential hypertension, scabies
Axis IV. Stress – moderate, no stable living arrangement – 4
Axis V. Level of functioning – grossly impaired – 7

Mr. P., on the emergency room bench, is the victim and also the victimizer of the mental health care system. After all the previous treatment failures, what should now be tried – a chronic care inpatient hospital? a chronic care day hospital? maintenance outpatient therapy? something else? After presenting an overview of these possibilities for maintenance therapy (see Table 1-5), we will return to what happened that night to Mr. P.

Chronic Care Hospital

The public (or at least some politicians and newspaper editorialists) periodically becomes irate because thousands of patients are maintained year after year in chronic care hospitals with only marginal efforts to mobilize them toward a more productive life (Talbott, 1978b). Although the advent of psychotropic medication has markedly reduced the number of patients in chronic care facilities, the unfortunate truth is that some psychiatric problems continue to remain refractory to all treatments and that for some patients the most suitable and comfortable existence occurs in the unstressful and structured setting of a chronic care hospital. In this environment, where the presence of severe psychopathology is tolerated, some patients are able to spend their days at work or hobby shops, enjoy recreational facilities, and establish superficial, but sustained, relationships with staff and other patients. Even those who are able merely to exist rather than fully participate in this setting can often live in a more humane way than is possible for them when they are pushed into the community. Without institutional asylum, they are likely to be abused by strangers and resented by neighbors. They often wind up sleeping on the street and are liable to suffer from exposure, starvation, and medical neglect.

Until recently, a number of states were attempting to close all of their chronic care inpatient facilities and to shift the burden of care for the patients involved into community facilities. This has turned out to be a mistake. We must recognize that even our improved acute treatment methods have limitations and that certain patients remain as much in need of custodial, asylum care now as if they lived in the 19th century. In fact, a renaissance of the "moral treatment" methods would certainly not be out of place for this population. The problem of many current custodial hospitals is that they have been dreadfully undersupported financially and have become deplorable places in which to live and to

TABLE 1-5

Differential Criteria for Treatment Setting When the Goal is Maintenance

Outpatient	Partial Hospitalization	Hospitalization
Relative Indications 1) Mental disorder of sufficient severity and chronicity as to require lifelong care, usually involving psychotropic medication.	*Relative Indications* 1) Patient has a chronic mental illness that would require custodial care or result in patient's isolation and deterioration in the community. 2) Patient requires a professionally organized and supervised social network. 3) Patient requires regular treatment, but behavior would deteriorate in a more active treatment program.	*Relative Indications* 1) Patient requires asylum because of chronic, severe and disabling mental disorder not amenable to treatment and impairing ability to survive in community. 2) Lack of family or community supports.
Enabling Factors 1) Ability to maintain oneself in community and/or presence of adequate family supports.	*Enabling Factors* 1) Patient must be able to attend and	*Enabling Factors* None
Relative Containdications 1) Patient improves sufficiently so that		*Relative Contraindications* 1) Patient has condition that might be

40

continuous care no longer necessary. 2) Problem severity requires more intense maintenance care.

form an allegiance to the program, and ensure that his financial and living arrangements will not interfere with treatment.

Relative Contraindications
1) Patient can be managed in less intensive outpatient program alone and is able to build a social network independently.
2) Patient is sufficiently impaired that symptoms require more intensive supervision (for example, inpatient treatment or intensive care partial hospital).
3) Patient has enough enabling factors to qualify for a rehabilitation partial hospital.

amenable to more intense treatment or managed in community.

41

work. A good chronic care hospital is a joy to behold and we need more of them.

Chronic Care Partial Hospital

Deinstitutionalization and shorter inpatient stays have led to the development of chronic care partial hospitals for patients who otherwise would be adrift without any regular daily activity. Like the chronic care inpatient hospitals, these partial hospitals have humble expectations, high symptom tolerance, and low staff/patient ratios. They are generally located geographically away from psychiatric hospitals. The treatment is often delivered primarily by paraprofessionals and is focused on buffering the stresses of everyday life and on providing a structured environment where patients can interact with others and can participate in various activities under supervision. For some, these hospitals become more than a place to play cards and take medication. The setting becomes an extended family and provides a social network comparable to that in an inpatient setting, but at far less expense and with greater patient autonomy and responsibility. For others, it is a nice place to drop in occasionally – a kind of sheltered social club.

Maintenance Outpatient Therapy

Some patients can be maintained at their current level of functioning without significant exacerbations so long as they are seen monthly for adjustment and renewal of medication. This can be done in individual or group treatment or in the setting of a psychopharmacology or medication clinic. Frequently, patients become attached to the clinic itself, feeling that the institution rather than any one particular therapist is looking after them. This is usually desirable because institutions generally stay while therapists may leave. Although such settings have been criticized for providing apparently perfunctory care, some patients actually cannot tolerate any involvement that they experience as too intense or intimate and instead respond more favorably to pleasant, though somewhat superficial, support, encouragement, and advice. Providing coffee and doughnuts is likely to increase patient compliance and morale. The use of long-lasting intramuscular depot medication also increases compliance and reduces rehospitalization ratio.

With these possibilities in mind, what should now be decided for Mr. P.? As opposed to the choices for Mrs. A. or Mr. B., the alternatives for Mr. P. all seem limited, perhaps hopeless, and certainly sad. With his dire past history, lasting benefit or even a reasonably humane existence in any setting seems doubtful. This prognostic pessimism diminishes interest in chronic patients and helps to explain why, until recently, chronic care facilities have not been carefully studied or even discussed.

The safest and most readily accessible choice for Mr. P. is to suggest yet one more admission to an acute care hospital. In an inpatient service, he can be bathed, fed, medically evaluated, and medicated before taking another half turn through the constantly revolving door back into the community. This acute setting offers temporary protection from exposure to cold or molestation in the park or a stabbing in the subway. While keeping Mr. P. in his holding pattern, the staff can attempt to make arrangements for an SRO and for aftercare at a day hospital or outpatient clinic. The problem with this disposition to an acute setting is that it is unlikely to address the long-range issues of how best to prevent constant relapses. Mr. P. will almost definitely return on a cold night to one or another hospital emergency room, never having followed any of the discharge plans that were made for him.

A second alternative is to refer Mr. P. back to the day hospital, where the staff is already familiar with Mr. P.'s response to different medications and is tolerant, even comfortable, with his ramblings, outbursts, gestures, and rituals. Of concern is the possibility that some adventitious event occurring outside the hospital — a stranger's remark on the bus, a fellow tenant's unexpected knock on the door or whatever — will rekindle Mr. P.'s suspiciousness leading him once again to take to the streets and to avoid the minimal social contact of the partial hospital setting.

A third, and probably least acceptable, option is to arrange for outpatient psychotherapy. Mr. P. has never responded to or even attended any of the many outpatient programs that have been recommended for him. When crisis intervention was tried in conjunction with rapid tranquilization, social service funding, and home visits, Mr. P. found the involvement too intense. After three weeks, he dropped out of sight for months. When less frequent outpatient care was arranged, Mr. P. never even showed up for an aftercare clinic appointment.

Unfortunately, the best choice for Mr. P. has become increasingly unavailable. He might be most comfortable and productive if he could be admitted for an extended period, perhaps the rest of his life, to a well-run custodial inpatient facility of the sort in which he has already spent the best 17 years of his adult life. Opponents argue that this option is old-fashioned, demoralizing, and neglectful of Mr. P.'s civil rights. Advocates reply that Mr. P.'s chaotic life in a predatory community is not an expression of civil rights, but rather presents an inability to accept the limitations of what certain people can be expected to achieve even with modern treatment methods. Some patients simply need "asylum" in the nonpejorative sense of this word. However, in recent years, under the theoretical aegis of community psychiatry and serving the practical financial function of reducing state budgets, many state hospitals across the country have "deinstitutionalized." They have redefined their function and now provide acute rather than maintenance care; they are no longer "asylums" for such individuals as Mr. P.

Considering these unappealing possibilities for Mr. P., the harried emergency room consultant decided not to decide, at least right away. After a psychiatric and physical examination, he ordered some screening blood tests and let Mr. P. sleep in the waiting room until morning. In the light of a new day, the situation seemed somewhat less gloomy. The consultant contacted the day hospital social worker, who for many years had been quite committed to Mr. P. She came to the emergency room, spoke at length with Mr. P., and escorted him to the day hospital, where he spent the day being bathed, fed, and medicated. She arranged for emergency welfare and living quarters and Mr. P. was taken that evening by a staff member to his new SRO. The following day another staff member was to stop by on the way to work to escort Mr. P. back to the partial hospital. When the staff member arrived the next morning, Mr. P. was nowhere to be found and attempts throughout the next three days failed to locate him. A week later he reappeared in the emergency room presenting exactly the same picture as described above.

Research Review

It is ironic that the plight of Mr. P. is at least in part the result of important advances made by psychiatry during the past two decades. Chronic inpatient custodial care has been challenged by the documented effectiveness of psychotropic drugs, brief hospitalization, day hospitals, and community-based treatment. Unfortunately, there has not been any concerted research effort to demonstrate that, for certain patients, custodial care remains the optimal form of treatment. This is an inherently difficult topic for study – symptom remission is more easily measured than is the evidence that further deterioration has been avoided or that life is being led more or less comfortably.

A number of studies have evaluated the cost-effectiveness of deinstitutionalization. Murphy and Datel (1976) compared institutional treatment with placement in the community. They first calculated the total cost for removing 52 mentally retarded patients from state institutions and providing them community care. The projected cost of housing, subsistence, and therapy over a ten-year period was far less expensive for community care. The study does have some methodological problems. The researchers concentrated on cost-effectiveness and not on patient benefit. Although they presented data on such things as marriage, normality of appearance, mobility in the community, and employment, they did not consider these factors sufficiently in determining cost/benefit ratios. Another problem with this study is that patients who refused placement in the community were considered treatment failures and excluded from the data analysis. A patient like Mr. P., who did not want community care but was forced into it, can over the long haul engender enormous costs in frequent hospitalizations, emergency room visits, social service time and money, and so on.

Cassell, Smith, Grunberg, Boan and Thomas (1972) studied 500 deinstitutionalized patients, mostly chronic schizophrenics, who had resided in mental hospitals for an average of 18.2 years prior to deinstitutionalization. They found that the cost of placing these patients in the community and providing welfare, follow-up, drugs and rehospitalization was almost 25% less than the cost of keeping them in the hospital. Although few of the patients would have been discharged if the deinstitutionalization program had not begun, 49% of the men and 38% of the women under age 65 were employed at least three months during the first two years after discharge; more than 20% of the men and 10% of the women were employed for at least 13 months during those first two years. Strikingly, medical care was actually less for the deinstitutionalized patients than would be expected for normally adjusted people in similar circumstances.

Studies of the type just reviewed have had a profound impact on the administration and policy of chronic care hospitals; however, they suffer from the limitations of a research design that is not experimental. For example, they did not consider that new treatments were simultaneously being introduced within mental hospitals and that the favorable response may have been due to the introduction of medication and not to deinstitutionalization. Furthermore, since a randomized control group was not used in these studies, it seems reasonable to assume that the patients who were deinstitutionalized may have been precisely those who were less disabled than those who remained in the hospital. The studies did not determine which subgroup of patients would do better if left in the hospital. In addition, although most studies try to calculate the total cost of discharged patients by including housing and maintenance expenses, a comprehensive accounting of community cost is far more difficult than figuring the total cost borne in a hospital. The relatively low cost reported for community treatment may be overly optimistic.

Weisbrod (1979) tried to do a more comprehensive and less contaminated study of the cost and benefits of community care. He randomly assigned patients to two groups. One group of 65 patients consisted of those who had been briefly hospitalized (usually less than one month) and followed at local mental health agencies with repeated hospitalizations over the next year. The 65 patients in the other group were placed in an alternative community-based program with relatively very little time in institutions; every effort was made not to hospitalize any patient in this group. Patients assigned to "community living" were required to take responsibility for problems which might in other circumstances have resulted in their return to an institution. Weisbrod's cost assessment of "community living" was comprehensive and included the expense of treatment, the financial burden on the family, and so on. The study indicated that community care was slightly more costly, but also more beneficial because those assigned to community treatment earned more from employment.

Despite the use of random assignment to a control group and comprehensive assessment of cost and benefits, Weisbrod's study does have important limitations that prevent its generalization to patients like Mr. P. First, although data were collected over a four-year period (1972–1976), each patient participated in the study for only 14 months. For chronic patients like Mr. P., that relatively brief time under study may not be sufficient. Second, Weisbrod studied fewer than 150 patients, all of whom came from the same geographic area – a group that may not be sufficiently representative of all those eligible for deinstitutionalization. Third, neither group contained patients like Mr. P., who had been institutionalized for many years and then placed suddenly and involuntarily back into the community.

Several studies have compared long-term day hospital care with outpatient treatment. Linn, Caffey, Klett, Hogarty, and Lamb (1979) compared the effectiveness of ten different day hospital programs to outpatient psychotherapy for chronic schizophrenics. As a group, patients treated in the partial hospital had superior outcome. Further, this study identified characteristics of good and poor outcome programs and of patients likely to be at high risk of decompensation in each particular treatment setting. Good outcome (as manifested by longer remissions, reduced symptoms, and greater alteration in attitude) was associated with programs that offered more occupational therapy, lower patient turnover, and relatively longer lengths of stay. Poor results were found in those centers with more professional staff hours, more group therapy, and high patient turnover. Interestingly, good outcome centers operated at significantly less cost than did poor outcome programs. Linn et al. were also able to determine which patients were at high risk in these programs. These tended to be patients who were anxious, guilt-ridden, motorically retarded, hyperactive, and disorganized. The greatest value of this study is that it suggests not only which patients do well or poorly in partial hospitals or outpatient treatment, but also what the qualities of the programs are that prove to be most beneficial to the patients. In short, the study helps determine not only who should receive the treatment, but how the treatment should be given.

Other preliminary attempts have been made to find out how patients in different diagnostic categories do in different settings. Guy, Gross, Hogarty, and Dennis (1969) also compared chronic patients treated in a partial hospital with those treated as outpatients. Both schizoaffective and chronic schizophrenic patients did better in the partial hospital setting; the improvement shown by those with schizoaffective disorders was greater than the improvement of those with chronic schizophrenia.

With such limited data regarding settings for maintenance therapy, no definitive conclusions can be made concerning the best disposition for patients like Mr. P. It is clear that many patients benefit from the combination of medication, deinstitutionalization, and community care, but available studies are not designed to separate a subgroup of patients like Mr. P. who require long-term custodial care. The momentum that swept patients out the hospital door may have gone too far when it deprived Mr. P. of his comfortable cubicle on Ward F.

SUMMARY

We have described three types of inpatient hospitalization (acute care, longer term rehabilitation, and custodial); three types of day hospital (acute care, longer term rehabilitative, and maintenance); and three types of outpatient care (crisis intervention, rehabilitative, and maintenance). For any given patient, it must be decided whether the goal of the treatment intervention is 1) to treat acute and urgent symptoms in a short-term setting, or 2) to help the patient change more deeply ingrained symptoms or behaviors in a longer term setting, or 3) to help prevent deterioration in what may be a lifelong, but less intense, treatment environment. For each goal, there must be a second decision about the most appropriate of three levels of care – inpatient, partial hospital, or outpatient.

A few important conclusions can be drawn from the available research:

1) Many patients who have received inpatient treatment for acute problems can probably be managed as well, less disruptively, and much more cheaply in acute day hospitals or by crisis intervention. Clinicians should probably think twice before recommending inpatient admission whenever these alternatives are available and should probably lobby and work toward making them more available.

2) Longer term rehabilitative hospitals probably serve a useful purpose for a selected group of patients, but this remains to be documented by research. Since the hospitals delivering such care are usually voluntary and dependent on third-party support, it seems crucial that they make every effort to initiate this research. Rehabilitative day hospitals have not been much studied or described in the literature but show great promise, particularly for those who might regress in a long-term inpatient hospital but who nonetheless require more structure than can be provided in outpatient treatment.

3) Although custodial care should certainly be provided at the least restrictive and least expensive level of care, this does not mean that long-term custodial hospitals can close up shop and transfer their patients in wholesale fashion into the community.

The reader will note that we have defined our settings not only by goal but also to some degree by duration and technique—issues that are separately covered in more detail in later chapters. This illustrates the fact, mentioned already in the Introduction, that it is impossible, and not really desirable, to completely keep separate all of the various steps of the treatment decision tree.

CHAPTER 2

The Format

After having chosen a therapeutic setting, the consultant must next make a series of decisions concerning the treatment format (e.g., group, family, marital, or individual), treatment orientation (e.g., psychodynamic, behavioral, cognitive, or systems), and the duration and frequency of the treatment that will occur within that setting. Although in clinical practice, these three decisions to some extent co-determine one another and are made together, for purposes of exposition we will consider each decision separately in each of the next three chapters. We will begin by discussing the clinical issues and relevant research regarding the selection of therapeutic format.

A GENERAL SYSTEMS APPROACH

A general systems approach (Schwartz, 1982) is a useful way to conceptualize the issues involved in choosing a particular format of therapy for a specific patient. Systems theory is based on the observation that nature is organized in hierarchies with smaller and less complex units subordinate to larger and more complex aggregates. Figure 1 places an individual within a condensed hierarchal scheme. Each level has its own distinctive characteristics and organization, but each level is also a component of a higher system. Every unit is both a whole and a part. Systems theory reminds us that nothing exists in isolation. Though each unit has its own unique properties and dynamics, at the same time each unit will be more or less influenced by supraordinate and subordinate systems. Systems theory also reminds us that neither a biological model of medical illness (the components shown below the "person" level) nor a familio-social model (the components shown above the "person") nor a

49

FIGURE 1

Society — Government
↕
Culture — Subculture
↕
Community — Organizations
↕
Friends — Relatives
↕
Immediate Family
↕
Spouse
↕
PERSON
↕
Nervous and Other Organ Systems
↕
Cells
↕
Molecules

psychological model ("the person") are by themselves sufficient. An integrative biopsychosocial approach is needed to conceptualize emotional problems and their treatment.

Although a general systems theory does not provide specific answers or remove the uncertainty inherent in choosing a therapeutic format, it is a useful way of conceptualizing the three steps involved when making this decision: 1) evaluating the intra-system problems; 2) evaluating the inter-system problems; and 3) deciding at what level or levels in the hierarchal system therapeutic interventions are most likely to be effective.

Evaluating the "Intra-system" Problems

The comprehensive evaluation of any patient requires the consultant to gather data directly or indirectly about each of the various systems. Moving "up" the hierarchy in sequence, this assessment would include information about physical disorders, psychological functioning, marriage, family background, friendships, professional and community interactions, culture, and nationality. Some evaluations of this kind provide data suggesting that one or perhaps two systems have played the most prominent, although not exclusive, role in causing or maintaining the current emotional problems. In such instances, the format of treatment should in all probability be directed at those systems that are most involved. For example, if a woman's sleeplessness, irritability, palpitations, and anxiety stem from hyperthyroidism, then an organ system (thyroid gland) will of course be the main focus of treatment and this will occur within an individual format. If an adolescent's truancy, defiance, and depression appear to be primarily the result of family battles and scapegoating, then the first choice would most likely be to treat the whole family system with the format of family therapy. And, if a man's embarrassment and fear of ridicule prevent him from establishing friendships or participating in age-appropriate social activities, the format of a heterogeneous group might be chosen to treat interpersonal inhibitions that arise within the community system.

Evaluating the Inter-system Problems

More often the emotional problems requiring treatment cannot conveniently be attributed to any one system. Instead, interactions among many systems are contributing to the problem. To place the origin in any one system would be unnecessarily reductionistic and is not in keeping with the biopsychosocial model. For example, a man depressed after a heart attack may at first glance appear to have a problem primarily arising from the person or organ or cellular system; but an inter-system evaluation might well reveal that his despair is not simply a personal and internal *reaction* to his disease but also a response to an *interaction* between his limited physical capacities and a failure to meet his wife's demands. The format of marital therapy rather than individual therapy or a combination of the two might then be the best choice to deal with this inter-system problem.

Although the necessity of such an inter-system evaluation is intuitively obvious, a wish to make a complex clinical situation more comprehensible and manageable may incline the consultant arbitrarily to confine a problem to one or two systems and thereby overlook information which may be helpful in deciding on a format. For example, when a woman in her late forties presents with signs and symptoms of a severe depression with melancholia the consultant might be tempted to restrict the problem to the cellular system and direct his attention to the use of antidepressants within an individual format. In reducing the problem for the purposes of management, the consultant might miss that the woman's despair was in part an inter-system problem — namely, the result of a complex interplay among factors like her feelings about aging, her hormonal status, her husband's middle-aged disillusionment and withdrawal, and her high school daughter's attractive vivaciousness. A marital or family format might be necessary and appropriate to treat and to alleviate a problem that had been too categorically regarded only as biochemical.

Deciding at What Level Treatment Will Be Most Effective

For most consultants, the first two steps (intra- and inter-system assessment) emerge quite naturally during the interview. The evaluation discloses those systems that figure most prominently in causing or maintaining the problem and the ways in which various interactions among systems are contributing to the problem. The third step is more difficult: deciding at what level therapeutic interventions are most likely to be effective.

Systems theory is helpful not only in conceptualizing what factors have contributed to the problem, but also in determining what therapeutic format will be most helpful. The theory holds that just as no one isolated system can sufficiently explain the cause of any given problem, a change in any one subsystem will necessarily have an effect on the workings of the general system. The consultant should therefore not feel pressured to find *the* one system from which the problem originated and to arrange a format to treat that system alone. Rather, the consultant can look for that system most amenable to constructive change and expect that any change will ultimately influence other systems as well. In short, *the selection of a reasonable format becomes less a decision about which system caused the problem and more a decision about which troubled system can best be treated and changed.*

Some examples will illustrate this point. A woman's obesity may have been "caused" by some combination of constitutional predisposition (cellular system), unconscious fears of sexual intimacy (person system), depression and overeating following fights with her husband (marital system), conditioned eating patterns in her family (family system) and even in part by economic and ethnic factors (community system and culture system); yet the format chosen for treatment – such as a homogeneous weight watchers group – may address most directly interpersonal issues not easily subsumed within any one of these etiological subsystems. General systems theory would sanction such a choice by explaining that if the interpersonal system is more susceptible to change and more immediately powerful in encouraging weight reduction, then this relatively peripheral system (from an etiological perspective) deserves to be chosen with the hope and expectation that improvement in any one subsystem will lead to alterations and improvement in other subsystems as well. In this sense, the theory is reassuring. Often a patient will not accept the recommended format (such as a heterogeneous group instead of individual therapy) or the preferred format cannot be arranged (such as family therapy with an adolescent child who refuses to attend). In these situations, the consultant need not feel defeated by an "unmotivated" patient if an accepted and acceptable alternative format can be found. Changes in one system will inevitably "spill over" and influence other more troubled but less accessible subsystems.

General systems theory can also be reassuring in those cases when both the consultant and patient might feel discouraged because the "basic" problem cannot be "cured." As long as positive changes can be made—even within systems not directly related to the core issues—treatment can be helpful. For example, a schizophrenic woman living in total isolation may have problems that arise most basically from the cellular system or person system and these systems may have proven refractory to change; nonetheless, a format of a homogeneous group therapy may be helpful and may prevent chronic discouragement and deterioration. The point is that even though the community system is not in any way primarily etiological, the most appropriate format for this patient may well be one that addresses this peripheral system and provides the patient an opportunity to share her dilemma with other chronically ill patients.

This optimistic application of systems theory does require a cautionary note. Although changes in one system will influence other systems, at times these changes are not necessarily the ones desired and may not be therapeutic. Changes in any one system can place stress on other systems, stresses which may be destructive rather than lead to constructive change. For example, if a chronically depressed man responds successfully to treatment of the person system, he may then be less willing to tolerate the infantilizing behavior of his family and spouse. They in turn may be quite distressed by his new capacity to assert himself and also to express resentment more openly. For this reason, the therapist must be alert to situations in which a change of format or combined format may be warranted; in this case, changing from an individual to a family format (or combining both) as the depression begins to improve might be necessary to address more directly problems which are arising secondarily in other systems.

One concluding remark about the application of systems theory to selection of a therapeutic format: We are fully aware that most of us do not instinctively conceptualize clinical problems in the way systems theory demands. To assimilate and comprehend the wealth of data presented in any clinical interview, we tend to narrow the focus and confine our formulations to one or two systems. Although this process makes the material more manageable, there is a danger that decisions will be based on too restricted a perspective. For a time during their inception, different formats – group, marital, family – were regarded by their advocates as *the* treatment of choice for the wide range of human misery and therapists were labeled by the formats they preferred – "family therapists," "marriage counselors," "group leaders," and so on. With the knowledge provided by accumulating clinical experience and controlled research studies, we are now closer to understanding that the benefits of one format over another are not easily discernible, perhaps because a change within any one system will affect supraordinate and subordinate systems as well. If any one system is amenable to change and can be approached skillfully, hopefully, and enthusiastically by the therapist, other systems will inevitably be influenced – for better or for worse. Although more bewildering and humbling than we would like, a general systems approach must be applied when selecting a format and assessing the results of any treatment. Put simply, general systems theory is a fancy model for confirming that there are many ways of skinning a cat.

To illustrate how a general systems approach can be used when one selects a therapeutic format, we will present a patient who might possibly benefit from any one of the various alternatives: individual psychotherapy, conjoint therapy, family therapy, heterogeneous group therapy, and homogeneous group therapy. After a description of these different possibilities, we will discuss what format was actually chosen for the patient and why. We will conclude by reviewing the relevant research to determine if existing studies would have supported the choice of format and would have predicted the outcome.

THE CASE OF THE UPROOTED SPOUSE

Mr. Y. is calling to arrange an appointment for his wife, whom he describes as increasingly seclusive and depressed. In the detached tone of a business letter, Mr. Y. laconically presents the facts: He and his wife are a Japanese couple in their late thirties and have two teenage daughters; he was transferred by his company from Tokyo to the United States three years ago; his wife has been unable to make the adjustment; their marriage is going sour; she needs help and has finally agreed to visit the consultant. He would also like to meet separately with the therapist – for reasons he does not explain. Is the therapist free to see him at 3:00 or 3:30 the day after tomorrow? And when would he like to meet with his wife?

Expecting the matter to be settled in this fashion, Mr. Y. sounds surprised at the suggestion that he and his wife be seen together for the first consultation and, again for reasons not made clear over the phone, he appears to find this possibility unseemly. Rather than lock horns over the issue (for it feels as though that is what would happen), the consultant agrees to make two appointments, one each to see Mr. and Mrs. Y. separately, but indicates that a complete consultation will probably require at least one subsequent joint visit. Without arguing, Mr. Y. schedules only the individual sessions for his wife and for himself, then right before ending the call, repeats one more time that his wife will never accept a conjoint session.

Mrs. Y. appears for her first appointment. She is an elegantly beautiful woman whose porcelain skin contrasts with the deep blue of her silk Japanese dress. Her features and manner are delicate, even fragile, like a thin vase meant to be admired, not touched. Speaking in an accented but idiomatic English, she admits blushingly that she has kept the appointment only to obey her husband. She would never knowingly go against his wishes, yet the notion that she requires help for her emotions is a profound humiliation from which she will not soon recover (and the consultant also senses that she will not soon forgive her husband for his insisting on the visit).

Throughout the interview Mrs. Y. remains refined and demure, but tells the consultant that she wishes to be cooperative and will answer questions as fully as she can. Yes, her husband is right, she has not adjusted well to New York City. Though always a bit shy and retiring, at least in Japan she had a close circle of cultured friends whom she had known since childhood. Now she is alone. The American neighbors near her suburban home seem brash and brazen. The Japanese affiliated with her husband's company have remained only superficial acquaintances — it makes no sense to get close to people who may be transferred unpredictably.

When asked how the move to the United States has affected other members of the family, Mrs. Y. stiffens, pauses, and becomes even more reluctant to expose such "private affairs." The silence breaks as Mrs. Y. reaches for a tissue and wipes away tears before they have in fact formed. Yes, if the truth must be known, Mrs. Y. is quite upset about how the move has changed her husband and children. In Japan they had been a tightly woven family with shared spiritual and aesthetic interests. Now, pursuing the immediate and forgetting their past, "certain ones" are losing their priorities, values, and heritage.

Mrs. Y. goes on to recall nostalgically how close she and Mr. Y. had been for so many years. They had grown up in the same neighborhood, attended the same schools, and as childhood sweethearts had decided to marry even before they were in their teens. But now the fairy tale has come to an end. Instead of living happily ever after in the home they had planned in their dreams and built with their love, she is now misplaced in a foreign land and watching her loved ones turn into strangers. As Mr. Y. continues his executive climb, he is either away on business trips or working long hours into the night at the office. Because he commutes from the suburbs into the city and is far away from their home, their traditional lunches together are no longer possible. And as for the children? They are "on their own," "liberated," "Americanized," and "dating every day or night." Mrs. Y. feels her previous bond with them is irreparably broken . . . "and there is more" – but having made this provocative remark, Mrs. Y. refuses to go on.

The consultant acknowledges that for both personal and cultural reasons, Mrs. Y. cannot easily reveal her private concerns to a stranger, even if he is a doctor. When she asks why she should, the consultant replies that while he certainly cannot guarantee that talking will be helpful, he is quite sure that her reticence will interfere with whatever help he might otherwise be able to offer. Only she can judge whether it is worth a try. After a long pause for reflection, Mrs. Y. proceeds with an unburdening sigh to tell "the rest of the story."

She has perceived a change in her husband's manners. The change is decidedly for the worse. In Japan his business associates were all male. His dealings with them were correct and formal. In the United States, his associates are now both male and female, and he has become informal and familiar in a way she finds offensive. In particular, Mr. Y. has developed a relationship that "lacks gentility" with a young American woman who is the representative of one of his subcontractors. He praises her, has lunch with her, even sends her Christmas gifts as if she were "a close friend." When asked if Mrs. Y. suspects there have been sexual intimacies, she bristles and looks at the consultant as if he had missed the point entirely. Of course the affair had never been "physical." She is convinced her husband would never be *that* indiscreet and assures the therapist she would know instinctively if he ever did betray her. The problem is not so much what he has done sexually or even what he might consider doing; the problem is that a closeness of whatever kind to another woman is in her view "unnatural."

Fearing that she herself may have also been indiscreet by airing such private concerns, Mrs. Y. abruptly ends the interview with the statement that she hopes the consultant will understand her position and forgive her openness. She adds, however, that any indiscretions that she may have committed will have been worthwhile if the consultant can convince Mr. Y. to sever his association with "the woman." The prospect of getting rid of "the woman" and returning the family to the status quo has clearly been the purpose of her visit as she conceives it. Having made her wishes known, Mrs. Y. cordially and gracefully departs.

The next day Mr. Y. arrives at the exact moment of his appointment. In contrast to his delicate wife, he is a robust and energetic man with an expansive confidence that fills the room with his presence. He begins the interview by asking what the therapist has in mind to help his wife adjust to their new living situation and, with this agenda declared, he implies that any other issues will be extraneous and a waste of time. His reasons for wanting a separate appointment are now stated directly. His wife, though she is a wonderful mother and woman whom he loves dearly, can be "something of a martyr" and "exaggerate everyday problems" until they (and she) become oppressive. Mr. Y. wants to correct any distortions before the consultant gets the wrong idea. Yes, he is indeed fond of his female business associate, but he is far more enraptured with a multi-million dollar merger he is orchestrating with the firm she represents. Now, at the very time that his career is at a crucial stage and just when he may achieve heights he had never before imagined, his wife is becoming a distracting nuisance and is unreasonably upset over what he regards as a perfectly legitimate professional relationship. She is being old-fashioned and has just got to be brought to her senses before her clinging and unreasonable behavior drives her and everyone else in the home crazy. Mr. Y. wants his wife "treated" so that she will learn and accept that business and personal affairs are conducted differently in the United States. Can the therapist teach her this lesson and help her adjust?

Despite his bullying manner, Mr. Y.'s genuine compassion for his wife is also shown during the interview as he tenderly reviews the loving times they used to have. Nevertheless, when the possibility of couple or family treatment is again mentioned to Mr. Y., he remains unenthusiastic and this time lists the reasons why it is a bad idea: 1) His wife is the problem and his presence would only prevent her from getting full attention; 2) his wife would never talk candidly in front of him; and 3) family treatment makes no sense at all because the children are fine and should be spared any embarrassment. He does believe, however, that one conjoint session would be a good idea because his wife will undoubtedly have some distorted notions that he may be able to help straighten out for the therapist.

The conjoint evaluation takes place the following week and begins with a stilted exchange of pleasantries. Mrs. Y. admires a picture in the consultant's office. She mentions that she had thought about the painting off and on all week and would have been complimentary during the first visit "but," she says, smiling graciously, "I was distracted." As if on cue, Mr. Y. then praises his wife's cultured taste and adds how she has brought the richness of the arts into their family life. With the same somewhat patronizing manner, Mr. Y. then thanks the busy consultant for arranging all the appointments so promptly.

After a few moments, the awkward cordialities can no longer contain the mounting tension in the room. When the consultant merely asks how things have been going at home, he is astonished as Mrs. Y. begins an uncharacteristic but uninterruptable attack on her husband for what seems to be an endless list of abuses related in one way or another to his female associate and their negotiations, dinner engagements, late nights, business trips, exchanged gifts, compliments, admiring glances, and other such indiscretions, all of which Mrs. Y. relates like a prosecuting attorney with the exact dates, places and other supportive evidence.

Mr. Y. at first responds by making a few rather meek attempts at explanation or denial, but then soon resigns himself to sit back and shrug off each new accusation with feigned indifference. In contrast to his inflated manner the previous week, he now appears no match for his wife's piercing attack. Mrs. Y. is now anything but demure. She reacts to her husband's retreat by becoming even more spiteful about "his infidelity of the heart," about his ruining a perfect marriage for "an unpruned rose," and about his more recent attempts to erode the moral values of their elder daughter by allowing her to "walk the streets." This last accusation strains Mr. Y.'s tolerance and he heatedly accuses his wife in turn of being too old-fashioned to understand their children and of clutching onto their younger daughter as if they were both frightened children adrift at sea. With that, Mrs. Y. begins shouting back in rapid Japanese and Mr. Y., now similarly oblivious to the presence of the consultant, begins his rebuttal in Japanese as well. Only when the consultant shouts "Stop!" does the couple stop ignoring him.

After everyone takes a minute to calm down, the therapist puts the obvious into words by stating that each spouse has been struggling to contain very strong anger towards the other. Mrs. Y. takes this statement as an accusation and guiltily explains she was only doing what she thought was expected by the consultant and her husband, that is, to express her feelings honestly. She issues formal apologies to her husband and to the consultant, promises to control herself, and whispers sulkily, "I can't even do *this* right." Mr. Y., again feeling frustrated and helpless, looks to the consultant for suggestions.

With only a few minutes left in the session, the consultant asks about happiness in the marriage. Just as the anger between the couple was surprisingly open, so is their obvious deep commitment and love for one another. The consultant then explains that he would like to give the problem some time for reflection before making definite recommendations about treatment. He mentions briefly the possibilities and suggests that the couple give the matter some thought before they all meet the following week to discuss what form of treatment would be most advisable. Mr. and Mrs. Y. agree and with the same controlled graciousness that had accompanied them into the room, they thank the consultant and leave.

Systems theory helps us conceptualize the many different levels of Mr. and Mrs. Y.'s problems:

Cultural System – Mrs. Y.'s poor adjustment to a new culture and her objections to her husband's and daughters' changed habits and manners as they have become westernized.

Community System – Mrs. Y.'s limited friendships, Mr. Y.'s preoccupation with professional pursuits and a long commute, the elder daughter's precocious dating patterns, the younger daughter's difficulties in school.

Family System – Mrs. Y.'s clinging to the younger daughter for support while Mr. Y. establishes the older daughter as an Americanized ally and encourages her to act against Mrs. Y.'s wishes.

Marital System – The mounting spite each spouse has for the other as Mrs. Y. resents her husband's possible affair of the heart and Mr. Y. resents his wife's alternating possessiveness and bitter withdrawal.

Person System – Mrs. Y.'s incomplete sense of an individuated self and her need to live through others rather than act autonomously (perhaps satisfying a DSM-III Axis 2 diagnosis of dependent personality disorder as well as an Axis 1 diagnosis of major depression without melancholia); Mr. Y.'s need for continuous success, admiration, and control to bolster self-esteem (perhaps satisfying the DSM-III Axis 2 diagnosis of compulsive personality disorder with narcissistic features).

Organ System – Mrs. Y.'s vegetative symptoms and family history of depression would suggest current neurotransmitter malfunction and constitutional predisposition.

The decision about therapeutic format for Mr. and Mrs. Y. will involve selecting that level or levels within the general system which will be most amenable to constructive change. We will describe the background and rationale of the five therapeutic formats under consideration – individual, conjoint marital, family, heterogeneous group, and homogeneous group (see Table 2-1) – and then, with this perspective, will return to what was actually decided for Mr. and Mrs. Y. and the results of that decision.

INDIVIDUAL THERAPY

An individual format would be an obvious choice for Mrs. Y. She is the declared patient, is clearly in despair, and is adapting poorly to changes in her husband, her children and her living situation. A one-to-one therapy could focus on these problems within the "person system."

Individual treatment is the most traditional and probably still by far the most prevalent of the psychotherapeutic formats. For thousands of years man has sought advice and relief from suffering by consulting privately with a designated authority – an oracle, shaman, witch doctor, priest, rabbi, village elder, or physician. This consultation has usually occurred within a "magic circle," a demarcated area invested with special powers and geographically or symbolically removed from the real world. The relationship between psychotherapist and patient in our own society maintains these elements of delegated omnipotence and confidentiality. A trip to the hospital, mental health clinic, or doctor's office is capable of stirring up in most people the same strange mixture of awe, fear, trust, and hope that has always been associated with entering a mysterious place that has been set aside from the day-to-day world.

Individual therapy has a number of advantages as well as certain definite disadvantages for situations like the one we have just described regarding Mrs. Y. In its favor, the individual format usually provides the smoothest induction into treatment with the lowest incidence of dropouts. Many patients are aware they have emotional problems and may even admit to themselves that they are in need of help, but they are easily intimidated, ashamed, and frightened about the very idea of psychotherapy. For them, the individual format may be the easiest to accept for several reasons:

1) Familiarity. In maintaining many of the features of the traditional doctor-patient relationship, the individual format is a familiar one that (for patients like Mrs. Y.) even succeeds in crossing cultural lines. She doubtlessly has had occasion in the past to see a doctor in Japan for advice, comfort, and relief of one or another physical problem. She may also have consulted a priest or other spiritual figure for suggestions and support. This familiarity based on tradition and personal experience makes the individual format less threatening than, for example, sitting down with a group of complete strangers to discuss intimate problems.

2) Role definition. Within the individual format, the patient not only knows what to expect, but has some idea about what is expected. In other formats (i.e., family or group therapy) the role of the therapist and patient has not been so traditionally defined or widely accepted, and patients must often struggle with greater uncertainty as they work out the kinds of interaction which will lead to constructive change. At least during the initial phase of individual treatments, the patient has some notion about what he or she is to do (to tell the therapist what is the matter) and some notion of what to expect in return (a suggestion, a pill, a reassuring phrase, or an interpretation). Despite cultural differences and personal inhibitions, Mrs. Y. was able to understand and to assume a defined patient role in the first session. When seen during the second session with her husband, Mrs. Y. had less sense of what to do. She vacillated between, on the one extreme, experiencing the encounter as a social exchange requiring compliments to the therapist stated in a stilted manner or, at the other extreme, experiencing the encounter as having no rules whatsoever so that she might feel free to lambast her husband while completely ignoring the therapist.

3) Confidentiality. For someone like Mrs. Y. who is exquisitely shy, embarrassed, and self-conscious, the issue of absolute privacy can be crucial. The presence of others – known or unknown to the patient – makes candid exposure too difficult for some patients.

4) Trust. The basic trust inherent in the individual format extends beyond the issue of confidentiality and derives in part from a transferential attitude related to early caretaking figures. The dyadic format in particular fosters a regression because it is reminiscent of the childhood experiences of being loved and nurtured by a strong, all-knowing, and protective parental figure. Accordingly, the individual therapist, even though a relative stranger, may be delegated certain powers and expertise by the childlike "helpless" patient. This initial positive transference can be used to overcome early resistances to therapy and to form the basis of an eventual working alliance. Despite Mrs. Y.'s cultural and personal reservations about revealing intimate concerns in the first session, the basic trust inherent in the individual format enabled her to expose potentially humiliating facts about herself and her family in the same way that patients will overcome their understandable embarrass-

TABLE 2-1

Relative Selection Criteria for Format: Individual, Family, and Group

Individual	Family/Marital	Group
Relative Indications	*Relative Indications*	*Relative Indications*
1) The patient's symptoms or character is based on firmly structured intrapsychic conflict that causes repetitive life patterns more or less transcending the particulars of the current interpersonal situation (e.g., family, job relationships).	1) Family/marital problems are presented as such, without either spouse or any family member designated as the identified patient; symptoms are predominantly within the marital relationship.	1) Patient's most pressing problems occur in current interpersonal relationships, both outside and inside family situations, such as:
2) Adolescent, young adult who is striving for autonomy.	2) Family presents with current structured difficulties in intrafamilial relationships with each person contributing collusively or openly to the reciprocal interaction problems.	(a) lonely, social and work inhibitions, excessive embarrassment with others, shy, feels unlovable;
3) Psychiatric problem is of such private and/or embarrassing matter that it needs the privacy of individual treatment, at least for the beginning phase.	3) Family has fixed and severe deficits in perception and communication:	(b) inability to share, needs excessive admiration from others, has difficulty understanding or caring about the needs of others;
	(a) projective identification so that each member blames the other for all problems;	(c) excessively argumentative, unable to cooperate, oppositional, authority problems;
	(b) family using paranoid/schizoid functioning; boundaries vague and fluctuating, parts of self readily projected onto other family members, trading of ego functions;	(d) excessively dependent, timid, unable to separate from family, unable to be properly assertive.
Enabling Factors	(c) a relentless fixity of distance maintained by pseudomutual and pseudohostile mechanisms;	2) The patient presents with problems that are significantly attributable to a specific disorder (e.g., alcoholism) for which a specialized group is available.
1) Comfortable in dyadic situation; able to handle the potential intimacy of the individual treatment setting.	(d) collective cognitive chaos and erratic distancing;	3) Patient has problems that are not predominantly interpersonal, but group indicated because:
2) Financial and temporal resources needed for individual treatment.	(e) amorphous, vague, undirected forms of communication that are pervasive.	(a) other modalities of treatment un-
	4) Adolescent acting-out behavior, e.g., promiscuity, drug abuse, delinquency, perversion, vandalism, violent behavior.	
	5) Another form of treatment is stalemated or has	

Relative Contraindications

1) Only issue of real importance is a family problem.

2) Patient regresses in individual therapy relationships.

failed, e.g., the patient has been unable to utilize intrapsychic mode of individual therapy or uses most of sessions to discuss family problems.

6) Improvement of one family member has led to symptoms or signs of deterioration in another.

7) Reduction of secondary gain in one or more family members is a major goal.

8) More than one person needs treatment, and resources are available for only one treatment.

Enabling Factors

1) Motivation is strongest to be seen as a couple or family, or an individual patient will accept no other format.

2) No family member has psychopathology of such proportions that family therapy would be prevented, e.g., extreme agitation, mania, paranoia, severe distrust, dangerous hostility, or acute schizophrenia.

3) Crucial members of a defined functional social system are available for family treatment.

Relative Contraindications

1) The presenting problem of the individual does not have a significant etiology in or effect upon the family system.

successful or reached maximum returns and further treatment needed.

(b) patient has a tendency to actualize the transference, to become excessively involved with and to persistently distort the relationship with an individual therapist.

(c) the patient is excessively intellectualized.

(d) patient cannot tolerate dyadic intimacy and is not motivated to change this characteristic.

(e) the patient typically elicits harmful countertransference responses from an individual therapist.

Enabling Factors

1) Patient is capable of participation in group treatment as evidenced by characteristics such as openness to influence from other patients, willingness to listen to others, willingness to participate in and maintain group process, etc.

2) Motivation for group treatment is at least adequate.

3) Availability or cost of treatment make

(continued)

TABLE 2-1 *(continued)*

Individual	Family/Marital	Group
		group referral desirable.
	2) Marital problems, if present, are chronic and ego-syntonic.	*Relative Contraindications*
	3) Defensive misuse of family therapy to deny individual responsibility for major personality or character illness.	1) There is an acute psychiatric emergency or crisis that requires more urgent, intense, specialized and individualized attention (e.g., acute depression, suicidal feelings, psychosis, mania, etc.).
	4) Massive but minimally relevant or unworkable parental pathology that indicates symptomatic child or adolescent should be treated alone.	2) The patient is likely to respond to brief therapy.
	5) Individuation of one or more family members requires that they have their own and separate treatment.	3) The patient refuses group treatment and his resistances are unmovable.
	6) Family treatment has stalemated or failed and has resolved what crises it can, and one or more individual members require additional individual treatment.	4) The patient manifests a condition that makes interpersonal relatedness disorganizing, impossible, or possibly harmful to the individual, group or both. Examples would include: patients with severe organic brain syndrome, severe impairment in reality testing, patients who are so dishonest, manipulative, suspicious, or explosive that it is impossible to form a therapeutic group alliance.
	7) There is a need for another modality of treatment prior to family therapy, e.g., detoxification, medication, individual sessions to establish trust.	
	8) Motivation to be seen alone, e.g., adolescents who state emphatically that they have personal problems for which they want individual help.	5) Group participation would be an acting out or an avoidance of another form of treatment that is more indicated.

ment and expose to a physician (who is usually a relative stranger) the most private aspects of body and soul.

5) Dyadic intimacy. Just as the individual format may be supported by the basic trust reminiscent of the child's attachment with parental figures, the format may also be the preferred choice when such trust is diminished and when the capacity for profound intimacy is absent. Individual treatment is often the preferred choice for patients who have no trouble forming superficial acquaintances, but who cannot form deeply emotional ties to others. As the relationship between therapist and patient evolves over time, it provides a model for intimacy and an opportunity to study difficulties in the development of sustained and deep emotional involvement.

6) Flexibility and specificity. A final and perhaps most important advantage of the individual format is that it provides the smoothest induction into treatment because the needs and demands of others can temporarily be put aside and the focus can be kept more or less exclusively on the specific requirements of the individual patient. This flexibility goes far beyond but is symbolized by the much greater ease in arranging mutually convenient appointments. Times are of course easier to schedule when only the patient and therapist have to be considered and not a family or a group. During the sessions, the therapist can direct full attention to the patient's problems, concerns, and sources of resistance without being constrained or distracted by the presence of others who may have different needs or therapeutic capacities. While maintaining this focus, the therapist can adjust his or her language and mode of interaction and thereby more effectively engage the patient. Some patients require a more affable, seemingly "casual" exchange, whereas others, such as Mrs. Y., would find a formal manner more appropriate and comfortable.

The individual format not only allows the therapist to adjust more easily to the needs and interpersonal style of the particular patient, but also allows the therapist more flexibility in adjusting the desired distance in the relationship. Some patients require considerable distance — spatially and emotionally — in order to feel comfortable. A patient with a paranoid personality disorder would be quite suspicious of a therapist who seemed too friendly; and a guilt-ridden patient might respond with increased guilt and feelings of unworthiness if the therapist seemed too helpful and concerned. On the other hand, an hysterical patient may respond to an overly methodical approach as cold and rejecting; and a schizophrenic patient may experience a therapist's neutrality as confirmation that the patient is incapable of interpersonal involvement. The individual format provides greater flexibility for the therapist to adjust intuitively the style and distance to meet the specific requirements of the individual patient.

In mentioning these advantages of the individual format – familiarity, role definition, confidentiality, basic trust, dyadic intimacy, flexibility and specificity – we are in no way suggesting that other forms of treatment cannot also sufficiently provide these aspects or cannot successfully deal with early resistances in therapy. Our point is that the individual format has certain inherent features that provide an easier induction phase for most patients. The task of explaining and demonstrating the value of other less traditional and immediately acceptable formats is too distracting and not worth the effort for some patients, especially when the patient's resistance is so strong that therapy might be rejected altogether. Apart from facilitating the induction phase, the advantages of the individual format are not so clearly evident either from the available research data or from accumulating clinical experience.

As we will discuss in the next chapter, certain techniques of therapy are associated with certain formats. For example, psychoanalysis and intensive exploratory psychotherapy have been conceptualized most often within the context of individual treatment. The question has not been answered as to whether the form changes the content, that is, whether the application of analytic techniques like interpretation of transference is quite different when used in the different environment of family or group treatment. The corollary question remains unanswered as well: Can the ambitious goals of certain individual treatments like psychoanalysis be reached through other formats? We will return to this question at the end of the chapter when reviewing research studies.

Because the individual format has particular advantages during the induction phase, many clinicians are inclined to proceed with this format without giving full weight to the disadvantages of individual treatment.

1) Distortion. The price of privacy and confidentiality is that the therapist receives incomplete data. Every patient to some degree consciously and unconsciously distorts the information presented to the therapist. These distortions arise because certain facts are omitted or denied (such as Mrs. Y.'s sexual frustration or her problems with her daughters). Moreover, in addition to obtaining a limited or incorrect view of the patient's life outside of treatment, the therapist sees only a limited range of patient behaviors within the treatment. Certain capacities, deficiencies, affects, and ways of interacting with others may not be included in the patient's relatively narrow repertoire of responses to the therapist and may occur only in the presence of others. For example, Mrs. Y. appeared a far more forceful and resourceful woman when seen with her husband who, in turn, retreated from her attack and no longer seemed the totally confident and controlling corporate executive. Extended exploratory individual treatments allow for a more thorough and diverse evaluation of the transference and therefore a wider range of patient behaviors, but even these exhaustive explorations fail to capture the versatility of reactions that patients show in family and group formats.

2) Isolation. The individual format tends to be the most isolated from the "real" world. Though this well-demarcated boundary connotes a protective, even magical air to the therapeutic situation, the resulting isolation can restrict the process. For example, in treating Mrs. Y. within an individual format, the therapist would be less able directly to influence the family situation and alter her environment; instead, the therapist would have to wait for changes within the patient to catalyze changes within other members of the family.

The increased control within the office situation provided by the individual format may mean less control of the environment outside the office. For example, suppose it turned out that Mrs. Y. poorly tolerates any confrontation by the therapist about the unreasonableness of her beliefs and her behavior. Within an individual format, the therapist would have to rely on others outside of treatment to make such a confrontation and hope that she will hear it. If Mrs. Y. were in marital, family, or group therapy, these confrontations would arise as a matter of course and might have greater impact and acceptability when made by someone other than the therapist. In addition, individual treatment can sometimes allow ego-syntonic problems to remain obscured from the patient's and therapist's view; inadvertently and unconsciously the therapist and patient collude to keep the problem out of the therapeutic field and only fortuitous events occurring outside of therapy may bring the difficulties to the fore. Mrs. Y. seemed like a perfect angel, not a bit spiteful, when seen alone. Family and group formats are far less dependent on outside circumstances to intercept unwitting collusions between therapist and patient.

3) Scapegoating. When any one person within a system is designated as "the patient," problems in others may become displaced onto the one in treatment who is simultaneously seen as the source of the difficulties as well as the hope for their resolution. Mr. Y. was scapegoating his wife in this way by attributing all the difficulties in the move and within his family to his wife whom he insisted should be the declared patient and treated for her depression. By excluding others and focusing only on the problems of one person, individual treatment can encourage such displacement not only by others but also by patients who erroneously come to view themselves as the cause and potential cure of all problems they encounter.

4) Infantilization. Individual treatment is the format most likely to foster regression. Patients tend automatically and unconsciously to assume a dependent stance and to delegate responsibility to omnipotent caretaking figures. The propensity for regression varies greatly from patient to patient. Even though the therapist (and the patient) may be well aware of the potential for this problem, a malignant infantilization sometimes develops and the patient becomes disproportionately reliant on the therapist rather than assuming a fair share of responsibility. Such patients experience themselves as if they were victims of a severe medical illness and were required simply to place themselves in the complete care of the lifesaving physician. The regressive pull of individual treatment can in some patients foster a near-total relinquishment of responsibility. Mrs. Y., for instance, could use individual treatment as no more than a surrogate marriage and begin living through and for her therapist in the same way that she had previously lived through and for her husband. In so doing she would never achieve a more autonomous and individuated view of herself.

Having considered the advantages and disadvantages of individual treatment, we will now proceed to a discussion of marital therapy.

MARITAL THERAPY

In considering the format of marital therapy, the consultant shifts the focus both of the problem and of its solution from an intrapsychic to an interpersonal point of view. This shift from a "person" to a "person-person" system is reasonable to consider for Mr. and Mrs. Y.: the initial phone call (Mr. Y. calling on behalf of Mrs. Y.) indicated that the emotional distress in one partner was interwoven with behavior in the other. Mrs. Y.'s depression was attributed to changes in her husband's professional life, and Mr. Y.'s tension was attributed, in turn, to his wife's despair, unreasonable demands, and emotional withdrawal. By insisting on seeing Mr. and Mrs. Y. together for at least one conjoint evaluation, the consultant introduced the importance of interpersonal as well as intrapsychic issues.

The idea that interpersonal difficulties contribute to an individual's emotional problems is, of course, anything but new and revolutionary. Confucius described how one spouse can inflict anguish upon another, and there can be no doubt that "bad marriages" predated even his early descriptions. What is relatively new is the establishment of a therapeutic format specifically designed to take into account such interpersonal dynamics. Marital therapy, as we recognize it today, began in the 1920s. Most of the early work was done by ministers, marriage counselors, and social workers. They did not publish descriptions of their clinical experiences in much detail and, as a result, the format did not receive much acceptance within the psychiatric community until 1929 when Karl Abraham and Hannah Stone started a marriage counseling center in New York City. This approach gradually received greater national recognition. In the 1930s Popenoe founded the American Institute of Family Relations which offered help to troubled couples and a decade later, in 1942, the American Association of Marriage Counseling was established.

Although psychoanalytically oriented therapists had supported the idea that interpersonal conflict could cause and maintain an individual's symptoms, they were hesitant to apply this belief by using a format other than individual therapy. In 1934, reporting in the *International Journal of Psychoanalysis,* Oberndorf described his experiences in treating a married couple; but despite publication in this prestigious journal, the paper was not given much notice. Fourteen years later, Mittelman (1948) wrote a more lengthy paper describing the concurrent analysis of marital couples in which the therapist saw each spouse separately. This paper created more of a stir. Although Mittelman agreed with the prevailing view that each spouse must be seen alone to develop and work through transference reactions, he also maintained that an advantage of seeing both partners was that the therapist could thereby better distinguish which problems were neurotic and which were determined by the actual situation.

Mittelman's introduction of external reality into the analytic field was quite controversial at the time, a controversy which now seems only of historic interest as the marital format has gained much wider acceptance and psychoanalytic theory has taken greater cognizance of reality (Gould, 1970; Wallerstein and Smelzer, 1969). Fifteen years after Mittelman proposed classification of marital interactions, descriptions of different marital formats began appearing prominently in the psychiatric literature: conjoint marital therapy (Brody, 1961; Haley, 1963; Satir, 1965); combined marital therapy in which spouses were seen individually and together (Greene and Solomon, 1963); collaborative therapy in which different therapists were assigned to each spouse separately and then the therapists conferred with each other (Martin and Bird, 1963); and also group therapy for marital couples (Boas, 1962; Leichter, 1962).

This development of marital therapy is not easy to distinguish from the concomitant development of family therapy. Once therapists began to enlarge the format in order to consider interpersonal as well as intrapsychic problems, varying combinations of different formats began to be recommended. At present, the decision to work with a marital unit instead of an entire nuclear family or even an extended family has not yet been resolved by research data or shared clinical opinion. Some advocates choose not to differentiate the two in theoretical discussions and, in practice, often combine marital and family formats including or excluding the children as the occasion warrants. Those with training and experience in child therapy are more often inclined to include the children in the therapeutic situation, whereas those who are more familiar in working with adults tend to exclude the children in arranging the format. Sex therapies, generally conducted in couples format, have flourished during the past two decades (Kaplan, 1974, 1979; Masters and Johnson, 1970). In making a recommendation for Mr. and Mrs. Y., marital therapy offers some clear advantages over individual treatment, but some disadvantages as well. Many of these advantages are related to the previously described disadvantages of individual therapy and need be mentioned only briefly here.

1) Less distorted data. Not only will information supplied by the spouse confirm, refute or elaborate data presented by the other partner, but the interaction between partners observed by the therapist will make material accessible for constructive change that might not be available in any other way. The process of finding different versions of "the truth" will, in turn, facilitate better communication between the two partners as they reach consensus rather than maintaining widely divergent views. For example, conjoint sessions will offer an opportunity to explore in some detail the meaning of Mr. Y.'s actual relationship with his female business associate, whereas in individual treatment for Mrs. Y., only her suspicions and fantasies about the relationship would be available for discussion.

2) Diminished scapegoating. By arranging to meet with both partners, the therapist explicitly and concretely indicates that Mrs. Y.'s problems are temporally and dynamically related to changes in Mr. Y. — and vice versa. The tendency of Mr. Y. to blame Mrs. Y. for all problems within the family is thereby short-circuited and similarly, the burden (actual and perceived) upon Mrs. Y. to resolve the problems of others is made less pronounced. The format of marital therapy decreases the use of coercion by the partners and encourages each of them to feel responsibility for both causing and resolving the problems. Paradoxically, by determining more precisely who is indeed responsible and to what extent for which specific difficulty, the boundaries between the two partners can also be more sharply demarcated.

3) Decreased regressive dependency. By defining the role of each partner not only as patient but also as responsible spouse, marital therapy generally limits the malignant regression and dependency which are more likely to occur in individual treatment. The patient is delegated a mature social role and not viewed as a helpless child. The presence of the spouse in the sessions serves as a constant reminder that the "real world" is waiting on the other side of the office door. In this way, the transition from treatment to everyday life is less abrupt and, accordingly, the therapist can influence one spouse to support and comfort the other partner during the times between sessions and at the end of treatment. For instance, Mr. Y. could be instructed on how best to handle rather than how to avoid his wife's demands; at the same time he might learn how to offer her comfort and companionship so that such demands are made less frequently. In the same way, Mrs. Y. could point out how her husband's provocative way of describing his female business associate contributes to her feelings of being excluded and betrayed. Exactly if, when, and how such statements would be made outside of the sessions would be determined in part by the techniques used by the therapist. The point to be emphasized here is that marital therapy offers a mode of influence that is readily translatable by the partners beyond the confines of the therapeutic hour itself.

4) Pre-formed transferences. The major transferences interpreted in marital therapy are those that each spouse has already developed toward the other — not the transference each patient might develop toward the therapist. Because the focus is more on the struggles between the spouses and less on the struggles between patient and therapist, objectivity can be maintained as the therapist acts as a more or less neutral "referee." Regressive, actualized transferences to the therapist are much less common as a problem in marital than in individual treatment. Moreover, couples begin treatment with ready-made transferences well in place, whereas in individual treatment if such transferences develop at all toward the therapist, they are likely to take considerable time to appear and to become accessible for a working through.

5) Limited reciprocal deterioration. The conjoint evaluation of Mr. and Mrs. Y. suggested that the cost of improvement in Mrs. Y. conceivably could be a reciprocal decline in the functioning of Mr. Y. As her depression lifted and she retreated less into a posture of helpless passivity, her bitter feelings toward Mr. Y. might become less contained and might cause Mr. Y. to become depressed himself and to become cowed by her escalating and harsh attacks. Marital therapy offers the therapist a chance to work with both partners concomitantly and fosters simultaneous change and growth so that such reciprocal deterioration is less likely to occur.

6) Cost-effectiveness. If both Mr. and Mrs. Y. need treatment and can be helped by working conjointly with one therapist, such treatment will obviously be more efficient for the therapist and less costly for the couple.

These advantages of marital therapy for Mr. and Mrs. Y. must be weighed against some significant disadvantages. As so often occurs in a discussion of differential therapeutics, the disadvantages of one kind of treatment run parallel to the advantages of another and vice versa. The following list of disadvantages of marital therapy will therefore repeat with different emphasis some considerations mentioned above regarding the individual format.

1) Lack of motivation. From the first phone call Mr. Y. indicated he was opposed to having sessions with his wife. Though he was willing to come for one conjoint evaluation, Mr. Y. now may adamantly refuse the format of marital therapy. A destructive power struggle and the loss of both partners to therapy may result from the consultant's insistence upon marital therapy, especially if he offers no alternative. Even if Mr. Y. reluctantly agrees, he may in a passive-aggressive manner subtly sabotage treatment to show he was justified all along in his opinion that couple therapy is a mistake. If this were to occur, neither he nor his wife would likely benefit very much from treatment – and Mr. Y. may use this one failure as an excuse not to proceed with another format or therapist and to blame his wife further for making his life miserable.

Patients can resist any form of treatment for countless conscious and unconscious reasons and thereby be labeled "unmotivated"; but an inherent disadvantage of marital as well as family and group therapies is that the resistance of one participant can force a delay in dealing with the needs of another patient who may be in more immediate distress and/or more accessible. This delay sometimes causes a quiet erosion of the treatment from underneath the surface, a process which becomes recognized only when the therapy suddenly stalemates or collapses and, for example, Mr. Y. announces unexpectedly that because his wife has not yet shown any substantial improvement, he has unilaterally decided to get a divorce and therefore has no intention of attending future sessions.

2) Lack of privacy. Some patients have a secret which they consider directly related to their problems but cannot imagine divulging to a spouse, a child, or even to a stranger in a group. For them, a choice of marital therapy means they will perhaps not ever have an opportunity to discuss the secret openly — or even worse, they forever experience in treatment the fear that the secret will be exposed to others against their will and better judgment. Perhaps Mr. Y. is reluctant to participate in conjoint treatment because he has in fact been having an affair with his female associate. Or perhaps Mrs. Y.'s depression derives in part from guilt over past relationships of her own or current erotic fantasies. Although trust and candor are eventual goals of many treatments, at times the fear of exposure is an insurmountable early obstacle to every format other than individual treatment (and certainly some secrets are well worth keeping rather than revealing, even in conjoint marital psychotherapy).

3) Impeded individuation. The form and the content of marital therapy tends to focus on interpersonal more than on intrapsychic issues. Although the growth and autonomy of the individual are expected to occur as an outcome of the therapeutic process, usually more emphasis is placed on the development and integration of the marital unit. As a result, those patients who are inclined to live through and for others and who have difficulty declaring their independence may not acquire a well-developed and autonomous sense of self if they are always seen in treatment with another. Mrs. Y. could, for example, use the format of marital therapy to restrict the main issue for discussion to her feelings about her husband and his behavior toward her; in so doing, she might never turn the focus of attention inward to examine her own wishes, memories, fears, fantasies, and dreams. If indeed a basic problem is Mrs. Y.'s lack of individuation or perhaps even a primary affective illness most amenable to psychopharmacotherapy and cognitive repair, the format of marital therapy could unhelpfully divert attention away from the more crucial "cellular" or "person" systems and into the interpersonal sphere.

4) Uncontained disruption. By catalyzing a more open exchange between partners, a marital format can backfire or even explode if the partners experience the treatment as a justification to express at last their long-suppressed resentment in an unrestrained, and perhaps cruel, manner. When the lid finally flies off, they may continue destructively to pick, prod, confront, and (perhaps worst of all) "analyze" each other long after the session is over and they have returned to what should be their everyday lives. Although the marital format does offer an opportunity for a couple directly to transport the content of treatment across the boundary of the therapist's office and into the outside world, each partner must be able to use discretion and not turn life itself into a disruptive and endless marathon encounter. For example, after the first conjoint evaluation of Mr. and Mrs. Y., the couple left the consulting room with considerable uncertainty about whether they could resume normal functioning after such an unexpected explosion. They wondered whether the rage, contempt, and bitterness would be even more extreme when not contained and channeled by the office setting and the presence of the therapist.

5) Exclusion of children. Since we will next be discussing the format of family therapy, we need only mention here as a preface that an additional disadvantage of marital therapy is that the children – who are apparently having problems of their own and who may also be contributing to their parents' problems – will be excluded from the treatment.

FAMILY THERAPY

The evaluation sessions with Mr. and Mrs. Y. had not explicitly indicated that the current problem extends very far beyond the "two-person" system to involve, in any significant way, cross-generational issues in the "family" system. In fact, Mr. and Mrs. Y. each made a point of stating how well their children were doing. Nonetheless, in the heat of the quarrel during the conjoint session, it seemed possible that the family was being split by fixed alliances with the older daughter allied to her father. Another possibility the consultant must consider is that the absolute denial of problems involving the children may constitute a form of protesting too much and that the current crisis between Mr. and Mrs. Y. stems in part from developmental changes within the family that have been displaced by them onto environmental changes outside the home. For instance, Mrs. Y.'s jealousy over her husband's professional "affair" may conceivably relate to jealousy over the older daughter's blossoming sexuality and closeness with the father; and Mr. Y.'s resentment of his wife may be related to unrecognized resentment about what he perceives to be the poor adjustment of his more fragile younger child. Family therapy, or at least an extended family evaluation, may be necessary to assess the presence and significance of these dynamics.

An appreciation of the role of the family in the development of an individual's problems is certainly not new. In our culture this concept can be traced back at least as far as the Bible and forms an important source of inspiration for Greek mythology which often attributed the struggles of an individual to the dynamics within "the house." A more recent conception is that an individual's problem can be viewed as a symptom of a troubled system—that Mrs. Y.'s "depression" is a manifestation and symbolic expression of pathological processes within the family unit. The obvious corollary of conceiving of the system as the problem is to treat the system directly and not make the individual patient the focus for intervention.

Although mental health disciplines have long believed that the workings of the family are instrumental in both the development and maintenance of individual psychopathology, they have been slow to apply this belief and to accept the wide use of a family format. Though Freud recognized that Hans' fear of horses on the street derived at least in part from family dynamics and parental reprimands, he treated the boy by working as supervisor to the boy's father and did not choose to include the child or other family members in the therapeutic format. Similarly, Frieda Fromm-Reichmann (1950) postulated (probably incorrectly) that a particular kind of pathology in the mother could induce schizophrenia in a vulnerable child, but she did not alter her format accordingly to directly treat the mother-daughter relationship; instead, she continued to see the patient primarily in individual therapy. For both Freud and Fromm-Reichmann, intrapsychic pathology might reflect family dynamics, but this then becomes structured and takes on a life of its own.

In contrast to the office-based psychoanalyst who during the first half of this century wrote extensively about family dynamics but rarely used a family format, practitioners who worked in child guidance clinics wrote less but were inclined actively to evaluate and treat the symptomatic child with other members of the family present. In the

1950s, there was an explosion of interest in the theory and practice of family therapy. A number of charismatic leaders emerged and established schools (or families) of family therapy: Nathan Ackerman (1966), who actively and often provocatively interacted as a surrogate member of the family unit; Lidz and Lidz (1949) who argued that the entire family environment contributed to schizophrenia and categorized the kinds of therapeutic interventions within such families; Bowen (1978), who provided detailed descriptions of treating "schizophrenic families" over time; Wynne, Ryckoff, Day, and Hirsch (1958), who correlated the occurrence of schizophrenia with particular kinds of faulty interaction and communication; and Bateson, Jackson, Haley, and Weakland (1956), who used communication and systems theory to understand the functioning of families. By the 1960s these pioneers had become acquainted with each other's work and bridges were built connecting the previously insulated family centers. The result was the establishment of the journal of *Family Process* and the wider acceptance of family treatment, not just for schizophrenia but for a broad range of less severely impaired diagnostic groups.

Before deciding whether family therapy should be suggested for Mr. and Mrs. Y., let us examine some of the advantages and disadvantages of this format. Because several of the considerations overlap with those already discussed in regard to marital therapy, we will focus upon those issues that concern whether or not the children should be included in the treatment (recognizing that many practitioners interweave marital and family treatment, at times including children, at others excluding them). We will begin with the possible advantages of including the whole family.

1) Increased data. The participation of the children in the sessions allows the therapist an opportunity to acquire invaluable information from and about the children. The therapist can observe firsthand the kinds of interaction that occur between and within generations. For example, is Mrs. Y. in fact clinging to her younger daughter as if they were both "drowning at sea"; and is Mr. Y. encouraging his older daughter to be excessively flirtatious and pseudoindependent? In addition, Mr. and Mrs. Y. may be consciously or unconsciously colluding with one another to deny certain facts, such as the extent of Mrs. Y.'s drinking or the fear hidden beneath Mr. Y.'s executive manner. The children often have less reason for such denial and may supply comments that challenge a collusive silence.

2) Consolidation of the family. By bringing the family together for problem-solving, the therapist conveys concretely as well as symbolically that he views the family as a unit with shared responsibilities and with individual as well as collective capacity to improve its modes of functioning. The presence of different generations helps place the current problem into the context of the family's history. What was previously experienced as an acute crisis may often be decompressed when it is seen within the broader perspective of the family's past and future. For example, with a reaffirmation of the family as a unit that has its own traditions, Mrs. Y. may feel less estranged and adrift. Once she feels her home to be a more secure base, she can begin to master the previously avoided anxieties experienced in her new environment. Also, the therapist can enhance this sense of the family's being an integrated unit by diminishing the splits that occur when different parents ally themselves with different children against other members of the family. Family sessions can sometimes dramatically eliminate such divisions when long-held secrets between certain members are disclosed. For instance, the older daughter might feel freer to divulge secrets about her father's condescending view of Mrs. Y. and how the father's attitude has increased the daughter's distance from her mother. Moreover, simply having the children present may help the parents to assume a more mature and consolidating role and prevent the kind of uncontrolled and potentially harmful outburst which occurred during the conjoint evaluation of Mr. and Mrs. Y.

3) Treatment of the children. An obvious advantage of including the children in the therapeutic format is that they themselves may require treatment. When parents are preoccupied with their own troubles, they may not notice the problems the children are having. Even if they do notice, parents may minimize the children's problems because such awareness increases the parents' sense of responsibility, helplessness, and guilt. The therapist may collude with this avoidance or minimization by not evaluating the children directly and by not including them in treatment.

The therapist may hope that once the parents' difficulties are resolved, the children in turn will improve. This approach can fail to consider that the children's problems may have developed an independent "life of their own" and may have become so severe that further delay is unwarranted. For instance, if the older daughter is acting out Mr. Y.'s illicit affair by becoming irresponsible and promiscuous, then she may experience possibly irreversible harm before the parents' differences are ameliorated. And, if the younger daughter's school difficulties are a result of a sympathetic identification with her despairing mother, then further failures may gather momentum during the crucial developmental period of her early adolescence, leading to a downhill course which will not be easily reversed if and when the mother's depression finally lifts.

4) Children as catalysts. Even if the children are having no significant problems of their own, their presence may provide insight and the therapeutic leverage necessary to make the system change. The adage about the wisdom that sometimes flows out of the mouths of babes accurately reflects the valuable therapeutic contributions often made by the youngest members of the family.

Many of the disadvantages of family therapy coincide with the disadvantages discussed above regarding marital therapy. We will therefore mention below those disadvantages which primarily involve the inclusion of the children in the therapeutic format.

A) Distraction. If the children are far removed emotionally and dynamically from the parental conflict, their inclusion sometimes constitutes a distraction that prevents treatment from focusing on more crucial individual and marital problems. Such distraction is more obvious and prominent with very young children, but even the presence of adolescents can at times dilute the material with irrelevant and personalized accounts. The parents in turn may foster these distractions so that more anxiety-laden subjects can be avoided. For example, Mr. and Mrs. Y. could use the presence of the children as an excuse for not discussing Mr. Y.'s "professional affair."

B) Loss of privacy. Certain intimate issues are best kept between marital partners and not discussed in front of children. If sexual difficulties have resulted from, or even partially caused, Mrs. Y.'s depression, this material would be hard to expose and treat with the children present.

C) Impeded individuation. Just as marital treatment can interfere with a partner's developing a more autonomous sense of self (see above), family treatment can interfere with an adolescent's developing an identity apart from the family. To include the older daughter in treatment at a time when she needs to separate from familial bonds may interfere with this crucial developmental task and place her too close to the bosom of the family.

D) Lack of motivation Family therapy has been suggested as a way of getting troubled children involved in treatment, especially if they have refused to participate in any other format, but many children are even more unmotivated to attend family sessions. If forced to come, their active or passive resistances may prevent any work getting done on other issues. The daughters may vigorously oppose any participation and sit sulking or may challenge every interaction. If their oppositionalism cannot be dealt with therapeutically, their inclusion in the therapy will prevent whatever might otherwise be worked out between Mr. and Mrs. Y.

E) Inexperience of therapist. Many therapists receive only limited training in work with children and are more temperamentally at ease working with adults. Of course, any format is at a disadvantage if the therapist lacks training and expertise, but this consideration may be particularly true regarding the therapist's decision to work with children.

HETEROGENEOUS GROUP THERAPY

Although very far from Mr. or Mrs. Y.'s original intentions, a heterogeneous group should be considered as a possible therapeutic format for Mrs. Y. Her self-consciousness, lack of assertiveness, and inability to establish new relationships can all be viewed as longstanding problems which extend beyond and become most manifest in systems other than the person, the marriage, or the family. Her more general interpersonal problems predate the current crisis and no doubt have contributed to it. A heterogeneous group format might focus on the predisposing difficulties she has had in interacting with others.

Heterogeneous groups have come from obscurity to wide acceptance during the last 50 years. In the 1930s, social theorists as well as psychotherapists began to examine closely the processes that are generated within small groups and to distinguish these processes from those that occur intrapsychically, dyadically, and in large groups. The study of the small group format was carried forth by individuals who came from radically different backgrounds: psychoanalysts (Burrow, Wender, Shilder, and later Bion, Foulkes, Slavson, Wolf, and many others), social scientists (most especially Lewin), and clinical innovators (such as Moreno with his interest in the theater).

Partly because theoretical contributions have been derived from many varied fields, heterogeneous groups have been based on widely different assumptions, methods, and goals. Furthermore, the format has been used not just for psychotherapy, but for education, organizational consultation, self-awareness, establishing community networks, promotion of social change, and so forth. Indeed, some have hailed group psychotherapy as a panacea effective for everyone. Others have used the format as a dumping ground for patients who cannot be accommodated in more expensive treatments or who scare off individual therapists. Because the form, content, and application of groups have been so varied, we will point out common themes present in most heterogeneous groups so that we have a clear idea about what we are actually considering for Mrs. Y.

These groups are called "heterogeneous" because the individual members do not share one particular symptom or situation and because they will differ widely in their problems, strengths, ages, socioeconomic backgrounds, and personality traits. In spite of these differences, a feeling of commonality develops and as a result, the patient realizes that he is not alone, uniquely strange, or crazy in his experiences. This realization reduces embarrassment, improves self-esteem, and promotes the sense of being acceptable.

Feeling more accepted, the patient is more able to disclose personal aspects about him/herself and to take interpersonal risks, first within and later outside the group. He learns to share the therapist and discovers that he can be helped by peers as well as helping them. The variety of interactions which follow afford the group member an opportunity to correct distortions about others, to discover how others regard him, and to alter maladaptive and repetitive responses.

Within this general framework, heterogeneous groups vary more in degree than in kind. For example, leaders trained in different schools of group therapy vary in the emphasis they place on group or dyadic or individual process. Some, such as Tavistock leaders, restrict their interpretations to the group as a system and avoid interpretations of individual behavior. Others, especially Gestalt therapists, focus on the individual and use the group mostly as a backdrop. Most therapists interpret group, dyadic, and individual process depending on the opportunities of the occasion, but some will emphasize the group, others the individual or dyads. The types of interventions are also determined by the goals of the group. If members are expected to strive for character change, then confrontation, insight, historical reconstruction, behav-

ioral modification, experimenting, and role-playing will be more emphasized. If members are merely expected to resume or maintain their usual
level of functioning, then advice, support, and a concentration on the
present will be more prominent. Despite these variations, when referring
a patient to a heterogeneous group, the consultant presumes that membership will be beneficial even if the patient's particular problems are
not the immediate focus of the group's activity and in fact may appear
to be completely unrelated.

With this brief overview of heterogeneous group therapy, let us now
examine the pros and cons of this format for Mrs. Y. We realize that
in the following discussion we have created an awkward and artificial
dichotomy between interpersonal and intrapsychic conflicts and that
every piece of behavior can (and perhaps should) be viewed from both
perspectives. We have found, however, that in clinical practice the
choice of a format is facilitated by sorting out the interpersonal and intrapsychic, insofar as one can. We will begin by discussing the possible advantages for Mrs. Y. of a heterogeneous group.

1) Focus on interpersonal relationships. Although both Mr. and Mrs.
Y. have concentrated on problems occurring within the family, the consultant's evaluation has revealed that Mrs. Y.'s difficulties extend
beyond the home and that except for a previously close relationship with
her husband, she has always been shy, dependent, easily embarrassed,
and socially inhibited. A heterogeneous group, while addressing and de-
sensitizing these chronic interpersonal anxieties and difficulties, might
also allow Mrs. Y. to realize that the distress over her husband and her
children is in part symptomatic of more general problems in understanding and relating to others.

2) Enhancement of observing capacities. So far, Mrs. Y. has not shown
any great capacity to recognize the way and the extent to which she
contributes to her problems. Instead, she attributes her despair only
to changes in others, such as her husband's new manner and professional involvements. In a group, some members might be able to confront
Mrs. Y. more directly, while others simultaneously offer the necessary
support. Such direct confrontations of previously ego-syntonic character traits are often more difficult in individual treatment, especially if
the alliance is fragile and the patient is prone to feeling criticized or to
use unproductive oppositionalism. In a sense, group members can assume ego-observing capacities not yet adequately developed in patients
such as Mrs. Y. and make comments that are perceived as less threatening than when made by an individual therapist.

3) Dilution of transference. Mrs. Y. had been inclined in the past to remain excessively attached to her husband. She is now likely to develop just this kind of relationship with the therapist and may experience the treatment as infantilizing in a way that would repeat, and not resolve, her tendency to establish and maintain hostile-dependent ties. A heterogeneous group, by being a more public and reality-validating format, can often prevent such a malignant regression with the treatment.

4) Dilution of countertransference. Mrs. Y. has already revealed certain masochistic character traits, such as her self-flagellation after berating her husband. A possibility in individual treatment is that she will alternate between harshly condemning herself for being so inadequate and then harshly condemning her husband and therapist for not meeting her needs. In reaction to this kind of hostile-dependent transference, the therapist may in turn alternate between feeling helpless and guilty that he cannot do more and being enraged at her unreasonable demands. These understandable but sometimes harmful countertransferential responses can be better balanced and neutralized in a group setting that dilutes the intensity of the transference and protects therapeutic neutrality.

The advantages of a heterogeneous group must be weighed against the formidable disadvantages of choosing this format for Mrs. Y:

1) Urgency of problem. The evaluation has not fully disclosed the severity of Mrs. Y.'s depression and the admittedly remote possibility of psychotic disorganization or of suicide if her depression is not soon relieved. A heterogeneous group would fail to give Mrs. Y.'s problems immediate enough attention and would not provide the intense, specialized, and individualized treatment such an acute crisis would require. A relative contraindication to heterogeneous group therapy is the presence of an acute crisis.

2) Responsiveness to briefer therapy. Group therapies deal with long-standing problems. They usually are open-ended and of relatively extended duration. Mrs. Y.'s depression may respond adequately and more rapidly if attention is given to her specific target symptoms in a briefer (individual or family or marital) treatment. Issues regarding duration and frequency of treatments will be discussed in detail in Chapter 4.

3) Avoidance of central issues. A heterogeneous group could, for a relatively extended period of time, not challenge Mrs. Y.'s view of her situation and could adopt Mrs. Y.'s view of herself as an estranged woman in a far-off land. She could then use the group as a home away from home and comfortably give her full attention to the problems of others, while avoiding her more central and pressing problems, such as her husband's rejection, her daughter's provocative behavior, and her own fears of becoming more assertive and less dependent. The group may allow some members to hide in the woodwork. This is fine if the intention of the recommendation is to provide a supportive environment.

4) Absolute intolerance to groups. As a result of Mrs. Y.'s profound depression, her cultural heritage, or her basic character, she may simply be unable to tolerate the group process – that is, she may be unwilling to listen to others, maintain confidentiality, change roles flexibly, and influence and be influenced by others. The consultant cannot simply label this intolerance as "lack of motivation" and push the patient into group. Some patients correctly assess that they are indeed too frightened or paranoid or schizoid or selfish to withstand the pressures and frustrations of group therapy. Such patients should not be asked to change embedded character traits even before the treatment for these traits begins.

HOMOGENEOUS GROUP THERAPY

Because Mrs. Y.'s problems have been presented by both her and by Mr. Y. as unique, the consultant may at first not appreciate that some of her difficulties are in fact shared by many others and that a homogeneous group might therefore be a helpful format. Different types of homogeneous groups have proven valuable for several of Mrs. Y.'s presenting problems, such as cultural estrangement, her distress over rearing adolescent children (Greenspan, Silver, and Allen, 1977), her resentment toward a husband she now considers chauvinistic and exploitative, her lack of assertiveness, and her timidity and embarrassment when with others.

Groups are called homogeneous because the treatment is targeted at a condition or situation shared by all members. Like heterogeneous groups, homogeneous groups can be placed conceptually in the "interpersonal system," but because the content and the process of these groups are focused on a specific problem area, the range of interactions among members tends to be more constricted. The focus may be on one of the following: an *impulse disorder* (such as obesity [Levitz and

Stunkard, 1974], smoking, alcoholism [Fox, 1962], drug addiction [Berger, 1973; Kaufman, 1973; Yablonsky, 1965], gambling, or criminal behavior [Aledort and Jones, 1973]); a *medical disorder* (such as cardiac ailments [Bilodeau and Hackett, 1971], ileostomy, terminal illness [Yalom and Greaves, 1977], or deafness [Pendergrass and Hodges, 1976]); a particular *development phase* (such as childhood and adolescence [Berkovitz, 1972; Slavson and Schiffer, 1975; Sugar, 1975], or old age); or a *psychiatric disorder* (such as agoraphobia [Teasdale, Walsh, Lancashire, and Mathews, 1977], schizophrenia [O'Brien, Hamm, Ray et al., 1972], somatoform disorder, homosexuality [Covi, 1972; Nobler, 1972], and many others).

Broadly conceived, homogeneous groups encompass a wide variety of shared experiences: expiation at religious communions, catharsis at Greek tragedies, and even abreaction at modern rock concerts. More narrowly defined, homogeneous groups originated with the work of a Boston internist, Joseph Pratt (Sadock, 1975), who in the early 1900s began speaking to groups of patients with tuberculosis. Pratt did more than provide a didactic lecture. He discovered that as he offered encouragement and support, the group began to have "a life of its own" and patients were able to help one another. Pratt's contribution went beyond simply noting that meeting with a group of patients was beneficial; many before him had recognized that. His major contribution was recognizing that the group process was psychotherapeutic in a way that meeting individually with patients was not. He documented what kinds of inspirational interaction were especially helpful in catalyzing a constructive group process. Lazell and Marsh (Sadock, 1975) soon thereafter applied these techniques to the treatment of psychotic patients in homogeneous groups. Before long, both within and outside of the psychiatric profession, homogeneous groups became tremendously popular for combatting alcoholism and drug addiction, for weight-watching and smoke-ending, for consciousness-raising, and for the wide variety of other disorders mentioned above. Although not labeled "psychiatric patients," more people are engaged in one or another form of homogeneous groups than in all other outpatient psychotherapies combined.

Like its individual members, each homogeneous group is different from another, but certain common characteristics can be found. Homogeneous groups all tend to provide a structured social network for individuals who previously felt they must suffer their problems in isolation. Within this integrated group community, members are given a defined role with specified procedures, duties, rights, expectations, and responsibilities. This role definition is in itself reassuring and relieves the tension of uncertainty and alienation. A sense of belonging develops with loyalty to the group and fellow sufferers. Some homogeneous groups, such as those used in drug rehabilitation programs and est, set up a hierarchy with a system of gradual promotion and the possibility of eventual leadership.

The advantages of a homogeneous group for Mrs. Y. overlap with those of a heterogeneous group discussed above and will not be repeated here. We will mention, however, two additional ways in which a homogeneous group might be helpful for Mrs. Y.:

1) Acceptance by the patient. Many homogeneous groups are considered outside the purview of the mental health professions (some are even "anti-psychiatry") and therefore the groups do not have the stigma attached to other forms of psychotherapy. Mrs. Y., with her reluctance to be revealing or introspective, might find membership in a homogeneous group more acceptable and less traumatic. For example, while rejecting all other recommendations, she might accept the consultant's encouragement to join a welcoming club at Japan House or to participate in an art appraisal and acquisition league supported by a museum of her interest.

2) Acceptance by the group. Homogeneous groups tend to accept and support new members promptly and graciously. In turn, new members tend to form an immediate group identification, feel engaged and committed, and are less likely to drop out before treatment has been given a chance. In contrast, heterogeneous groups often confront or ignore new members. The heterogeneous group has its own momentum and agenda and may find the problems presented by the new patient a distraction, or worse, an unwanted intrusion (similar to the arrival of a new sibling). Mrs. Y.'s lack of confidence in interpersonal situations might increase temporarily if she sensed that the group was not particularly interested in her difficulties or comments. Homogeneous groups, by providing the sense of commonality and of fighting a shared problem, can offer immense support and self-validation. Because contact among members outside the group are encouraged and often required, the benefits spill over into everyday life and decrease the day-to-day isolation experienced by patients like Mrs. Y.

The disadvantages of homogeneous groups also overlap with those of heterogeneous groups described above and need not be elaborated in detail, but before recommending a homogeneous group format, the consultant should consider two formidable disadvantages for Mrs. Y.

1) Avoidance of other problems. Because the chosen homogeneous group is likely to focus only on a specific situation (such as Mrs. Y.'s cultural acclimation) or a specific symptom (such as her resentment toward her husband and the woman's role), other important areas are likely to be avoided. Mrs. Y. might, for example, follow the consultant's suggestion and join a nonprofit homogeneous group to raise funds for a museum. Although her social isolation would improve, she might be diverted from dealing with her feelings about her husband and children and with intimate relationships in general. She will therefore be deprived of achieving more ambitious goals.

2) Limited psychiatric influence. Some homogeneous groups pay a price for avoiding the stigma of being "psychiatric," especially when members require a form of psychiatric treatment that the group itself cannot offer and may even disparage. Mrs. Y.'s depression, for instance, may require psychopharmacological intervention and more specialized care. In addition, homogeneous groups tend not to explore resistances. Unmotivated patients are simply not accommodated unless they change their point of view. Mrs. Y. might discontinue a homogeneous group and destructively retreat further into herself without receiving any further follow-up from the group or the consultant.

Given the possibilities and the pros and cons of each therapeutic setting, what format was actually chosen for Mrs. Y. and how was this decision made? The consultant believed that the available data did not make one choice clearly superior to the alternatives. Based on his preliminary assessment, he felt that Mrs. Y. did not have a specific enough situation or symptom to motivate her to join a homogeneous group; would flatly reject a heterogeneous group as being too intimidating and culturally unacceptable; would see no reason to involve the children in family therapy; might use marital sessions only as an opportunity to attack her husband without examining the causes of and solutions to their difficulties; and might use individual sessions only to complain about her husband and become too attached to the therapist. All things considered, he concluded that the individual format would probably have the best chance of promptly and specifically dealing with her resistances while he learned more about the causes and severity of her depression and its effect upon others. After an extended consultation, the decision about a more permanent format could then be made with greater knowledge.

The consultant, realizing that his preference was not particularly superior to possible alternatives, adopted the consulting strategy of sharing the decision-making with his patients (we will discuss this process of negotiation further in Chapter 9). He outlined to Mr. and Mrs. Y. the choices of format and, just as we have done, explained their rationale, advantages, and disadvantages. This process allowed Mr. and Mrs. Y. to become informed consumers and to participate in and take responsibility for the decisions made. Mr. and Mrs. Y. discussed the treatment possibilities and agreed that the previous session was helpful, even if distressing, for both of them. They decided to continue meeting together with the consultant. While Mrs. Y. firmly declared this "mutual" decision, Mr. Y. sat quietly nodding in agreement.

Without challenging their decision, the consultant asked in what ways the previous visit had been helpful. Mr. Y. was not sure. All he knew was that his wife was less depressed and more like her old self. She hadn't complained once all week about his "professional association." Mrs. Y. interrupted: *She* had not mentioned the woman because *he* had not mentioned her either. What then evolved during the rest of the session was that previously Mr. Y. had indeed been more than just casually mentioning the "other woman"—he had, in fact, been waving the relationship in his wife's face and broadcasting the other woman's virtues in front of the children and friends.

Mr. Y.'s reasons for humiliating his wife in this way only became clear in subsequent conjoint sessions. He flaunted the professional affair whenever he felt threatened by his wife. In recent years Mrs. Y. had been less and less the shy, self-effacing woman he had married. More confident, she had started to become outspoken at dinner parties about her political beliefs. This growing confidence also had its effect closer to home. Mr. Y. felt threatened by his wife's intellectual pursuits, by her desire and at times demands for more frequent sex, and by her high aesthetic, spiritual, and professional expectations for him and for the children.

Further marital sessions disclosed an irony not at first seen. It was Mrs. Y.'s growing confidence and not her depression that had initially thrown the marriage off balance. Mr. Y., in part because of an identification with an ineffectual father, felt threatened by women throughout his life: first, by his intrusive mother and successful older sister and later, by adolescent girls who matured more rapidly than him. In contrast, until a few years ago, Mr. Y. never felt intimidated by his loving and hero-worshipping wife. Although at times "too sensitive and affectionate," she had at least always let him wear the pants. Ever since their romantically idealized moments together as childhood sweethearts, Mr. Y. had felt that he could count on her always being behind him, beside him—but never in front or on top. Then, several years before their move to the United States, as her children required less moment-to-moment care, Mrs. Y. began to pursue cultural interests outside the home. In reaction, although not fully aware of it at the time, Mr. Y. felt a potential loss and suddenly began to undermine his wife's changing behavior and threatening autonomy. For example, Mr. Y. would suddenly encourage his younger daughter to cling to her mother and demand that she spend every moment around the home. In this way, Mr. Y. would not "lose" his wife either.

Weekly marital sessions over the next few months helped Mr. and Mrs. Y. reach a higher level of understanding. The therapist would point out how Mr. Y. would interrupt and thereby put down his wife whenever she was making an important point, and how in turn Mrs. Y. would not challenge this interruption and instead retreated into a hurt and sullen position. The couple came to realize that Mr. Y. covertly kept his wife down and depressed because he was threatened whenever she was more assertive, and that Mrs. Y. preferred to sulk and, in this passive manner, get back at her husband by making him feel guilty and frustrated. She was wary of confronting him directly, partially because she sensed that *he* might not be able to take it.

With these realizations, the conflict over the professional woman faded into the background. Mr. Y. saw that the relationship with this colleague was indeed more than a business matter and was motivated in part by his wish to have a woman waiting in the wings to buffer the potential loss of his wife. He had flaunted the other woman's virtues to diminish his wife and thereby be less intimidated by her. A similar dynamic operated closer to home. Mr. Y. was encouraging his older daughter to be sexy and outspoken in part to have her help him keep Mrs. Y. in her place, and in part so he could in a counterphobic way learn to master the anxiety he had felt toward sexy, assertive women during his adolescence.

The marital format appeared to be well-suited to Mr. and Mrs. Y. They were able to work with the material constructively and examine how the process within sessions applied to their interactions outside. Mrs. Y. was learning that she did not need to dissolve into a masochistic position in order to protect herself or her husband, and Mr. Y. was learning that he did not need to keep his wife depressed in order to have her around. Before this work was completed, however, Mrs. Y. found out that her father in Japan was dying of incurable lung cancer. Without a second thought, she took her children out of school and within a few days flew to Japan to care for her father, leaving her husband behind in the United States. On that note, treatment ended. Mr. Y. did not call the therapist during her absence, and Mrs. Y. did not contact the therapist as they had arranged before she departed.

A year later, Mrs. Y. wrote a letter to the therapist, apologizing for leaving so abruptly but explaining she "had to do it." Her father died within a few weeks after her return home; her older daughter was on the Dean's list in an Ivy League college; her younger daughter was away at boarding school and "managing"; her husband had been promoted so they would be staying in the United States for at least another four years; and as for Mrs. Y., she had insisted that they sell their suburban home and move into an apartment in the city, where she was now working as a translator and appraiser for a distinguished auction house. At the end of the letter she talked about how she and her husband have lunch together now almost every day: "We no longer need to be together, but we still want to be. Thank you. Sincerely yours, Mrs. Y."

COMPARATIVE RESEARCH REGARDING THERAPEUTIC FORMATS

The preceding discussion illustrates the many considerations involved in choosing a therapeutic format and the difficulty in knowing afterwards whether the right decision was made. Although conjoint therapy appeared to be helpful in relieving Mrs. Y.'s depression, Mr. Y.'s insecurities, and the family's distress, the possibility remains that another format would have achieved equal or better results.

The available outcome research does not cast a guiding light on the choice of format. Most studies comparing formats have resulted in tie scores. One exception is the finding in a number of studies that marital or family therapy may be superior to individual therapy in the treatment of marital or family problems. If one considers Mrs. Y.'s presentation as primarily a marital problem, then comparative research supports the decision to treat her in a marital rather than in an individual format. Gurman and Kniskern (1978) summarized data indicating that conjoint marital treatment is superior to conjoint plus individual therapy, concurrent therapy, or individual therapy. They also found that individual treatment for marital problems has twice the rate of deterioration than conjoint, group, and concurrent collaborative marital therapies. Their review of the outcome literature reinforces Hurvitz's (1967) view that doing individual therapy with only one spouse can actually be harmful for a marriage.

Family treatment is equally effective. In a review of the available comparative data on family therapy, Gurman and Kniskern (1978) concluded that in all seven studies, family treatment was at least as good as other formats and at times even better. The choice between marital and family treatment has not been studied.

Just as one can find support in the research literature for choosing either marital or family therapy for Mrs. Y., one can also find support for using a heterogeneous group. Reviews of the literature by Luborsky, Singer, and Luborsky (1975) and Parloff and Dies (1977) indicate that with mixed groups of psychoneurotics group treatment offers no discernible advantage or disadvantage when compared with individual treatment. A patient like Mrs. Y. is generally suitable for both treatments. In Luborsky's "box score" review, only in one study did the group format show a clear advantage and that was with schizophrenic patients. As Grunebaum (1975) noted in his paper entitled "Soft-hearted Review of Hard-nosed Research on Groups," health, high social class, education, developed object relations, impulse control, ability to tolerate frustration, reality-testing, intelligence, verbal skills, and motivation all correlate with successful treatment in either individual or group therapy and are not of value in choosing one over the other. Nor have age, sex, marital status, or diagnosis been found to discriminate those who do better in group or individual therapy. Because so many patients do equally well in both, Yalom (1977) comments that it is easier to identify the characteristics that weigh against admission to group therapy than to establish clear and differential indications for it. In their most recent review of group outcome studies, Bednar and Kaul (1978) conceded the same point. All in all, the research indicates that group therapy works, but it does not yet indicate for whom it works best.

Homogeneous groups have rarely been compared to other formats, but the differential efficacy of these groups seems likely given their success with problems that have resisted other formats. The enthusiastic endorsement of the disciples and the many thousand successful graduates of homogeneous groups (Alcoholics Anonymous, Weight Watchers, Smoke Enders, etc.) is convincing even in the absence of well-controlled investigation.

We have saved for last mentioning an exhaustive study done by Smith, Glass, and Miller (1980). They reviewed 475 psychotherapy outcome studies by means of a meta-analysis and concluded that the current evidence does not document any differential effectiveness for any particular format—one format appears to be as effective as another, whether it be individual, group, or family psychotherapy. The importance of these conclusions as well as their limitations and the innovative methods used to reach them require further elaboration. We will therefore return to meta-analysis in Chapter 8 when discussing in more detail the research methods that have been used to establish guidelines for differential therapeutics.

In spite of the failure of available research to document differences, we believe the therapeutic format does make a difference and sometimes all the difference. A group therapy probably instills the notion that conflicts are best resolved in an interactional process with other people, whereas individual treatment probably conveys that introspective strategies are more important. We do not agree with Haley's (1973a) provocative suggestion that only inexperienced family therapists worry whether the other members of the family are present in the flesh or only conceptually. The differences among formats may be too subtle to be tapped by available research designs and instruments but the methodological limitations prevent us from assuming that the differences are unimportant especially in the face of clinical judgment to the contrary. In this chapter we have discussed only a few of the many co-variables that influence a consultant's and patient's choice of format. We must continue to rely on clinical judgment while we await further research to clarify which of these variables are the most crucial.

SUMMARY

We have discussed how systems theory is a helpful conceptual framework in choosing amongst various treatment formats. Individual treatment is most directed to the person subsystem while marital, family, and group therapies are addressed at increasingly extended networks of interpersonal relationships. Although available research does not yet document differential effectiveness for the different formats, clinical experience indicates that there are certain advantages and disadvantages of each.

The individual format has the great advantage of widespread patient acceptance (since it is so much like other more familiar healing relationships) and widespread clinician expertise (since most training programs in psychotherapy focus on teaching individual rather than group or family treatment). The individual format is also the most flexible, most specific to the patient's perception of problems, confidential, and the most likely to uncover and treat problems involving dyadic intimacy. The disadvantages of individual treatment are the relatively limited slice of behavior and incomplete information about the patient it affords, as well as the greater tendency to promote regression and actualized transferences and the possibility that the individual patient will be scapegoated.

Marital and family treatments are usually superior to the individual format when the presenting problems pertain to difficulties in marital or family relationships, because the problems can be directly recreated in the treatment setting and also because transferences are already in place and do not require an extended time to develop toward the therapist. In addition to being more cost-effective, these formats protect the therapist's technical neutrality and reduce regressive pulls and scapegoating. The disadvantages of marital and family treatment include the possibilities that they may reduce autonomy, cause even more family disruption, impose on needed privacy, and distract attention from necessary individual interventions.

There are no clear indications favoring the choice of the marital or the family format and this decision often depends on the training of the therapist, i.e., child psychiatrists tend toward family work, while adult psychiatrists prefer marital therapy. Many therapists combine the marital and family formats and include or exclude the children depending on the exigencies of that particular moment in therapy. The advantages of including the children are that their presence provides increased data on how the family interacts and important therapeutic leverage for change. Inclusion of the children may also help consolidate the family and may uncover problems the children are having that require attention. The disadvantages of including the children are that their presence may cause distraction, loss of privacy and frankness, and may impede their own individuation from the family.

Heterogeneous group therapy has achieved outcome successes equivalent to those of individual therapy in studies that compare the two formats. This group format is particularly useful for patients who present with interpersonal problems. It has the additional advantage of allowing the therapist to observe the patient's behavior in a variety of transferential relationships, of diluting transferences and countertransferences between the patient and therapist, and of increasing the patient's ability to observe, empathize with, and help others. The format of heterogeneous groups has the major disadvantage of relatively low patient acceptance and high dropout rates. The group has its own agenda and process and may have trouble adjusting to new members and addressing their specific concerns. This format is also not a treatment for a severe crisis.

Homogeneous group therapy, targeted to a specific problem, symptom or behavior, has the advantage of greater acceptance by the patient and warm acceptance by the group toward most new patients. This format also helps to reduce the patient's sense of isolation and demoralization and allows him or her to be helpful to others. These groups are also inexpensive and often deal with problems for which there is no other available effective treatment. The major limitation of homogeneous groups results from their narrow focus, which may allow other important issues and possible treatments to be missed.

CHAPTER 3

The Orientation

Each school of psychotherapy has applied its theories and methods to a wide range of patients in all kinds of settings and formats. For example, behavioral therapy has been used for hospitalized women with severe anorexia nervosa as well as for outpatient family therapy with a stuttering child; client-centered psychotherapy has been used for chronically hospitalized schizophrenics as well as for homogeneous groups of corporate managers; psychoanalytically-oriented treatments have been used for borderline characters in long-term reconstructive hospitals as well as for students in college counseling programs; and the possible combinations of settings, formats, theories, and methods go on an on.

Members of the many separate psychotherapeutic schools might politely express some disagreement about which setting or format the consultant chooses, but the choice of therapeutic technique is likely to be contested more sharply. Such controversy arises in part because therapeutic technique – what one actually *does* with a patient – is often based not just on one's training and professional expertise, but also on one's own personal view of the human condition and the causes and cures of emotional problems.

Selection of therapeutic technique is not only controversial, but also confusing because there are so many possibilities. Therapeutic procedures derive from a rich array of theories, experiments, professions, philosophies, innovations, assumptions, prejudices, and charismatic personalities. The list of alternative methods described in the literature seemingly grows with each publication. In trying to document separate schools of psychotherapy, Parloff (1980) counted over 250 contenders for the honor of being the most effective treatment. Some authors have suggested satirically that a moratorium be declared by the mental health profession: No more new techniques should be allowed until those already in existence have been studied sufficiently.

The proliferation of therapeutic techniques makes their categorization difficult. No method is completely satisfactory. Techniques cannot be easily subdivided into a manageable number of neat and mutually exclusive groups. In one attempt, Smith, Glass, and Miller (1980) listed 29 specific therapies which could be further condensed into 18 groups and then ultimately clustered into two large classes: behavioral therapies and verbal therapies. The behavioral class included systematic desensitization, flooding, and modeling techniques; the verbal class included psychodynamic, cognitive, and humanistic techniques. In another attempt, Luborsky, Singer, and Luborsky (1975) used two comparisons: 1) behavior therapy vs. psychotherapy; and 2) client-centered therapy vs. traditional therapies. Both Smith et al. and Luborsky et al.'s attempts at categorization have proved to be valuable for reviewing outcome research, but they are not particularly helpful in choosing a therapeutic technique.

At present, no one knows how or why therapists do what they do and what exactly influences their daily choices of methods and goals. Some therapists tend to concentrate their therapeutic efforts on only a few defined and specialized methods, such as psychoanalysis, biofeedback, psychodrama, or reciprocal inhibition with desensitization. Other therapists tend to use a variety of overlapping methods; applying an eclectic approach, they choose a particular technique after some assessment of the patient's changing needs. This comprehensive approach means that the various components — a little of this and a lot of that — are blended judiciously on the basis of the individual patient's capacities, desires, and goals.

The challenge for the referring consultant is to distinguish a thoughtfully titrated blend of different techniques from a mindless concoction which allows therapists complacently to convince themselves that whatever they happen to be doing in their offices is appropriate and sufficiently effective. We cannot simply rely on intuition. Nor can we rely on the nonspecific influences cited by Frank (1978), namely, a confiding relationship supported by myth, hope, privacy, and presumed expertise. Though these "common elements" may be helpful in all psychotherapies, some uncommon elements may be beneficial or detrimental depending on the particular patient. Even if we cannot yet document who will do better with focal therapy as opposed to rational therapy or reality therapy or Gestalt therapy or direct-decision therapy or orgone therapy or logotherapy, we must acknowledge that these methods *are* different (at least in some ways) and that differences count (at least for some patients). Psychotherapy is not an innocuous procedure. As Parloff, Wolfe, Hadley, and Waskow (1978) point out in their review of 700 published and unpublished controlled studies of treatment effectiveness, about 10% of patients who enter some form of psychotherapy may be harmed rather than helped.

Until more definitive information is available, the responsibility falls upon the consultant to apply clinical wisdom and incomplete scientific data when recommending specific therapeutic techniques. We have found it useful to conceptualize this complex task by determining which of three major mental functions should primarily be addressed during the process of therapy: the patient's understanding, behavior, or emotion. If the aim of treatment is primarily to increase the patient's understanding of his/her problems, then the therapy will be *exploratory* or *cognitive* in nature. If the aim is primarily to help control or decondition maladaptive behavior, then the therapy will be more *directive* in nature. And if the treatment is primarily intended to allow the patient to express and share feelings, then the therapy will be *experiential* in nature.

Table 3-1 illustrates how these three broad categories of techniques relate to aim, source of data, therapeutic stance, maneuvers, and different psychotherapeutic schools, with representative therapists and references for each school. This categorization is similar to that proposed by Karasu (1977), who divided psychotherapies into psychodynamic, behavioral, and experiential. As will become more clear later in this chapter, we prefer our terms because some "exploratory" therapies, such as transactional analysis or rational therapy, are not predominantly based on a psychodynamic (psychoanalytic) model and because some "directive" therapies, such as problem-solving or simply giving advice, are not based on behavioral (learning) models.

Like other attempts at categorization, ours has many shortcomings. The functions of the mind are so interrelated that any major function (such as emotion) will inevitably both affect and be affected by every other function. Accordingly, many psychoanalysts or behavioral therapists would be rightfully surprised by any implication that only experiential therapists use emotional sharing as part of their repertoire. The distinctions we are suggesting must be considered a matter of degree and not absolute. In addition, even if one category of psychotherapy is used during one period of treatment, we realize that another category may be indicated later on, perhaps even later in the same session. For example, experiential maneuvers may be required during the induction phase as the patient relates long-suppressed embarrassing feelings; after a trustful alliance is established, exploratory or directive techniques might then be indicated to treat the underlying defensive structure or maladaptive behavior.

Despite these limitations, we have found our categorization a helpful guide for the consultant and the therapist, both of whom must decide which specific maneuvers will be most beneficial for this particular problem with this particular patient at this particular time. Such decisions are never clear-cut, but some choices can be made more easily than others. For example, an elderly and lonely schizophrenic man would probably profit more from experiencing a supportive relationship than from understanding his problems in an exploratory treatment or from being systematically desensitized to the many anxiety-filled situations which by now pervade every aspect of his life. A young man with many friends and no isolated symptoms would more likely be placed in an exploratory treatment to understand his inhibitions about success than be given advice in a directive treatment or offered a corrective emotional experience. An uninsightful and guarded woman with a fear of flying and no other troubling symptoms would more readily accept a directive therapy than a probing exploration of the symbolic meaning of her problem or an intimate sharing with another.

Even these decisions are subject to questions and discussion and, unfortunately, most patients raise issues that are far more complex and indeterminate than the oversimplified examples we have just given. To illustrate some of the quandaries that arise, we will present a patient in detail and then discuss the many considerations regarding selection of therapeutic technique. We will elaborate on the development and rationale of various kinds of exploratory, directive, and experiential therapy. After addressing the relevant issues of the actual clinical situation, we will first describe what in fact happened with the patient and then discuss whether the consultant's decision would be supported by existing research studies.

THE CASE OF THE PANIC-STRICKEN SCHOLAR

The call to make an appointment is in itself revealing. When the consultant answers the phone, a Mr. T. quickly introduces himself and says, "Are you there, dear?" Mrs. T., apparently on another extension, answers her husband with a tentative, "Yes, I'm still on," but says no more. Mr. T. breaks the silence, "Well, tell him, dear. Tell the doctor what's the matter. . . ." Another silence follows, then a click. Mrs. T. has hung up, leaving her husband to explain: During the past few weeks something has come over Mrs. T. She's just not been herself. It began innocently enough. One evening she uncharacteristically canceled an invi-

Table 3-1

Table 3-1
Therapeutic Techniques

Category	Primary Aim	Sources of Data	Therapist's Stance	Techniques Strategies Maneuvers	Subcategories and Representative Therapists
Exploratory	Increase understanding of intrapsychic conflicts	Developmental history Unconscious derivatives: dreams; fantasies; parapraxes; free associations Transference Resistances	Transference figure Neutrality Abstinence Anonymity	Observations Clarifications Interpretations Genetic reconstructions	Psychoanalysis (Greenson) Psychoanalytically-oriented psychotherapy (Langs) Focal therapy (Sifneos) Time-oriented therapy (Mann)
Directive	Change maladaptive behaviors (including psychophysiological responses and covert behavior such as depressive thoughts) Increase or learn adaptive behaviors (e.g., social skills, assertiveness, problem solving)	Symptom-focused history Sequences: habits; patterns; Behavioral analysis Cognitive analysis	Expert Advisor Teacher Parental surrogate	Desensitization Hierarchal construction Graded exposure Flooding Modeling Positive reinforcement	Reciprocal inhibition (Wolpe) Strategic psychotherapy (Haley) Direct decision (Greenwald) Sex therapy (Kaplan) Reality therapy (Glasser)

				Techniques	Therapies
				Contingency contracting Assertive training Cognitive preparation Strategic assignment Suggestion Manipulation Advice Directives Relaxation training Paradoxical injunction	Hypnotherapy (Spiegel) Biofeedback (Ray) Stress Innoculation (Meichenbaum) Desensitization (Marks) Cognitive therapy (Beck) Rational emotive (Ellis)
Experiential	Experience and sharing feelings	Ahistorical Here-and-now-experiences Empathic awareness	Symmetrical Non-authoritarian	Abreaction Empathy Sharing Identification Imitation Confrontation Exhaustion	Client-oriented therapy (Rogers) Gestalt therapy (Perls) Logotherapy (Frankl) Primal Scream (Janov) Corrective emotional experience (Alexander) Orgone therapy (Reich) Est (Erhard)

tation to a dinner party at the last moment because she was feeling "out of sorts." A few days later they had orchestra tickets for her favorite ballet, but she refused to go for the same reason. Then, as Mr. T.'s soiled shirts accumulated without being taken to the laundry and as Mrs. T.'s research books were not returned to the library, Mr. T. realized that his wife was *never* going out, day or night. While he was at the office, she was staying in the apartment. He now understood why she had recently been asking him to do other small chores, like picking up a few items at the drug store or dry cleaner's on the way home from work.

Last month when he confronted her about all this, she admitted that the idea of going out, especially alone, was now unimaginable. She was sure she'd have a heart attack and collapse in the street. With Mr. T.'s urging, she agreed to see their family internist, but then backed down. The doctor made an exceptional house call, examined her fully, and declared Mrs. T. perfectly fit. Her breathing problems were all in her imagination and he advised her to get psychiatric help, but until now she has refused even to make the call and agreed today only if Mr. T. stayed home with her when she did.

Their daughter was home for Thanksgiving from college and has decided that her mother has "completely flipped out" and that her father is a fool for putting up with such craziness. She cannot understand why he agrees to accompany her mother on short walks around the block or to cancel important business trips so that Mrs. T. will not be alone. If it weren't for his daughter's prodding, Mr. T. admits he might not even have insisted on the call today. He hates to get his wife upset about anything. It throws her into such a panic; he's afraid she will faint, or maybe even something worse will happen. What should he do?

The consultant suggests to Mr. T. that he ask his wife to return to the phone although she can be assured that she need not talk if she so chooses. When Mrs. T. picks up the extension, an appointment is made for the following afternoon. Ten minutes before the scheduled time, Mr. T. calls from the apartment. Mrs. T. refuses to get in the taxi even with her husband along for support and protection. The consultant can hear Mrs. T. gasping for breath on the other line. He briefly explains the effects of hyperventilation and advises Mr. T. to call back as soon as the immediate panic subsides so other arrangements can be made. Nearly a month passes before Mr. T. calls again. The daughter is now home for the December holidays and has pressed for another appointment With her daughter as a companion, Mrs. T. is willing to make another try to get to the office.

This time she makes it. Mrs. T. is a strikingly attractive woman who might have stepped out of the pages of *Town and Country* magazine.

Even without makeup, she looks much younger than her 40 years. She greets the consultant in a poised and cordial manner, but after leaving her daughter and husband in the waiting room and walking into the private office, she becomes overwhelmed with anxiety the moment he shuts the door. The consultant's attempts to reassure her are without effect and her hyperventilation continues until she becomes dizzy. Only after her husband is asked to come in and sit beside her is Mrs. T. able to proceed. Fifteen minutes later her initial sophisticated manner has returned and she is considerably calmer and ironic about her "crazy spells." Yes, she had always been unusually wary of heights, elevators, and flying, but her fears had never kept her from doing what she had to do. She sees this whole mess as "frighteningly ridiculous."

The consultant is able to obtain only a rough sketch of Mrs. T.'s life: She's been married for almost 20 years; their other child, a son, is now at a boarding school in Europe because of some disciplinary problems last year in a local school; and her husband, several years older than she, recently became a senior partner in a prominent Wall Street law firm and too often must be out of town for days at a time. Mrs. T. has also been quite successful in her own career: She is a respected researcher and ghost writer for college professors and has published her own freelance articles in prominent newspapers and magazines. At present she is working on a piece about agoraphobia — which of course she can only do in her apartment. Mrs. T. is amused by the irony of it all and committed to keeping her appointment three days later even though her daughter will by then have returned to college.

During the next session Mrs. T. leaves her husband in the waiting room and comes into the office alone. Although her husband still believes the problem has been going on for only a few weeks, the first panic attack actually occurred four months ago when Mrs. T. was in a taxi one evening headed to a charity dinner for which she was already quite late. Although the occasion was for couples, her husband was delayed on a business trip and planned to join her at the dinner when his flight arrived. In the taxi Mrs. T. imagined what it would be like walking into the hotel ballroom where the affair was being held. Everyone else would have started dinner. They would look up from their soup and quietly watch her walk in late — and alone. What would they think? Would people notice how nervous she was? Her flushed face? Her heavy breathing? What if she tripped or became dizzy and fainted? The gossip about her would go on for weeks and she would never be able to face those people again.

As Mrs. T. recalled what had happened in the taxi that night, she reexperienced in the consultant's office the very same symptoms that had become so unbearable in the cab: her heart was pounding, her chest was tight, she felt light-headed, and she had tingling in her fingertips and around her lips. She interrupted her account to ask the consultant if she could possibly be having a heart attack. In reply, the consultant repeated an explanation about how anxiety can cause overbreathing which changes the blood gases and causes the characteristic symptoms she was describing. He indicated that this could be corrected simply enough by switching to abdominal breathing. Mrs. T., feeling momentarily relieved, then assumed the manner of a prodding journalist and began asking about the consultant's "fascinating professional life." The consultant responded that the more immediate task was to understand what happened after Mrs. T. felt so anxious in the cab, and he encouraged her to continue. Smiling in agreement and taking a deep breath, Mrs. T. went on:

Mrs. T. had decided in the cab that she was simply too anxious to attend the dinner. She went back to the apartment, left a message for her husband at the airport and by the time he returned home, she had calmed down, taken a nap on the couch, felt much better, and assumed that was that. Several days later, however, she was in a department store trying on lingerie and had a similar episode in the dressing room. She felt the walls were closing in on her and that she would suffocate. This episode lasted only a few moments and cleared as she left the store to return home. A more terrifying episode occurred the following week while she was waiting in line at the supermarket. She felt so trapped that she was compelled to leave her full cart of groceries and flee the store. She returned to her apartment and has since had all of her groceries delivered.

Too ashamed to discuss these three panic attacks with her husband or anyone else, Mrs. T. was determined at first not to let them rule her life. Her first response was to go to a medical library and read everything she could find about agoraphobia, claustrophobia, vertigo, panic attacks, psychotropic medication, behavioral therapy, and psychoanalysis. She found some relief in learning how many people shared her symptoms, but despite her knowledge of the incidence, etiologies, and proposed treatments of the disorders, her avoidance of potentially anxiety-provoking situations continued nonetheless. Many hours of the day were spent planning disguised strategies or negotiating with her husband or friends so that she would not have to leave the apartment alone. She would invite a friend for lunch and then go shopping with her, or she would order fresh fish delivered to the apartment and then tell her husband they would have to eat at home that night rather than meet at a restaurant. If circumstances absolutely forced her to go out alone, she attempted to restrict her range to the few blocks surrounding her apartment. If circumstances forced her to go into an enclosed area, she would calculate in advance the location of all the exits in case she needed to make a fast getaway.

One night her ability to conduct strategic planning broke down. Mr. T. was out of town and there was no answer when she placed her evening call to him at his hotel, which was their routine when he was away on business trips. Soon she imagined that robbers might enter her apartment and find her defenseless. She realized that the chances of this happening were remote and yet she could not remove the thought from her mind. She paced the apartment frantically and only after four stiff drinks and several more phone calls to her husband was she able to reach him and finally fall asleep. Since that episode she had not left the apartment at all. Eventually her husband realized what was going on.

When asked, Mrs. T. says she has refused to seek psychiatric help because she is so embarrassed about her behavior and besides, people should be able to solve their own problems and not become dependent on a crutch. She admits, however, that even before these panic attacks, she was curious about how her unusual childhood might have affected her personality and wondered if a psychoanalysis might be "interesting."

Mrs. T. was raised by servants in an exceptionally wealthy New England home. She recalls these many servants fondly, but has only vague memories of her parents who died in a private plane accident when she was nine. She became the legal ward of an aunt and uncle who lived on the same estate, although servants actually shared most of the parenting responsibility until she was old enough for boarding schools and college. She believes that the shifting of caretaking figures had some effect on her even before her parents' death as evidenced by her terror during the first day of school and the constant vague aches and pains that reduced her attendance throughout grade school. Bedtime has always been difficult for her. She was frightened of the loneliness, the monsters under the bed, of recurring nightmares in which she was chased and attacked, and of being frightened that she might suffocate and die during the night. She especially dreaded the prayer, "Now I lay me down to sleep, I pray the Lord my soul to keep; if I should die before I wake, I pray the Lord my soul to take." She smiles at the childishness of this fear but then adds, "I married my husband right after college. I guess I haven't had to lie alone at night for some time, except of course when he is away on business."

In contrast to the panic that occurred at the beginning of the first session a week ago, Mrs. T. comments how comfortable she now feels with the consultant; and she seems reluctant to leave the office at the end of the second session. She explains that except for her husband and children she has no truly close relationships, so the sharing of feelings during these visits has been quite a unique experience for her. In her own opinion, the paucity of intimate relationships in her life has stemmed from her shyness and insecurities, although, ironically, others believe she is simply cold and intellectual. Walking out the door, Mrs. T. turns back toward the consultant, smiles warmly and says that she will look forward to meeting with him the next week to hear what he has decided regarding her treatment.

Mrs. T.'s five-axis DSM-III diagnosis is:

Axis I.   300.21 Agoraphobia with panic attacks.
Axis II. 301.82, 301.60 Avoidant and dependent personality disorder.
Axis III. Mitral valve prolapse.
Axis IV. Minimal stress – daughter leaving for college – 2
Axis V.   Highest level of functioning during the past year – very good – 2

The psychiatric literature would support a number of quite different alternative psychotherapy techniques for the treatment of Mrs. T. The consultant could recommend one of the many *exploratory* treatments to help her understand the unconscious or preconscious basis for her irrational fears with the expectation that this understanding would also then lead to a change in her avoidance behavior and panic episodes. Or the consultant could recommend one of the *directive* treatments to teach Mrs. T. how to breathe properly and relax muscle groups, to desensitize her fear of frightening situations or extinguish her overwhelming anxiety by in vivo flooding, and to help her master self-deprecating thought patterns and shyness. Or the consultant could select an *experiential* treatment which could give Mrs. T. a chance to ventilate her feelings in a reassuring and supportive relationship that would in effect replace the loss of her daughter and husband as confidants and possibly increase her social skills and self-confidence. Any one of these alternative treatments (see Table 3-2) could be combined with the use of psychotropic medication. To keep the focus of this chapter on the selection of psychotherapeutic technique, we will defer until Chapter 6 a discussion of the issues involved when combining psychotherapy with psychopharmacotherapy and other somatic treatments.

Before describing what therapeutic technique was chosen for Mrs. T. and the ultimate outcome, we will first present the development and rationale of the three alternative categories and will outline the advantages as well as the disadvantages of each regarding Mrs. T.

EXPLORATORY TECHNIQUES

Psychoanalysis

The development of psychoanalysis over the past 100 years established the techniques used today in most exploratory psychotherapies. Prior to this development, psychopathology was viewed by psychiatrists as primarily ideopathic, constitutional, or hereditary. The strange ideas of the emotionally disturbed were considered, like fever, the *result* of an "infliction"; the ideas were not seen as the *cause*. Sigmund Freud found that irrational ideas led to symptoms and, furthermore, that these ideas were linked with memories and dreams and fantasies which the mind kept out of awareness in the "unconscious."

The notion of the unconscious was of course not new; Plato discussed the concept in *The Republic*, and many philosophers and psychologists after him have been intrigued by the dark side of the mind. What *was* new, indeed ingenious, was the discovery that unconscious ideas were not passively buried in deep recesses of the mind, but instead were actively and constantly influencing behavior. The mind had to work to keep forbidden wishes and fears from full awareness and expression. This work, called "repression," was a continuous, but not totally successful, mental activity. In everyday life the repressed wishes and fears were only partially disguised and found expression in the form of dreams, fantasies, myths, symbols, slips of the tongue, jokes, memory lapses, art, and so on. And sometimes unconscious ideas – in particular those motivated by sexual and aggressive conficts – were expressed more maladaptively by means of psychiatric symptoms.

The concept of the dynamic unconscious helped explain various kinds of psychopathology. An example will illustrate this point. A young woman on the eve of her marriage to an older man suddenly develops numbness and paralysis below the waist which cannot be explained neurologically. Psychiatric consultation suggests that for this woman the marriage to a much older man represents both a wish for father and a guilty fear of acting on such unconscious incestuous impulses. The anxiety generated by these conflicting wishes and fears was converted into a somatic symptom. This conversion reaction resolves the conflict, albeit maladaptively, by expressing the wish through illicit attention given to "private parts," by expressing the fear through preventing the "incestuous" union, and by expressing the associated guilt through the "punishment" of a somatic ailment. Other seemingly irrational kinds of behavior can also be explained by the concept of the dynamic unconscious, such as, obsessions and compulsions, unsubstantiated suspiciousness, or excessive despair.

TABLE 3-2

Selection Criteria for Treatment Techniques and Strategies

Psychodynamic	Directive	Experiential
Relative Indications 1) Patient's problem can be understood as a manifestation of an intrapsychic conflict. 2) Goal of treatment is character change, as opposed to simply symptom reduction, in at least one area of conflict. *Enabling Factors* 1) Patient is motivated to change his behavior and to understand himself better, not merely to attain symptom relief. 2) Patient is willing to make sacrifices (e.g., time, money) in order to participate in the treatment. 3) Patient is honest about himself and his motivations.	*Relative Indications* 1) Problem under control of environmental (e.g., family) contingencies? 2) Clear, definable symptoms or problem behaviors (e.g., phobia, compulsions). 3) Goal is symptom reduction and/or behavior change. *Enabling Factors* 1) Willingness to take direction from others. 2) Motivation to do homework assignments. 3) Willingness to expose oneself to	*Relative Indications* 1) Existential angst, feelings of emptiness, lack of identity, and self-alienation. *Enabling Factors* 1) Ability to be emotionally involved with a therapist and yet accept the boundaries of a therapeutic relationship. *Relative Contraindications* 1) Presence of specific problems more amenable to change by more specific techniques.

4) Patient has psychological mindedness, and is eager to study his behaviors and feelings, including those that occur during the interview in regard to the therapist.
5) The patient has the ability to experience, tolerate and discuss painful affects.
6) The patient has relatively high ego strength as evidenced by educational, work, and sexual performance, and the ability to accept responsibility.
7) The patient is intelligent and able to communicate verbally his thoughts, feelings and fantasies.

Relative Contraindications
1) Specific symptoms (e.g., phobia, depression, sexual dysfunction) that demand immediate attention dominate the presenting picture.
2) Discussing unconscious conflicts has resulted in destructive regression and/or actualized transference in previous treatments.

anxiety-provoking situations.
4) Willingness to accept the focused and limited goals.

Relative Contraindications
1) Patient feels the goals are too limited, and techniques are too concrete.

2) Tendency to substitute therapy for life.

The concept of the dynamic unconscious may also be used to explain Mrs. T.'s "irrational" behavior. Her repressed wishes (e.g., to be cared for, to have illicit sexual experiences, to exhibit herself grandiosely) and her repressed fears (e.g., abandonment, punishment, shame) are symbolized and displaced onto relatively harmless external circumstances. Mrs. T. might thereby come to fear being trapped in situations that might deprive her of help (e.g., elevators) or that symbolically encourage wishes to be sexual and exhibitionistic (e.g., dinner parties without her husband). An internal conflict is displaced onto tangible external situations which can then be avoided. Intrapsychic anxiety is contained at the price of making fearsome what is in fact a harmless external situation.

Because at first Freud believed that repressed wishes were the cause of his patients' symptoms, he designed a treatment to bring the forbidden desires into awareness. Initially, he used hypnosis, prodding, and encouragement to make the unconscious become conscious, but he found these methods were not widely applicable, at least in his hands. Despite his efforts, the resistances and defenses mounted by many of his patients were simply too strong. He then learned that "free association" was a more useful technique. He instructed patients to say whatever came to their minds. Given time, tolerance, and facilitating interpretations, patients gradually could overcome and understand their censoring, their repression. Through dreams, memories, and other associations that derived from internal fantasy, the unconscious material could be revealed and analyzed. The techniques for such a psychoanalysis included "clarification," in which various associations were organized and made explicit, and "interpretation," in which inferences were made about wishes and memories that had not quite reached consciousness but on the evidence of accumulating associative trends could no longer be denied.

In addition to producing previously repressed material, many patients developed an intense relationship with the analyst that was reminiscent of earlier real or imagined relationships with parents and significant others. The need to transfer this past relationship onto the therapist also provided data for analysis. To enhance the formation of this transference neurosis and to prevent the analyst from interfering with full disclosure of the patient's latent wishes and fears, Freud made rather stringent suggestions about the analyst's stance:

1) He recommended the analyst remain a relatively unknown figure (anonymity) so that the patient's view of the analyst would be predominantly a product of the patient's regressive fantasies and not represent the reality of the situation.

2) He recommended that the patient's desire for approval, support, love, and reassurance not be gratified by the analyst (abstinence). The resulting frustration was designed to increase the intensity of the underlying needs and thereby make them more obvious and capable of being understood.
3) He suggested that the analyst not take sides with any of the forces involved in a given conflict (neutrality). If the analyst did not favor one agency over the other, all aspects of the confict – the wishes, fears, guilt, defenses, and reality of the situation – could all come into view and be analyzed.
4) In order to facilitate the regressive process of freely associating without distraction and to make abstinence, anonymity, and neutrality more feasible, Freud recommended that patients lie on a couch with the analyst out of view. If patients were sufficiently motivated and capable of examining the unconscious material and the transference distortions as they emerged, then infantile conflicts could be "worked through" in a more adaptive and less symptomatic manner.

From the wealth of data produced by free association, regression, and transference neuroses, Freud and other psychoanalysts constructed many theories about human behavior, such as those involving dream processes, defensive mechanisms and character formation. In the early years of psychoanalysis, special attention was given to elucidating instinctual development (libido theory). Later the focus shifted to ego psychology, i.e., understanding how anxiety and other symptoms stemmed from intrapsychic conflict among different hypothetical structures of the mental apparatus (id, ego, superego, and perceptions of external reality). Psychoanalysts next became most interested in object relations theory, i.e., a way of understanding how the infant's relationship with early caretakers became distorted, internalized, and structured to form the basis of identity, character, and symptoms. Recently, the psychoanalytic literature has been especially interested in self psychology, the healthy and pathological interest in oneself (narcissism) and the ways by which the self is structured and self-esteem is regulated.

As various psychoanalytic theories have evolved over the years, some (like the Oedipus complex) have by now become generally accepted and even taken for granted. Others have been completely revised, are still debated, or have been discarded altogether. Because of the pervasive influence psychoanalytic theory has had on understanding all human behavior, an unfortunate confusion has developed between psychoanalytic *theory*, psychoanalytic *treatment*, and psychoanalytic *technique*. Although they "grew up" together, they are not the same. For the consultant deciding whether an exploratory treatment is indicated for a given patient, psychoanalytic theory must be distinguished from psychoanalytic treatment and technique. The failure to make such a distinction has caused a misunderstanding among many patients and some therapists, and also has caused some confusion in the literature regarding differential therapeutics.

Many patients consider themselves to be "in analysis" no matter what kind of treatment they are receiving. Although some may be in a type of exploratory psychotherapy, only a very small number (less than 1%) are in psychoanalysis as traditionally conceived, that is, four to five sessions per week for an indefinite period of time (usually at least two years) and working through a well-established transference neurosis as the main therapeutic strategy. Similarly, patients often use the terms psychologist, psychiatrist, therapist, analyst, and psychoanalyst interchangeably, whereas only a small fraction of those in the mental health profession have had a training analysis and have met the requirements of an approved psychoanalytic training institute.

This confusion among patients and among the general public probably does little harm. The confusion is potentially more harmful if therapists themselves fail to distinguish the use of psychoanalytic concepts from the use of psychoanalytic technique. While conducting peer reviews and while supervising psychology interns, social workers, psychiatry residents, psychiatry nurses, and medical students, we have found that therapists often automatically assume a psychoanalytic stance and introduce psychoanalytic maneuvers with all kinds of patients in all types of psychotherapies without fully appreciating that these techniques have specific indications and can be ineffective or even damaging if not judiciously applied. For example, a schizophrenic patient given little structure or direction and simply told to "free associate" may produce no more than psychotic ramblings or, even worse, may become frighteningly disorganized. A borderline patient placed on the couch may respond to the regressive situation by developing a strongly actualized or even psychotic transference if no reality confrontations are used to bring the heightened fantasies back down to earth. An obsessive patient may use premature genetic interpretations to increase rather than diminish rigid intellectual defenses and may secretly view with defiance and disdain the therapist's attempts to reconstruct childhood struggles. A medically ill, depressed patient may perceive the therapist's anonymity and abstinence as cold, rejecting, and further evidence that the physical deficit makes the patient undesirable.

Regarding phobic patients like Mrs. T., Freud himself noted that a therapist cannot remain completely neutral and refuse to "take sides." The phobic patient should be encouraged and must somehow enter the feared situations; otherwise, the analysis itself becomes a comfortable retreat, expiation, and means of avoidance not only of the feared situation, but also of change (Freud, 1955a).

These examples of how psychoanalytic maneuvers can be inappropriate or harmful have been presented to illustrate the importance of distinguishing theory from technique. In every clinical situation, the therapist benefits from a psychodynamic understanding of the patient – the schizophrenic's "denial" and "projection," the borderline's "splitting" and "identity diffusion," the obsessive's "isolation of affect" and "punitive superego," the physically ill patient's "loss of self-esteem" and "unobtainable ego ideal," and the phobic's "displacement" and "separation anxiety." These and many other psychoanalytic ideas have become so intrinsically interwoven into our understanding of all human behavior that at present it is difficult or impossible for anyone (including psychopharmacotherapists and behavior therapists) to see any patient without at least some psychodynamic observations. The point is that the therapist can use psychoanalytic theory to understand a patient's psychodynamics and *not* use psychoanalytic techniques as a means of treating them.

Freud himself was well aware of this distinction and applied psychoanalytic understanding to certain categories of patients (such as schizophrenics, severe narcissistic characters, and psychopaths), while recommending that one not use psychoanalytic techniques. As described in his own case studies, Freud himself was often anything but an anonymous, abstinent, and neutral therapist. He used directive and experiential techniques when he believed they were indicated. In fact, a psychodynamic understanding of the patient may at times help to make clear why psychoanalytic techniques are not feasible or advisable. The consultant seeing Mrs. T., for example, might decide that her tendency to regress in order to be taken care of and to avoid separation would make psychoanalysis unproductive, potentially infantilizing, and harmful. The consultant might use a psychodynamic assessment to recommend a treatment with less chance of a malignant regression, such as one of the less intensive exploratory psychotherapies or one of the directive or experiential psychotherapies, which we will discuss later in this chapter.

Although psychoanalysis offers the possibility of a relatively uncontaminated working through of embedded personality problems, its lack of structure may also be harmful for patients who do not have the capacity to form a trusting relationship with the analyst, to tolerate the frustration inherent in the analytic situation, or to analyze constructively the distortions that develop within the transference relationship. In response to such concerns, a number of analysts have searched for ways of widening the applicability of psychoanalysis. They have suggested that limitations in the patient need not preclude analysis, although they may prolong the treatment and increase its difficulty.

When a patient does not meet the strict enabling factors for analysis, some have recommended either another less demanding treatment as a first step or a "trial analysis," a period of assessment to determine if the impeding factors are too severe for the analysis to proceed. Eissler (1953) broadened the applicability of analysis by introducing "parameters," necessary deviations from traditional analytic technique that can later be analyzed when sufficient repair and growth have occurred. Kohut (1971), in an attempt to make the benefits of analysis available to those with narcissistic characters, has suggested modifications in analytic technique: The analyst does not prematurely intercept the patient's projections of omnipotence onto the analyst nor the patient's contempt; instead, the idealizing and mirroring transferences are permitted full development before being interpreted as phase-appropriate behaviors from the past that are unadaptive in the present. The induction into analysis of these patients with more severe psychopathology is considered worth the risk and efforts because psychoanalysis for selected patients may be the only hope when all other treatments promise little.

Psychodynamic Psychotherapy

Psychoanalysis is of course not the only kind of exploratory psychotherapy, but most treatments in this category derive from psychoanalytic concepts and techniques. Accordingly, they have been labeled "psychoanalytically-oriented psychotherapy," "long-term psychotherapy," and "psychodynamic psychotherapy." These exploratory psychotherapies, like psychoanalysis, use clarification and interpretation to resolve intrapsychic conflicts that are causing symptoms and maladaptive behavior. The resolution of conflict is expected to improve self-esteem and interpersonal relationships and to facilitate character change.

Although the psychodynamic psychotherapies are not as precisely defined as psychoanalysis per se, the patient generally comes one to three times per week for at least a year, faces the therapist, and is encouraged to speak freely without dwelling on any preselected area. Because a full transference neurosis is considered neither necessary nor desirable, the therapist interprets transference phenomena whenever they serve as resistances or are related to the patient's problems. The therapist is not concerned that these interpretations might inhibit the development of a more regressive transference experience. Similarly, because the goal is not a complete character analysis, the therapist may choose to influence the patient by offering some structure, suggestion, education, and support as indicated.

Advocates of the psychodynamic psychotherapies believe that the rigid selection criteria for a traditional psychoanalysis exclude many patients who benefit from a sustained psychodynamic therapy and that equivalent benefits may be obtained by a treatment that is not as costly, intensive, or prolonged. They point out that regression may be detrimental for some patients and that many patients lack the time, money, motivation, and necessity for understanding the more subtle aspects of their character. They argue as well that because psychodynamic psychotherapy can be tailored to the needs of the individual patient, it can have a wider applicability than psychoanalysis and can be more efficient.

Focal Therapy

As we will discuss in the next chapter regarding the duration and frequency of treatment, not all exploratory psychotherapies are long-term. A case in point is "focal therapy," a brief dynamic psychotherapy developed by Malan (1963, 1976). In contrast to the ambitious goals of psychoanalysis and to the variability and flexibility of psychodynamic psychotherapy, focal therapy is designed to achieve limited goals within a structured format. The therapist quickly constructs a working formulation, focuses the patient on one particular conflict, and directs interpretations to that area. As treatment proceeds, additional data may compel changes in the initial formulation, but generally the focus remains fixed on a specific conflictual area throughout treatment, which usually lasts between 12 and 50 visits. Some authors recommend that a date for termination be set at the beginning of treatment to highlight issues surrounding separation; others suggest a more flexible approach in choosing both the focus and termination date. Proponents of focal therapy believe that it can provide not only symptomatic improvement but also sustained character change within the circumscribed area.

Most exploratory psychotherapies are closely related, at least in theory, to psychoanalysis – but some are less so. For example, although transactional analysis is designed to remove symptoms by increasing a patient's understanding, the underlying theory developed by Eric Berne (1961) is to some degree dissociated from psychoanalytic concepts.

Cognitive Therapy

Cognitive therapy is another example of a treatment that is exploratory in nature but also quite different from psychoanalytic theory and techniques. The intention of cognitive therapy is to uncover, make explicit, and change previously automatic, preconscious cognitions that cause maladaptive feelings and behaviors. Although this kind of exploration was developed in part by psychoanalytically inclined therapists, the techniques used in cognitive therapy are highly directive and reflect the strong influence of learning theory and behavior therapy. We have therefore included our discussion of cognitive therapy in the directive techniques discussed later in this chapter, even though we recognize that the techniques of cognitive therapy straddle the boundary between exploratory and directive treatments.

Having pointed out how the consultant can use psychoanalytic concepts and not recommend a psychoanalytic treatment or technique and, conversely, how the consultant can reject psychoanalytic theories and still recommend an exploratory psychotherapy, we will now consider the advantages and disadvantages for Mrs. T. of a kind of treatment primarily designed to increase an understanding of her crippling fears.

Most kinds of exploratory treatments would resonate with Mrs. T.'s intellectual approach to life. As her character style, choice of profession, and reaction to symptoms indicate, she gains a sense of mastery and confidence by understanding complex problems. Her research project on agoraphobia could be presented to her as the first step toward a more thorough, personal, and specific investigation of her own psyche. In addition to appealing to her interests and temperament, uncovering psychotherapies would reinforce her expressed curiosity about the effects of an unusual childhood on her chronic fears of being alone and her ways of "putting people off."

Not only would Mrs. T. be inclined to accept a recommendation for an exploratory treatment, but she would also most likely be able to participate in such a choice and may even have the ego strength for an intensive and prolonged treatment like a classical psychoanalysis. For example, she is intelligent, psychologically-minded and self-observant. She realizes her panic episodes are irrational ("crazy") and also perceives subtle aspects of her personality as ego-dystonic and maladaptive, such as her reserved and shy manner. Throughout her life she has shown a capacity to withstand frustration, control impulses, modulate affect, and establish at least some close relationships. She has the time, the money, and apparently a husband and children who could accept changes in her character. During the consultation, despite her initial anxiety and then her intellectual control, she was able to engage the interviewer and establish a relatedness on which a therapeutic alliance could be built. Although her current panic attacks are serious and interfering with important aspects of her life, she is not in such an overwhelming crisis that she would be incapable of reflecting thoughtfully on past and present conflicts. Finally, she has none of the obvious contraindications to those treatments primarily designed to increase understanding: She is not acutely psychotic, profoundly depressed, mentally retarded, or sociopathic, and she does not suffer from drug or alcohol abuse.

But even if Mrs. T. has the motivation and the capacity to undergo a psychoanalysis, the question still remains whether this would be the best recommendation. An important distinction must be made between *enabling factors* and *indications*, otherwise the consultant may be tempted to suggest an intensive and extensive psychoanalytically-oriented therapy simply because the patient is willing and able. A primary indication for a psychodynamic treatment is that the symptoms arise from intrapsychic conflicts and not from environmental pressure, role assignment, known biochemical imbalance, or ignorance. Mrs. T. appears to meet this requirement. An understanding of her conflicts might therefore be helpful not just in relieving the current panic episodes, but also in resolving persistent characterological problems, such as her fears of being alone as well as her reluctance to be more open with others. Mrs. T. might also learn how her intellectualization and isolation of affect were used during her childhood to defend against the pain of many traumatic separations, how she continues to protect herself from the anguish associated with both attachment and loss, and how her early defenses are no longer adaptive. The ambitious goal of a psychoanalysis would be to work through these developmental conflicts within the context of a transference neurosis.

The advantages of an extended exploratory treatment must be balanced against possible disadvantages and even risks with such an approach. As noted before, Mrs. T. could make therapy simply an intellectual exercise. She might examine at length the many conscious and unconscious reasons why she was anxious, without ever actually confronting the anxiety-laden situations. Therapy would become an indulgence, a retreat, and would thereby only enhance rather than resolve her tendency to avoid those things which make her uncomfortable, whether they be elevators or close relationships.

Another risk is that after a prolonged probing inquiry dredged up the many painful events of her youth, Mrs. T. might use this knowledge only as an excuse to be the way she is – she would now feel entitled to have her problems because of the misery she endured. Furthermore, a destructive negative transference might emerge if the repressed bitterness toward her rejecting parents were displaced onto the "cold" therapist. The therapeutic alliance might not be strong enough to weather such a rageful storm; Mrs. T. might not be able to appreciate her distortions and to realize that the therapist's abstinence, anonymity and neutrality were part of the treatment and not part of the therapist's character. Under such conditions, harmful countertransference problems might also ripen and fester.

Even if a prolonged negative therapeutic reaction did not develop, an infantilizing regression might. Having contained her dependency yearnings for so many years, Mrs. T. might latch onto the therapist, overidealizing his compassion and understanding. This possibility is already suggested by the rapidity with which Mrs. T. felt close to the consultant. Although on the surface the exploratory treatment would appear to be examining, for example, the intricacies and ramifications of an erotic transference, the treatment would actually be supplying dependency needs under the guise of a sustained uncovering inquiry.

Considering the deprivation of Mrs. T.'s early years, an in-depth analysis also runs the risk of unearthing a malignant core: a borderline personality disorder may be lurking beneath Mrs. T.'s intellectual facade. If this were the case, rather than a strong negative transference or an overly dependent transference, Mrs. T. might then develop a near-psychotic hostile-dependent relationship with the therapist. Unable to keep her primitive reactions contained within the treatment arena, she might begin to act on these intense feelings with her husband, children, and others and, as a result, show more impairment than if the purulent abscess had never been drained. A knowledgeable therapist can of course be on guard for these and other transference reactions and try to keep them from spilling onto others outside of treatment; but when selecting an exploratory treatment, the consultant must consider the propensity of some patients to develop masochistic, overly dependent, or even psychotic transferences that can strain the skill and wisdom of even the most expert and experienced therapist.

Although such dreadful consequences of a psychoanalytic treatment would seem unlikely for Mrs. T., one way of offering some protection would be to recommend an exploratory treatment with less regressive pull. As we will discuss in more detail in the next chapter, a time-oriented therapy, while exploratory in nature, might short-circuit destructive dependency by sharply circumscribing Mrs. T.'s unrealizable expectations and by making separation problems the focus of treatment.

Mrs. T. meets at least two of the rather stringent enabling factors for this demanding treatment: She has a circumscribed conflict around separation and has shown a desire to change herself and not merely obtain symptom relief or have a forum to voice her complaints. It is not yet clear, however, whether she has the capacity to focus on one isolated area of conflict or the capacity to quickly analyze transference distortions and then relinquish a meaningful relationship with the therapist. Furthermore, a limited exploration might short-change Mrs. T.; by focusing on only one area, she may fail to resolve many other chronic and significant difficulties in her life, such as her rigidity and shyness which may or may not revolve around separation conflicts.

In discussing the pros and cons of an exploratory treatment for Mrs. T., we have so far only mentioned those treatments based on psychoanalytic principles. There are other exploratory treatments that are "nonanalytic" but use understanding as the primary mode of change; for example, Ellis' rational-emotive therapy and Berne's transactional analysis. Treatments that deal predominantly with conscious and pre-conscious conflicts may give Mrs. T. an intellectual handle on her problems, a handle strong enough to support her during panic episodes. But because Mrs. T. is reflective and intellectual by nature, she may find that these treatments do not get to the root of her problems; she may therefore reject such treatments — and their therapists — because they seem superficial and ineffective.

Where then does that leave us in terms of an exploratory treatment for Mrs. T.? On the positive side, she appears to have many of the enabling factors and indications with no obvious contraindications; therefore, the most compelling reason for not recommending an uncovering inquiry might simply be that another method — directive or experiential — would be more efficient and effective. To assess this possibility, let us now examine the development and rationale of these alternative techniques.

DIRECTIVE TECHNIQUES

Throughout history attempts have been made to get those with emotional problems to "behave themselves," but very often this has been to no avail. For years the emotionally ill were defined as those who remained refractory to the usual directive techniques of advice, instruction, and discipline. The insane and disturbed did not respond as expected to the customary methods that were used in child rearing, social conditioning, and education. They could not "learn from experience" or "be reasoned with." This pessimistic view has been modified in recent years. We now know that directive techniques can be very effective in helping the mentally ill; the trick is to find the right directive and the right technique for a particular problem.

At the beginning of this century, while Freud was developing psychoanalysis in Vienna, Thorndike in the United States and Bekhterev and Pavlov in Russia were developing principles of learning theory and testing them with animal and human experiments. Except for some scattered and uninfluential reports, the findings of these researchers were not applied clinically to behavioral disorders until the 1950s when Joseph Wolpe and Arnold Lazarus began publishing their impressive results. Since then, behavioral as well as other directive techniques have been increasingly accepted as valuable additions to the profession's psychotherapeutic repertoire. We now have scientifically-based, systematic methods of helping patients control specific maladaptive behaviors, most especially those relating to anxiety and phobias, but also stuttering, tics, smoking, overeating, sexual dysfunctions, drug abuse, delinquency, marital discord, obsessive thoughts, disparaging ideas, and exaggerated psychophysiological responses.

Unlike psychoanalytic techniques, directive techniques did not evolve primarily from one school of thought. They emerged from many different kinds of experiments, philosophies, and clinical studies; and they are still in the process of becoming more integrated and comprehensive.

If a consultant decides that a patient's treatment should principally be designed to change or control behavior, he must then decide which of the many directive techniques would be potentially most helpful (Table 3-1 provides only a partial list). To help the consultant in this complex selection process, we will briefly review the background and rationale of four representative kinds of directive techniques: 1) systematic desensitization and flooding; 2) positive reinforcement; 3) cognitive therapy; and 4) problem-solving psychotherapy. We will then discuss the pros and cons of suggesting any of these directive methods for Mrs. T.

Systematic Desensitization

Joseph Wolpe (1958) developed this procedure on the basis of his experiments with cats. In the tradition of classical (Pavlovian) conditioning theory, Wolpe first made cats fearful of a cage in which they had received electric shocks; he then "systematically desensitized" the cats by bringing them gradually closer to the cage in a series of discrete steps *and* feeding them at each step. He reasoned that feeding the hungry cat psychophysiologically inhibited their acquired fearfulness ("reciprocal inhibition").

Wolpe's clinical technique was a logical extension of these experiments. By doing a careful behavioral analysis, he would determine the discrete situations that made the patient increasingly anxious. For example, the first anxious "step" for Mrs. T. would be imagining her husband getting ready for work in the morning while she watches vigilantly; and the tenth "step" would be for her to imagine pacing the bedroom all alone on a stormy night while her husband's away for a three-week business trip.

After Wolpe had constructed a hierarchy of scenes (antecedent stimuli) which made Mrs. T. more and more anxious, he would find some method of psychophysiologically inhibiting this anxiety. Instead of using food as he did with the cats, he would use progressive relaxation of muscle groups. Others since Wolpe have used hypnosis, biofeedback, transcendental meditation, and adjunctive use of drugs, such as bensodiazepines or a rapid-acting intravenous barbiturate. According to Wolpe's procedure, Mrs. T. would imagine the first frightening scene in the hierarchy and de-condition her anxiety by pairing it with the relaxation response. When a sufficient number of repetitions had been performed to minimize the anxiety, he would systematically proceed to the next graded step until even the most terrifying situation had become tolerable.

In considering a program of systematic desensitization for an anxious patient like Mrs. T., the consultant should realize that some modifications of Wolpe's original methods have been developed in recent years. Although they do not precisely parallel Wolpe's laboratory model, they have demonstrated advantages for some patients. For example, *graded exposure* is an effective alternative. Instead of imagining the frightening situation, the patient actually approaches the "stimuli" through a series of small steps. No specific relaxation training is involved; the anxiety extinguishes in the first situation and the patient is then encouraged to go on to the next step. Mrs. T., for instance, might be told to stand alone outside her Park Avenue apartment until this no longer makes her anxious. When her anxiety was sufficiently reduced, she would then be instructed to go to the corner and remain outside the sight of the doorman, and so on.

Because procedures conducted in real life (in vivo) instead of in the imagination tend to be faster and more reliable, graded exposure is a potentially more effective technique for those who are afraid of their own panic symptoms and willing to undergo exposure in order to extinguish their anxiety. A disadvantage of graded exposure is that the patient does not learn a systematic method of relaxation which can be used in the future to reduce excessive muscular tension and emotional arousal. For patients with tension headaches, asthma, neurodermatitis, ulcers, colitis, hypertension, and the like, relaxation training is often a valuable component of directive treatments because the benefits extend beyond mastering a specific situation and can be applied more generally. Moreover, less motivated patients may accept systematic desensitization, but refuse graded exposure.

An even more rapid procedure for extinguishing anxiety is *flooding*. The patient is instructed to place himself in the most terrifying situation and withstand the anxiety at its full intensity for an increasingly prolonged period of time. For example, Mrs. T. might be taken by her husband to a supermarket and then left there on her own. As she experiences a panic attack upon his departure, her inclination would be to run home, but if instead she manages to persevere and remain exposed to her anxiety, it will gradually decrease during the next few hours and will eventually extinguish. This clinical finding, though perhaps intuitively used for years, is supported by animal experiments: A conditioning response (like Mrs. T.'s anxiety) will gradually be extinguished if it is not reinforced by avoidance or escape. Though flooding is the most effective treatment for phobias, it often is not feasible because the patient simply refuses or has a physical condition (such as a heart problem) that would make the stress contraindicated.

Graded participant modeling is a possible alternative for those patients who either will not approach the frightening situation alone or have trouble imagining a frightening scene and tolerating the associated anxiety. Children and extremely apprehensive adults often fall into this latter group, and very intellectual patients like Mrs. T. also often have trouble letting their imagination go freely. The modeling procedure, based on imitative behavior in animals and elaborated for clinical use by Bandura (1977; Bandura and Walters, 1963) involves first having the therapist calmly go through the series of feared events while being observed by the patient, then having the patient and therapist take each step together until the patient can handle the final predetermined situation with equanimity and confidence. Mrs. T., for instance, might first observe and then eventually ride in an elevator with the therapist for longer and longer periods of time and to higher and higher floors, until she could push the emergency stop button at the top floor and remain reasonably calm before releasing the button and returning to the ground floor.

In presenting this condensed review of techniques based on classical conditioning and modeling theory (systematic desensitization, graded exposure, flooding, and graded participant modeling), we may have been misleading. We do not mean to imply that the only real factor to consider when recommending these procedures is the patient's premonitory willingness and that the choice of therapist is less important. On the contrary, although the literature on directive approaches emphasizes the therapeutic technique more than the therapeutic relationship, the skill and artistry of the therapist may make all the difference. Even when a treatment manual describes what should be done and in what order, the patient is not simply plugged into a series of robotic procedures. The therapist must be able to engage the patient and form a working relationship. In this regard, directive treatments share a common bond with exploratory and experiential approaches.

As well as being empathic and engaging, the behavioral therapist must also be able to extract a precise behavioral pattern from what at first may appear to be a diffuse and unfocused chief complaint. The therapist must then consider the personality and motivation of the patient when constructing a hierarchy that will be acceptable to the patient and that will address the subtleties of the frightening situation. If the situation cannot be easily reproduced in vivo or in the imagination, then the therapist may need to use symbols, pictures, videotapes, or even actors as surrogates. The creativity, charisma, optimism, intuition, and encouragement of the therapist, though not easily relatable to the animal model, are important, and perhaps essential, "reinforcers."

Many therapists, even those who consider themselves to be exponents of a particular exploratory or experiential school of psychotherapy, use directive techniques much more often than they appreciate, albeit much less directly and consciously than behavior therapists. As patients repeatedly try to "understand" or "share" their fears in a comfortable setting, a kind of desensitization, reciprocal inhibition, graded exposure, and extinction inevitably occurs; and as patients increasingly identify with the therapist, a kind of modeling takes place as well. An advantage of directive treatments is that anxiety-reducing procedures can be designed more systematically and efficiently. In addition, because the goals of treatment are explicit and observable, the patient gains the confidence of having mastered a specific task, rather than vaguely "feeling better about myself." For this reason, as we will discuss at the end of this chapter, outcome studies also tend to be tilted toward directive treatments: If the results obtained by a technique are more easily measured, the effectiveness of the technique is more easily documented.

Positive Reinforcement

Animal experiments have shown that if a behavioral response is consistently followed by a reward, such as food, stroking, praise, or absence of pain, then that "positively reinforced" behavior will occur more vigorously and more frequently. On the other hand, if a certain behavior is followed either by punishment ("an aversive stimulus") or by no stimulus at all ("extinction"), then the response tends to occur weakly and less frequently under similar conditions in the future. These laboratory findings correlate with our everyday experiences: We reach again for another piece of pie if it tasted good; we don't reach again for a stove if we got burned. Extensive research has shown that complex behavior can also be shaped by a combination of subtle responses in the environment. B. F. Skinner (1938), for example, arranged an elaborate system of positive reinforcements and extinction to make pigeons perform colorful and outlandish feats. Skinner was the pioneer of "operant conditioning" in which behavior is determined by its environmental *consequences* (as opposed to classical conditioning discussed above in which behavior is determined by environmental *cues*).

Because operant conditioning requires arranging the environment to respond to behavior in a particular way, its clinical use was at first reserved primarily for patients in institutions where positive reinforcement and extinction could be programmed systematically into the setting. One of the first such applications was designed by Ayllon and Azrin (1968) who improved the eating habits of chronic psychotic patients. Instead of having the staff inadvertently reinforce the patients' bad eating habits by giving them more attention if they were tardy, sloppy, or refusing to eat, the staff was instructed to ignore these problems. For instance, if patients were late, they simply didn't eat (extinction and punishment). The time previously spent criticizing and cajoling these patients was now available for more praise, encouragement, and support on the ward (positive reinforcement). Within only a few days, the disruptive behavior around mealtime diminished markedly.

Encouraged by this study, the same researchers then designed a more consistent and concrete system of reward and punishment, the *token economy*. Severely impaired, institutionalized patients received a token for responsible behavior (e.g., bathing or making beds), and lost tokens for obstreperous or assaultive behavior. Tokens could be used to buy special treats or privileges (e.g., additional TV time). The token economy not only reinforced or diminished specific kinds of behavior, but it also had a more general effect: The tokens helped repair the social breakdown syndrome which commonly occurs among chronically hospitalized patients who are deprived of social experiences like making and spending money. The success of this technique led to a broader application with other kinds of patients, such as the acutely psychotic, the mentally retarded, the autistic, young adults with anorexia nervosa, and juvenile offenders in community facilities.

In the past few years positive reinforcement has been advocated in the treatment of those who are outpatients and are less severely ill. Instead of the institutional staff arranging the environmental consequences, the therapist and patient collaborate to find an adequate reinforcer and to establish a contract. This contract defines precisely what the reward will be and under what circumstances it will be given. For example, Mrs. T. and her therapist might agree that for every ten minutes she spent alone outside the home, she could spend ten minutes preparing a free-lance article – a source of great satisfaction for her. Under no circumstances could she write unless she had met these conditions. A more complicated *contingency contracting* might include her husband, who would be trained to ignore her anxiety spells entirely but who would consistently offer praise for those periods she spent alone outside the apartment.

When considering the various techniques of positive reinforcement for a given patient, the consultant must determine if it is feasible to arrange the environment so that the rewards or punishments can be provided appropriately and systematically. Operant techniques are difficult to implement in complicated and diverse settings. For example, an acute medical ward has so many different and rotating staff members responding to the varying demands of patients that reinforcers would be hard to apply in a controlled and consistent fashion. Similarly, one could not hope to "arrange" one of Mrs. T.'s dinner parties so that she would receive only positive reinforcement. On the other hand, operant techniques may be successful with a well-integrated and motivated family who can learn to reinforce behavior in a systematic manner.

Some patients are more willing to accept a program of positive reinforcement than others. A sophisticated and intelligent woman like Mrs. T. might view such procedures as mundane and demeaning. The consultant can point out that she has not on her own found better ways of "breaking bad habits" and that sometimes the simplest method is best. In fact, some of the symptomatic improvement may come from reducing a complex and confusing problem into smaller and more comprehensible units. Mrs. T., for instance, might feel less overwhelmed if her pervasive fears and shyness were broken down into more manageable components, like crossing the street, going grocery shopping, walking into a cocktail party, and so forth.

As a general rule, because positive reinforcement requires that the patient be able and willing to do the behavior so that it can be rewarded, these techniques are better suited for situations in which the goal is to diminish maladaptive behavior (such as heavy drinking or nagging) or to increase motivation for a new behavior (such as doing homework). When patients present with paralyzing phobias or with sexual dysfunctions like vaginismus or impotence, they may be too anxious even to attempt the desired task and therefore cannot be positively reinforced. In such cases, systematic desensitization is often a necessary alternative.

Cognitive Therapy

When conditioning theories were first applied to clinical situations, the focus was more on what the patient did and less on what the patient felt or thought. The goal of treatment was for the patient to *act* differently. Of course, therapists recognized that patients changed their feelings and their thinking as they mastered designated tasks. They had a more positive regard for themselves and they had less distorted views about frightening situations, but these intangibles were first considered at best "secondary reinforcers."

Before long, behavior was not so strictly defined to include only "the organism's skeletal muscle activity." The use of relaxation training for systematic desensitization led to an interest in psychophysiological responses — heart rate, blood pressure, hormone changes, and so on. These responses were themselves now viewed as a kind of behavior, and therapists searched for effective techniques to alter these responses when they were maladaptive, i.e., in the etiology of tension headaches, hypertension, asthma, ulcers, colitis, rash, pain, bed-wetting, and even cancer. As a result of this growing interest in psychophysiological "behavior," techniques such as biofeedback, self-relaxation, hypnosis, and transcendental meditation were added to the clinician's therapeutic armamentarium.

In the past few years, behavior has become even more broadly defined and includes not only psychophysiological activities emanating from "the black box," but activities *within* the black box as well. Throughout this century, the "peripheralist" psychologists have been opposed to examining mental processes that must be inferred and that are not easily observed or measurable. Other behaviorists have argued that humans differ from experimental animals precisely because their central cognitive functions have an important influence on their behavior; this school of thought has insisted that "covert behaviors" like thinking cannot be ignored. The impetus for cognitive therapy arose partly out of this school's persuasive argument, but only partly. Cognitive therapy also borrowed heavily from the psychoanalytic belief that changing ideas could alter behavior.

Because cognitive therapy can trace its roots to several different academic traditions, it cannot easily be grouped with only behavioral therapies. We have placed it in this section because the *techniques* of cognitive therapy are predominantly directive, that is, the therapist actively instructs the patient what to "do" and when and how to do it. Though many have contributed to the development of cognitive therapy, we will focus on the work of Aaron Beck (1976) because he has been so influential in popularizing this treatment, refining it, and testing its effectiveness.

Beck documented how cognitions are influenced by the systematic application of directive techniques. Borrowing from the behaviorists' clear description of methods and empirical verification, Beck devised a strategy to modify a neurotically depressed person's mode of thinking. Though psychoanalytically trained, he concluded from his clinical work that patients are depressed not because of some deep unconscious conflict, but because they have acquired—have "learned"—misconceptions about themselves and about the way the world is. This negative view of themselves, of the world, and of the future—the cognitive triad—has inherent internal and external reinforcements that perpetuate the depression: "I'm no good so I can't do this, and the fact that I just failed goes to show you that I'm bad, and the situation is impossible, and the future is hopeless, so what's the sense of trying?"

Since Beck considered neurotic depression to be primarily cognitive in origin, he believed treatment should aim at correcting cognitive distortions rather than exploring their etiological roots. Moreover, he believed that the most efficient method of changing the misconceptions of depressed patients was by using the well-documented directive techniques of the behavioral therapist. He designed a precise blueprint delineating each therapeutic maneuver, including graded task assignments, homework assignments, cognitive rehearsal, cognitive reappraisal, and so on, carefully documenting the effectiveness of each step as well as the overall therapeutic outcome. The results have been quite promising (Rush, Beck, Kovacs, and Hollon, 1977; Rush, Khatami, and Beck, 1975).

There are certain limitations in this approach. Not all depressions are primarily based on cognitive misconceptions. Beck underestimates the impact of psychobiological and social factors; and his assumptions about the etiology of depression run counter to the psychoanalytic contention that neurotic depressions persist because intrapsychic conflicts arise from relatively fixed "structures" in the mind.

Another limitation of cognitive therapy is that depressed patients often refuse to withstand the frontal assault against self-derogating attitudes. They are unable to take an active role in suddenly changing life-long trends of passivity. For example, although Mrs. T. emphasized her panic attacks during the consultation, she also mentioned that she had been feeling "depressed." Is this depression based on a negative cognitive triad, or is it really based on an understandable loss of self-esteem now that she cannot leave the apartment alone? Would she view a cognitive therapist's remarks as confronting and punitive and would she be too frightened even to begin the program? Would she end up feeling a failure and even more depressed because she could not participate in the treatment? These questions would need to be addressed by the consultant before recommending cognitive therapy for Mrs. T.

Some techniques used in cognitive therapy have been an implicit part of the therapeutic armamentarium since the beginning of psychotherapy. Therapists have often confronted patients on the irrationality of their beliefs and have then suggested ways to change, but these tactics have not always been applied in a consistent and systematic way. Psychoanalytically-oriented psychotherapists may have at times not been aware (or at least not acknowledged) that they were actually directing patients to change their attitudes. Beck explicitly describes and legitimizes some of the common components of directive treatments: 1) assuming an authoritative stance; 2) clearly defining the target symptoms; and 3) designing a specific program to be followed in order to change the overt or covert behavior.

Although rational-emotive therapy as developed by Albert Ellis (1962) shares many of the features of cognitive therapy, Ellis places greater faith in change through understanding, whereas Beck emphasizes that activity and a systematic program are necessary. In this sense, the two approaches straddle the border between the "exploratory" and "directive" categories we have suggested. In making a subtle (and perhaps nonexistent) distinction between the two treatments, the consultant might choose rational-emotive therapy for intelligent patients who are autonomous and not severely disturbed and for whom new insights alone will be sufficient for change, whereas cognitive therapy would be recommended for those who will require explicit directions and practicing in order to change.

Problem-solving

Edward Bibring (1937), attempting to define exactly what a psychodynamic psychotherapist could do to effect change in patients, concluded there were five essential therapeutic maneuvers: clarification, interpretation, abreaction, suggestion, and manipulation. Under our system of categorizing therapeutic techniques, clarification and interpretation would primarily be designed to increase understanding and would therefore be exploratory; abreaction would primarily be designed to express feelings in the here and now and would therefore be experiential; and suggestion and manipulation would primarily be designed to alter behavior and therefore would be directive.

By the technique of suggestion, Bibring meant more than the therapist suggesting outright that a patient do this and not do that. He meant that by using a psychodynamic knowledge of human behavior in general and of the patient in particular, the therapist could carefully time and phrase certain statements in such a way that they would imply – and in that way "suggest" – what would or should happen. This maneuver has a covert and magical quality. For example, when an anesthesiologist says to an apprehensive patient preoperatively, "After you awaken from surgery, you'll feel groggy and confused in the Recovery Room," the implicit reassurring *suggestion* is that the patient will in fact awaken from surgery and not die on the operating table. In the same way, a psychotherapist might maneuver and encourage Mrs. T. by saying, "After you return home from grocery shopping alone, you will feel slightly light-headed but relieved and proud of overcoming one of your basic fears." The implied message is that Mrs. T. will arrive home safely and will not have collapsed from a panic episode while feeling entrapped in the store. When used authoritatively in the context of a positive transference, such a suggestion offers an almost magical reassurance and, in addition, might be most effective if Mrs. T. did not fully appreciate how she was being influenced.

By manipulation, Bibring meant that after acquiring a dynamic knowledge of the patient and deciding what would be in the patient's best interests, the therapist could take a particular stance or make a particular statement that would influence – would "manipulate" – the patient. As with suggestion, the patient might not know how he was being influenced at the time. In its most benign and simple form, manipulation is no more complicated than a mother placing a bandaid on a child's cut to "make it all better," or a consultant matching suitable personalities in selecting a therapist for a patient and thereby privately manipulating the therapeutic environment.

But manipulation can be a more subtle, complex, and tricky maneuver and has been criticized for being presumptuous, patronizing, infantilizing, coercive, and abusively authoritative. For example, after several sessions with Mrs. T., the therapist might conclude that Mrs. T. was always afraid of being alone and abandoned but that because of her early marriage and her close relationship with the children, these fears were not so apparent. She developed a symptomatic agoraphobia when her children "left" her and when she feared her husband, on whom she now depended all the more, might also leave for another woman (as he became more successful and she became less attractive). The therapist might also conclude that Mrs. T. unconsciously displaced these fears onto situations where she herself might be found desirable and where she might be tempted to act on her own impulses to be unfaithful (e.g., arriving alone at a dinner party). By avoiding such situations and viewing them as terrifying, she is able to deny her own and her husband's potential extramarital affairs, the possible disruption of their marriage, and the ultimate loss of the one on whom she now so desperately depends.

But, having privately arrived at this dynamic formulation, the therapist might then choose to manipulate Mrs. T. by telling her something quite different. He might say, for instance, that her fears of being alone have developed because of "a second wave of sexual desires" and that her panic episodes are unconsciously intended to make her husband dissatisfied with her and to drive him away so that she will be free to have numerous and varied sexual encounters. This maneuver, based on a dynamic understanding of Mrs. T. and counter to the therapist's actual beliefs, would be specifically designed to reduce the panic episodes. Each time Mrs. T. felt anxious she would think that she was expressing a desire to leave her husband and to act on forbidden sexual wishes (whereas in fact the opposite was the case). Because of this paradoxical maneuver, she would be coerced into stopping the panic to show the therapist and herself that she was not unconsciously trying to leave her husband.

Whether suggestion or manipulation would be effective maneuvers for a patient like Mrs. T. is debatable. The point here is that they represent attempts to alter a patient's behavior by directive or paradoxical methods. For purposes of differential therapeutics, these methods must be distinguished from techniques intended to increase understanding by exploring the underlying reasons for symptoms. They must also be distinguished from those techniques intended to foster an emotional exchange. Both suggestion and manipulation are examples of problem-solving techniques.

Problem-solving techniques are now associated with the writings of Jay Haley (1976) and Milton Erickson (see Haley, 1973b), but they are shared by many different kinds of psychotherapists who have described innovative ways of influencing behavior. In his book *The New Psychotherapies,* Harper (1975) indicated how a list of all the new techniques could become encyclopedic. Frank (1973) has pointed out that many of the so-called contemporary methods for solving problems may not be inventions but rather inheritances from our predecessors. Faith healers, witch doctors, spiritual advisors, and physicians, using their delegated authority, doubtlessly applied skill and wisdom to influence behavior, but without defining or perhaps even themselves realizing what directive techniques they were utilizing.

From the viewpoint of differential therapeutics, this lack of documentation is compounded by the fact that problem-solving techniques did not emerge from any one school of thought, but rather by accumulating knowledge from several different sources (especially systems, crisis, and communications theory, hypnosis, and common sense). One cannot review psychoanalytic or behavioral or existential theory to trace the development of problem-solving techniques. But, as Karasu (1977) has eloquently suggested, one can see how the recent emphasis on problem-solving techniques mirrors important trends in our society – our concerns, values, and conflicts.

Just as the currently accepted zeitgeist helps define what constitutes a problem, it also prescribes preferred methods of solving them. An interest in more directive techniques arose in part out of a disenchantment with individual psychotherapy which was often long, expensive, questionably effective, and unavailable to most who needed help. The interest in directive methods also arose from the 20th century's commitment to new technology and action rather than to history and understanding, and from the concomitant belief that problems could be "outmaneuvered." Also, the interest in problem-solving approaches arose in part from the success of one kind of directive technique, namely, "behavioral therapy."

Because most problem-solving techniques have not been well described or studied and because they arose from so many different philosophical, cultural, and social forces, a special burden is placed on the consultant who must decide if a problem-solving technique would be the preferred method of treatment for a given patient. In actual clinical practice, most consultants in making a referral often select the therapist and not the technique, relying on the judgment of the chosen therapist to determine if, when, and what directive approaches should be used. Deferring the decision to the therapist does not of course resolve the dilemma, but only makes it more isolated and idiosyncratic. Unfortunately, at present we learn about many problem-solving strategies only through faddish or controversial books or from anecdotes passed on among colleagues either informally or during supervision and at professional meetings. These various clever "ploys," though colorful in the telling and dramatic in the reported outcome, are often viewed skeptically by more traditional and conservative therapists. These unique problem-solving strategies need to be more carefully described and scientifically studied.

We are dissatisfied ending this discussion of representative directive techniques on such an ambiguous note. Having begun with an account of how laboratory experiments led to the use of systematic desensitization and having described the more precise methods of positive reinforcement and cognitive therapy, we are reluctant to conclude by mentioning the poorly defined techniques of problem-solving, techniques that are flexibly and privately tailored to the individual and that are at this point supported by the presumed wisdom of the therapist and not by any one theory or controlled study. But even though these directive techniques are not well documented, they encompass some of the most common maneuvers a therapist uses in his day-to-day practice and they must therefore be acknowledged. By analogy, child rearing is not usually based on any one theory or on well-defined methods, yet clearly the child's behavior is influenced by more than exploring reasons or sharing feelings. Advice, limit-setting, persuasion, suggestion, manipulation, discipline, and other direct problem-solving maneuvers are used every day and have a profound, though not easily measurable, effect. The question remains which maneuvers are most effective for which patients and how can they be used most efficiently.

Finally, the rationale for labeling this category of techniques "directive" rather than "behavioral" should now be apparent. The current approaches used by therapists to influence behavior extend beyond the theory and practice of behavioral therapy. Just as psychoanalytic approaches represent only one group of exploratory treatments, behavioral therapies represent only one group of the many directive approaches. We believe that labeling all directive methods as behavioral (as suggested by Karasu and others) is too specific and more confined than current clinical practice would warrant. We believe that directive connotes the range of maneuvers in which the therapist focuses attention on a particular piece of overt or covert behavior and attempts to influence behavior in a particular way.

Let us now examine the advantages and disadvantages of directive techniques for Mrs. T. From the evidence presented, some types of behavioral treatment would appear to be an excellent choice for Mrs. T. Although she has experienced mild characterological difficulties over the years, her most severe problem — agoraphobia with panic episodes — is of recent onset and perceived as ego-dystonic. The well-circumscribed target symptoms should make a precise behavioral analysis feasible. All phobic patients are by definition hesitant about approaching anxiety-laden situations, but Mrs. T. appears more willing than many to confront her problems directly, as evidenced by her continuing in the past to take planes and use elevators despite her fears, and by her willingness to return to the consultant a second time and enter his office alone despite her anxiety attack during the first session. Graded exposure or in vivo flooding would be the treatment of choice if enough trust can be built up for Mrs. T. to confront her anxiety directly. These techniques are the treatment of choice for agoraphobia; systematic desensitization is useful for simple phobias.

Other directive techniques also might be considered for Mrs. T. Regarding positive reinforcement, she has the conscientiousness and discipline to follow whatever contract might be arranged between her and her therapist, and her husband has already shown a concern and willingness to participate in the event that a contingency contract is also deemed helpful. Regarding cognitive therapy, though Mrs. T.'s primary symptom is not depression, a similar approach of cognitive reappraisal and task assignments could be designed. She already appreciates that her ideas are "crazy"; a systematic cognitive approach could reinforce the realization that her fears are irrational. Such a diligent and didactic technique might appeal to her "scholarly" approach to life.

Regarding problem-solving techniques, Mrs. T.'s attitude during the consultation indicated a willingness to delegate authority to another. In the context of this dependent and even magical relationship, she could be influenced explicitly or implicitly by problem-solving maneuvers, such as advice, prodding, encouragement, paradoxical injunction, suggestion, and manipulation.

A major disadvantage of directive techniques is that the chosen method may be too specific and thereby too limited. Whereas the panic episodes might respond to treatment, other underlying difficulties might persist. An opportunity would then be lost to achieve more ambitious goals, such as making Mrs. T. less timid, less dependent, less self-conscious, and less frightened of being assertive. The theoretical notion that a phobic symptom, once removed by directive methods, would be replaced by other symptoms has not been substantiated by clinical practice; however, there is a risk that Mrs. T. will not achieve true autonomy if only directive methods are used. Instead, she will have her dependency on others reinforced: "I could not solve or even understand my problems; I had to have someone else direct and support me." For this very reason, Mrs. T. might herself reject the recommendation for a directive approach, feeling that such techniques would be demeaning and not give her sufficient intellectual control. The consultant would then have to decide whether her refusal was based on objections to the technique itself or whether she would once again be simply avoiding rather than trying to confront anxiety-provoking situations.

EXPERIENTIAL TECHNIQUES

Exploratory, directive, and experiential techniques are always combined to a greater or lesser extent in clinical practice; in theory, however, each approach represents a quite different view of human nature and how to change it. For example, unlike the directive techniques discussed above which developed out of a faith in experimentation and technology, many of the experiential techniques developed as a reaction against that same technology. Instead of seeing man as the potential beneficiary of technical accomplishments, experiential psychotherapists often regard technology and direction as the cause and not the cure of man's ills.

In the opinion of experiential therapists (e.g., Gendlin, 1978; Perls, 1969; Rogers, 1942), we have all been subordinated to mechanistic forces, which in turn have led to our depersonalized and dehumanized existence. In their view, we are living in an age of alienation, meaninglessness, and boredom. Accordingly, any therapy which imposes directive and mechanistic methods only contributes to the basic problem rather than solves it. Indeed, a leading proponent of this view, Carl Rogers (1942), originally called his mode of treatment "non-directive psychotherapy."

Many experiential psychotherapists have not only rejected technology as the basis of psychotherapy, but some have rejected reason as well. Their position, stated most extremely, is that "thinking" has done little to enhance what is truly valuable. They therefore distrust intellectual solutions and place greater emphasis on spontaneous feelings and immediately experiencing events to acquire a sense of personal authenticity.

The importance of expressing feelings is of course not new. Aristotle spoke about the cathartic value of drama; and an important aspect of all psychotherapies through the ages has been to provide a situation for those who are troubled to "get things off their minds." In this sense, shamanistic rituals and Catholic confessionals share common features. Mesner and Janet, and Breuer and Freud (particularly in *Studies in Hysteria*, 1955c) appreciated the therapeutic value of abreacting, i.e., ventilating feelings which had not been given direct and full expression. Abreaction continues to be a recommended therapy for traumatic neuroses, adjustment disorders and delayed grief responses, and is the essential ingredient of funeral rituals that facilitate the mourning process.

Some new schools of experiential psychotherapy advocate more than empathic understanding and abreaction. At their most extreme, these schools view all psychopathology as the result of dampened feelings. Emotional problems are not caused by one's inheritance, constitution, biological inflictions, or developmental trauma; they are caused by not realizing – not actualizing – one's potential. Anxiety is conceptualized as the tension between what one is and what one can become. Those with emotional distress are therefore no different than the rest of us and should not be labeled as sick; they should not be "diagnosed." Indeed, anyone may benefit from a therapeutic experience and, since the goal is to reach a universal consciousness, there are no limits to how much can be accomplished by such an encounter. This spiritual orientation of psychotherapy can be traced to Oriental religions and to Western existential philosophies.

The ideas of the existential philosophers were not confined to theoretical discussion in the parlor armchair or sidewalk cafe. They were specifically and logically applied to therapeutic techniques and, in turn, affected the stance, the maneuvers, and the goals set by existential therapists. Along with rejecting the medical model of classifying psychiatric diseases, the experiential schools reject the authoritative and patronizing stance implicit in the doctor-patient relationship. Patients are clients, not helpless children, and should be treated as equals rather than infantilized. The psychoanalytic position of anonymity, abstinence, and neutrality is rejected as well. The therapeutic relationship should not be obscure, abstract, or asymmetrical, but rather a real encounter between two persons that will change and actualize both of them. The therapist should be genuine, have unconditioned positive regard for the client, and, as opposed to withholding gratification, should provide the support, affection, and praise that would naturally emanate from a personal friendship.

Because many experiential schools have disdain for the past or, at the very least, view it as irrelevant, representative therapists do not dwell on a developmental family and personal history as is characteristic of exploratory methods; nor do they perform a behavioral analysis of trends and habits as is done with many directive treatments. Instead, experiential therapists prefer to approach the client with no preconceived notions based on the there and then, while treasuring the potential worth of the here and now. And since intellect is devalued along with the past, the therapists do not strive to have clients recall their childhoods, verbalize their concerns, or articulate their insights. Therapeutic change is the result of the emotional experience itself; putting that experience into words is not necessary. In order to heighten that experience and to break through and break down defenses, the therapist may use confrontation, sensory motor tasks, encounters, and even physical and emotional exhaustion.

Experiential therapists usually choose to leave the goals of treatment unspecified. Since social and parental pressure to achieve are seen as contributing to unwarranted anxiety, every effort is made to deemphasize achievement such as character change or symptom removal. Instead, the client should only strive to experience the therapeutic encounter as fully as possible. By not struggling but simply allowing it to happen, the client will automatically take another step toward self-awareness, cohesiveness, and actualization.

For purposes of exposition, we have presented the more extreme and contemporary experiential view. In fact, psychoanalysts such as Alexander and French (1946) years ago described the therapeutic value of a "corrective emotional experience," Winnicott (1965) conceived of the therapeutic situation as a "holding environment," and most psychotherapists have realized the healing process of the "real" relationship with patients (Greenson, 1967). The history of man indicates that changes in character usually take place in the context of a real or imagined relationship with another, whether that person be mentor, guru, or some other significant person.

Because experiential therapies are designed to have the client experience feelings in the here and now, the techniques tend to be defined less sharply than the interventions used for either exploratory or directive therapies. Indeed, some proponents of the experiential method would oppose any definition of techniques, feeling a description might be regarded as a rigid rule that would limit the necessary flexibility required to be as open and receptive and unbiased as possible when interacting with a client. Nevertheless, some experiential therapies have been articulated and, as we have done above in discussing exploratory and directive techniques, we will now present some better-known kinds of experiential therapies to illustrate their development, methods, and rationale.

Client-centered Psychotherapy

As originally developed by Carl Rogers (1942) at Ohio State University in the 1940s, the central hypothesis of this treatment is that the person has vast internal resources for change and that these resources can be realized in the process of a nonjudgmental and nondirective relationship. The term "client" rather than "patient" is used to indicate that the process is not based on a medical model, a model that by implication is hierarchal, manipulative, and demeaning.

The techniques of client-centered psychotherapy reflect the belief that the encounter is not designed for "treatment" but for "growth." Therapeutic *maneuvers* are seen as potentially destructive; instead, the emphasis is on therapeutic *attitudes* – empathic understanding, unlimited positive regard, and genuineness. These attitudes establish the proper climate and nurturance for growth.

With Mrs. T., for example, the client-centered psychotherapist would first convey an unqualified acceptance despite her incapacitating fears, her reluctance to seek treatment, and her shy demeanor. This external acceptance would make Mrs. T. more willing to appreciate that her irrational fears must have an internal source. She would then spontaneously pursue this internal source by relating memories and fears and previously unspeakable fantasies. Through this process, she would begin to assume more responsibility for her difficulties – responsibility for both their cause and their solution. No longer would she simply blame the past for causing her fears, nor would she depend on her husband rather than on herself as a source of support. The next stage of therapy is seen as crucial: Mrs. T. would recognize a disparity between the actual self she experienced in the therapeutic relationship and the frightened and shy self she had experienced throughout her life. The realization of this disparity with its emotive and psychophysiological concomitants would catalyze a process of growth. Mrs. T. would have shaken and then discarded the former structured view of herself and, ideally, would be less constricted by internal threats in other relationships and in the way she evaluated herself. Unlike many other experiential approaches, client-centered psychotherapy has attempted to trace its theoretical roots, to describe its specific methods, to delineate the stages of change, and to document its results through outcome research.

Gestalt Therapy

As developed by F. S. Perls (Perls, Hefferline, and Goodman, 1951), in New York in the early 1950s, this approach is based on the theory that the best adaptation requires a full awareness of physiological and psychological needs. Maladaptive behavior will inevitably arise when those needs are kept out of awareness, i.e., when they are repressed by the forces of society. Treatment thereby attempts to bring the various parts of oneself into total awareness. This holistic view – the Gestalt – will give meaning to one's different ideas and feelings and experiences.

The techniques are designed to overcome those barriers that prevent an individual from being totally aware of his or her needs. Both psychological and sensory motor exercises are used. With Mrs. T., for example, the Gestalt therapist might actively confront her sexual inhibitions by requesting that she describe in dramatic detail what it would be like for her to go to a dinner party alone in a low-cut dress and seduce an attractive, available man. Or, to break through her intellectualization and shy demeanor, the therapist might prescribe a series of "exercises" in which Mrs. T. would be asked to convey by facial expressions and bodily gestures, but not words, what she was feeling – in particular, her feelings of wanting to be loved and her fears of being abandoned. The aim of these techniques would be to make Mrs. T. less inclined to displace these repressed yearnings and concerns. Her irrational fears would thereby be resolved.

The results of Gestalt therapy, though quite vivid and impressive when related at workshops, have not yet been systematically studied.

Psychodrama

As developed by Jacob Moreno (1946) first in Vienna in the 1920s and later in New York, this approach attempts to provide greater self-awareness by having the patient actually enact those situations where conflicts are likely to arise. The role-playing is designed to have the individual experience the problem; the goal is for the individual to understand the problem as well. Interpretations are used for this purpose. In this sense, psychodrama is also related to the exploratory approaches.

The techniques derive from impromptu theater. Mrs. T., for example, might be instructed to enact – rather than just imagine – an evening at a dinner party. Another patient might play the role of Mrs. T.'s auxiliary ego and comment "off stage" what Mrs. T. might self-consciously be thinking in such a situation: "Stop flirting . . . you better go home to your husband . . . your slip is showing . . . that man wants to use you. . . ." Meanwhile, the director (the therapist) might set the scene with other "actors" to elicit the patient's worst fears and thereby make them more accessible to consciousness and understanding.

Like other approaches that are most easily categorized as experiential – such as est, radical therapy, the human potential movement, existential psychotherapy, sensitivity training, and encounter groups – psychodrama emphasizes emotional experience as the therapeutic mode, but this method certainly uses exploratory and directive techniques as well.

As we have tried to stress throughout this chapter, this overlap of techniques is inevitable. Therefore, the consultant cannot be expected to choose one category of techniques to the exclusion of all others, but rather to determine whether understanding, behavior, or emotional involvement will be the *primary* focus. In this regard, let us now consider whether an emotional experience in the context of a facilitative therapeutic relationship should be the main emphasis of treatment for Mrs. T.

Experiential techniques might break through Mrs. T.'s intellectualization and reserve. During the process of expressing her dependent fears and desires, she could establish with the therapist the kind of empathic and intimate relationship she has sought throughout her life. This primal bond with another, unavailable in her youth and unobtainable in her marriage, could then be internalized and could give her the reassurance to overcome not only her agoraphobia, but also her fears of being alone and of being more open. During the consultation she has shown the potential, perhaps even the craving, to construct such a close and trusting relationship. By her occasional free-lance writing, she has also shown the drive to be more creative in her own right and less dependent on the needs and demands of others. In addition, she does not have the fragile character structure which would contraindicate a confrontational approach and the emergence of intense feelings.

A major disadvantage of an experiential approach would be the possibility that as a close relationship was gradually evolving between Mrs. T. and her therapist, the panic episodes and avoidance patterns would continue and consolidate, making them even more refractory to treatment. Mrs. T.'s professional and marital life would no doubt be strained and suffer while the agoraphobic symptoms continued. Another possible disadvantage is that Mrs. T. would keep the intimate sharing with the therapist confined to the sessions and not take the risk of applying such openness to others in the real world. The distance between her and her husband and children might widen rather than diminish if she constantly compared the closeness during treatment with the formal reserve of her other relationships. Experiential treatment would then become only an isolated event in her life with no relevance to her fears, her professional ambitions, or her significant relationships. Experiential treatment would become merely "an experience."

The consultant appreciated that many of the alternative techniques might be helpful for Mrs. T. After some deliberation, he chose a program of graded in vivo exposure. He based the decision on the well-documented effectiveness of this approach for agoraphobia, on the apparent eagerness of Mrs. T. to master her fears strategically, and on the monosymptomatic nature of her problems with the lack of serious premorbid difficulties. Mrs. T., having herself read extensively about behavioral procedures, agreed with the decision and left the third consultative session graciously and gratefully.

Since Mrs. T. could afford the very best, she was referred to a leading expert in behavioral therapy. During the first hour she found the behavioral therapist crass and abrasive, resented his cold manner, and before a behavioral analysis could even begin, she stormed out of the office (and into her husband's awaiting arms). She waited two weeks, then called the consultant, explained what had happened, and asked for another referral. Although the behavioral therapist in question was not generally viewed as brusque or paternalistic in the way Mrs. T. described, the consultant complied with her request and selected a kindly older female therapist who was also experienced in behavioral procedures. Again Mrs. T. was dissatisfied. This time the problem was just the opposite; the female therapist seemed too "wishy-washy" without any confidence or style.

Rather than discuss the matter over the phone, the consultant made another appointment for Mrs. T. She again arrived with her husband, but this time wore a low-cut provocative dress which she claimed parenthetically to have just thrown on in a rush. After only a few minutes into the session, the consultant realized that a source of Mrs. T.'s resistance regarding the referrals was an erotic dependent attachment to himself. When he asked Mrs. T. directly about this, she became flushed, anxious, and defensive, but then finally confessed that although nothing sexual had entered her mind, she had not stopped thinking about the consultant since they parted and wondered if, now that the consultation was over, they could become friends. The consultant replied that since Mrs. T. did not even know what he was like outside the office, her wish for an involvement must be based more on fantasy than fact. He added that the severity of her current symptoms must take precedence over exploring such fantasies, which might even delay addressing her immediate symptoms. The longer the symptoms persisted, the more intractable they might become. Mrs. T. again accepted the consultant's remarks graciously and decided to return to the first referral.

The second time around, the therapy proceeded splendidly. During graded in vivo exposure, Mrs. T. attacked each step of the hierarchy vigorously. After ten sessions she was able to take a taxi to a movie alone at night and sit in the middle of the row (as opposed to an aisle seat for a quick escape). Flooding techniques were then introduced and after 20 sessions and three months, Mrs. T. felt "free as a bird" and, as the ultimate achievement, flew to Switzerland alone to enjoy a spring vacation with her son at a ski resort.

The consultant learned about this outcome from the behavioral therapist at a professional meeting. Along with describing the treatment, he mentioned good-humoredly that in spite of several billings, Mrs. T. had never paid for her last session. Since she clearly had the money, he wondered why.

Two years to the day after the initial consultation, Mrs. T. again called for an appointment. She was planning on leaving her husband

and wanted to discuss the matter before making a final decision. She arrived for the appointment alone and looking as glamorous as ever, though with a touch more makeup. Mrs. T. succinctly and matter-of-factly outlined her life since behavioral therapy ended: The panic episodes had not returned and no other symptoms had taken their place. The recurrent nightmares of being chased or lost seemed possibly more frequent or at least more noticeable, but not overwhelmingly troubling. During the spring ski vacation with her son she had met a friendly widower and had had her first extramarital affair, which was "awkward but enjoyable." No longer afraid of flying, she had started taking business trips on her own and had fallen in love with a divorced college professor, who was her husband's age but more of a family man. She felt more comfortable with him than she could ever remember and pictured a life of corduroy coats, Dunhill pipes, Gothic arches, scholarly pursuits, and stability. She then laughingly asked for the consultant's "permission."

The consultant replied that he was pleased that Mrs. T. now felt more free, but added that her request for consultation reflected some doubt about her decision. Since many of the consequences could be irreversible, he suggested that Mrs. T. explore the matter before making any definite decision. He also mentioned that in view of her early childhood Mrs. T. might consider that her wish for stability was based more on the past than on the future.

Mrs. T. was referred to a reputable and renowned psychoanalyst and after an extended evaluation of several sessions, she began a traditional psychoanalysis. That was four years ago. From another source the consultant learned that Mrs. T. is still married and in analysis. There is no further information.

REVIEW OF OUTCOME RESEARCH REGARDING THERAPEUTIC TECHNIQUE

Clinical research would support the consultant's choice of behavioral therapy for Mrs. T.'s panic attacks and agoraphobia. Many studies have shown that behavioral techniques are effective for the treatment of phobic symptoms, but the advantage of behavioral methods over other techniques has not yet been well documented. In the mid-1960s, when behavioral techniques were being greeted enthusiastically, Gelder and Marks (1966) compared them with conventional psychotherapy. As is too often the case their studies did not precisely define the nature of the "conventional psychotherapy," but it probably involved some mixture of exploratory, experiential, and nonbehavioral directive techniques. Gelder and Marks (1966) found no statistically significant difference between behavioral therapy and psychotherapy for phobic patients. In a later report (Gelder, Marks, Wolff, and Clarke, 1967), they found a slight difference favoring behavioral treatment, but in a two-year follow-up this slight difference was no longer apparent.

In contrast to these studies by Marks and Gelder, three reports have shown a more decided advantage of behavioral techniques for patients like Mrs. T. In 1961, Lazarus used desensitization methods for groups of agoraphobic and claustrophobic patients and found this technique superior to nonbehavioral group therapy. Studies favoring behavioral techniques were then supported by the work of Gillan and Rachman (1974) who found that for multiphobic outpatients, desensitization was better than either relaxation training or psychotherapy immediately after treatment and at three-month follow-up.

Luborsky et al. (1975), as well as Kazdin and Wilson (1978), have reviewed in detail the research comparing behavioral techniques with other methods. The consultant should keep in mind an implicit conclusion from these two more extensive reviews: Despite many myths to the contrary, the documented advantage of behavioral techniques for phobic patients has not been impressive. The number of comparative studies is few and the design of the studies is often poor (for example, not defining more precisely the alternative "psychotherapy"). Although the consultant can honestly reassure patients like Mrs. T. that psychiatric treatment has a good chance of helping relieve her symptoms, the consultant cannot state with the same scientific support that a particular approach will remove the symptoms faster or will last longer or will be more beneficial to areas other than the phobia itself. These issues have not yet been sufficiently examined.

Once the consultant chooses a behavioral approach, the next problem is to decide *which* behavioral technique will be most effective: desensitization in fantasy? desensitization in vivo? flooding? graded exposure with the therapist present? graded exposure without the therapist? or, as with Mrs. T., some combination of these different techniques? Marks (1978) critically reviewed studies of various behavioral approaches and concluded that those methods which directly exposed patients to the feared stimuli were most effective. In another review of the behavioral research literature, Linden (1981) set up a "box score" for the different techniques and also found that in vivo techniques were slightly preferred. Of the four reviewed research studies, two favored in vivo exposure and two were tied.

Because of some methodological problems, no study comparing exposure in fantasy with exposure in vivo can be considered definitive.

For example, Emmelkamp and Wessels (1975) arranged three types of behavioral treatment and found that graded exposure in vivo was better than either flooding in fantasy or flooding in fantasy followed by graded exposure. But the study did not provide *graded* exposure in fantasy nor did it consider that some phobic patients simply will not confront the actual frightening situation until some desensitization in fantasy has occurred. The prognosis might be better for any patients willing from the start to meet the dreaded situation in real life. In another comparative study, Mathews and his associates (1976) treated 36 agoraphobic women like Mrs. T. with one of three treatments: exposure in vivo, exposure in fantasy for eight sessions followed by exposure in vivo for eight sessions, and exposure in fantasy followed during the same session by exposure in vivo. Although no significant differences were found among the three groups, the results are suspect because *all* patients were strongly urged to practice in vivo exposure between sessions. Perhaps the favorable outcome for the three groups was primarily a result of this self-exposure *between* sessions and the different techniques *during* sessions were far less important.

Regarding the selection of a behavioral treatment for Mrs. T., we can so far conclude that outcome studies do indicate that behavioral techniques are effective for her kind of phobic symptoms, but that behavioral methods have not proven clearly superior to other techniques and that in vivo graded exposure holds only a slight edge over other behavioral procedures. The question then arises whether any particular kind of in vivo exposure is most effective. Two studies (Emmelkamp and Wessels, 1975; Mathews, Johnston, Lancashire, Munby, Shawn, and Gelder, 1976) compared a gradual approach to the feared stimuli (graded exposure) to a maximal exposure from the start (flooding) and found the methods to be equally effective. Whether the therapist should or should not be present during the in vivo exposure is also undecided. The same study by Emmelkamp and Wessels found that results were better if a patient like Mrs. T. took control of her exposure, but again such patients willing to take charge on their own may be inclined to do better no matter what technique is used.

We will defer a discussion about the concomitant use of psychopharmacotherapy until Chapter 6 when we will consider in more detail the complex issues concerning combined treatments. But, having already discussed in Chapter 2 the selection of the therapeutic format, we should point out that some behavioral therapists have studied whether group or individual exposure is more effective. Hafner and Marks (1976) exposed groups of four to seven patients to the frightening stimuli four different times during a two-week period and compared the results with patients who had been exposed for a similar length of time but in the presence of a therapist rather than a group. After six months, both sets of patients maintained improvement. The results were not quite as favorable for the individually treated patients, but only on measures of nonphobic areas. Other similar studies (Hand, Lamontagne, and Marks, 1974; Teasdale, Walsh, Lancashire, and Mathews, 1977; Watson, Mullett, and Pillay, 1973) also suggest that in vivo group treatment is at least as effective as in vivo individual treatment — and obviously less expensive.

Among the few studies which have attempted to compare different techniques, the best designed was conducted by Sloane, Staples, Cristol, Yorkston, and Whipple (1975). Patients at a university outpatient clinic who had either personality disorders or psychoneuroses were assigned to either a behavioral (directive) or psychodynamically-oriented (exploratory) therapist, or they were placed on a waiting list as a nontreatment control group. The three groups of patients were comparable in terms of age, sex, and severity of illness, and the therapists were comparable in terms of extensive experience in their respective traditions. Furthermore, random samples of actual treatment sessions were used to see if the experts did indeed use the techniques they represented. Patients were assessed by independent evaluators before and after treatment in terms of target symptoms as well as occupational and social adjustment.

Immediately following the termination of treatment (after an average of 14 sessions) or at the end of a trial no-treatment period, all three groups had improved significantly in that their target symptoms were less severe, but both of the treated groups had improved more than the waiting list control group. There was no significant difference in improvement between the group treated with behavioral as opposed to dynamic techniques; and there was no significant difference in improvement among the three groups regarding work or social adjustment. At follow-up after one year, both treatment groups had maintained or continued improvement and the control group had caught up sufficiently so that no significant difference among the three groups was now apparent. These follow-up reports, however, are more contaminated than the original assessments because many patients had other therapeutic experiences during the intervening year.

Although Sloane's study can be praised for its careful design and controls in terms of selecting a technique for patients like Mrs. T., his work unfortunately did not measure the more subtle aspects of treatment and outcome. In Mrs. T.'s case, for example, when she returns two years later, the consultant is far less concerned about whether Mrs. T. will continue to work and far more concerned about whether she will find an adaptive way of dealing with her unrequited dependency needs. Sloane's study, which deals with more measurable and immediate issues and with the response to a relatively brief treatment, does not directly deal with these more inferential, intrapsychic aspects. In addition, the "dynamic therapies" were once again not clearly defined in terms of technique and included a blurring of exploratory, experiential, and nonbehavioral directive maneuvers under the label of "interpretive statements."

The work of David Malan (1976) is an illustrative contrast to that of Sloane. Malan's study wrestles with the subtleties and ambiguities which Sloane chooses to ignore but it suffers from design problems. For example, the study tries to distinguish between symptomatic and characterological change, and they emphasize the differences between various kinds of nonbehavioral techniques. Malan's outcome measures are idiosyncratic and his statistical methods are suspect in ways that will be discussed in more detail in Chapter 8. Nonetheless, the results are interesting. Positive outcome at the end of a relatively brief treatment held up for many years and was related primarily to motivation for change and to the ability of the patient and therapist to engage in an uncovering inquiry with a focus on transference and early parental relationships. Though Malan's studies lack the scientific crispness presented by Sloane, they represent a good first try at examining whether character change can be used as an outcome measurement and whether psychoanalytic techniques (used during Mrs. T.'s second phase of treatment) can be correlated with therapeutic results. Whatever the final answer will be, Malan can be credited for defining some of the issues for future investigation and debate.

Many other studies have been performed comparing techniques for patients who are like Mrs. T. Luborsky et al. (1975) summarized this comparative research and found that *in general* "behavioral" were superior to "verbal" techniques in six studies and not significantly different in 12 others. He concluded that behavior and verbal therapies were more or less equivalent in their results, with a slight tilt toward behavioral techniques for circumscribed phobias and toward verbal techniques for psychosomatic symptoms. In a similar kind of general review, Kazdin and Wilson (1978) found behavior therapy more effective overall and specifically in the treatment of neurotic depression, addictive behaviors, and institutional management of psychotic disorders.

An innovative general comparison has also recently been completed by Smith et al. (1980). Using a procedure called meta-analysis, they have compared over 400 outcome studies. We will review this ambitious work in more detail in Chapter 8 on research methodology; for now we will only summarize their conclusions regarding therapeutic technique. They found the most effective techniques to be (in declining order): cognitive, hypnotherapy, cognitive behavioral, systematic desensitization, dynamic eclectic, and eclectic behavioral. They found the moderately effective techniques to be (again in declining order): psychodynamic, Adlerian, client-centered, and Gestalt. Some of their results were quite surprising and do not match with intuition; for example, they found psychodynamic techniques were most effective for psychotic patients. They also found that when variables such as patients' age, sex, severity of illness, and diagnosis were controlled, no significant differences between dynamic, behavioral and experiential treatments could be found. They conclude that even with an extremely large available data base, there is insufficient information to answer the question of which technique is best for which patient. Clinical wisdom must still prevail.

The only study comparing different kinds of exploratory techniques was conducted at the Menninger Clinic and reported in the early 1970s by Kernberg and his associates (1972). The 42 studied inpatients and outpatients were as a group more severely disturbed than Mrs. T., but like her, they were involved in a long-term exploratory process conducted by an experienced therapist. One group of patients had undergone psychoanalysis and the other group was placed in a psychoanalytically-oriented psychotherapy. The average psychoanalytic treatment was longer (835 sessions) than the psychoanalytically-oriented (289 sessions) one. Each patient was assessed before and after treatment in terms of work status and social function as well as given a score on the health/sickness rating scale.

The global rating showed that both groups improved with no measurable difference between the two types of exploratory treatments. More specifically, patients like Mrs. T. who possessed high ego strength and sustained interpersonal relationships did better than average in both treatments, but the psychoanalytic approach with the focus on the transference material was even more productive. On the other hand, patients who, unlike Mrs. T., had low ego strength improved more when the treatment was supportive/expressive (directive/experiential) with a structuring of the current life situation and a focus on the here-and-now therapeutic relationship. Appropriately enough, patients assigned to therapists with the highest skills and experience (like Mrs. T.'s psychoanalyst) did better in both treatments, but, interestingly, the lesser skilled therapists did better with psychoanalysis than with the supportive psychotherapies. This suggests that supportive psychotherapies are more difficult to do and require more experience.

This study at the Menninger Clinic has been criticized for its naturalistic approach, for its unusual statistical procedures, for its small number of patients and large number of hypotheses, for its absence of a control group, and for rating the therapist's skills by those who knew the therapist and knew the therapeutic outcome (Malan, 1973; May, 1973; McNair, 1976). Nevertheless, even the harshest critics have applauded the attempt to study the results of different long-term exploratory treatments on a heterogeneous group of patients. The Menninger project stands in contrast to the majority of studies which typically test a very brief psychotherapy with relatively healthy patients or even normal college students with minor complaints.

SUMMARY

What can we conclude? Certainly no study (or even the review of many studies) indicates the absolute choice or clear superiority of any one technique. Each study reminds us that the quality of change must be distinguished from the quantity of change: If Mrs. T. had been placed in a study of behavioral therapy, she would be considered dramatically improved, but the factors being measured (such as taking an elevator without anxiety) might be much less important to her than the more subtle and less easily measured changes in self-esteem that might only accrue from experiential or exploratory techniques (Heine, 1953; Klerman, Dimascio, and Weissman, 1974). Rather than feeling discouraged and jaded, we can leave this discussion of therapeutic technique and Mrs. T. with an appreciation of just how unique each clinical situation may be and how complex choices must be tailored to the individual.

CHAPTER 4

The Duration and Frequency

In preceding chapters, we have suggested ways in which the consultant can receive some guidance through the complex decisions about therapeutic setting, format, and technique by focusing on particular variables: that is, when selecting a setting, the consultant focuses on the *goals* of treatment; when selecting a format, the consultant determines what *system* is most amenable to intervention and change; and when selecting a technique, the consultant considers whether the process of treatment should primarily be directed at influencing *behavior, thoughts, conflicts, emotion, or the social system.*

The decision regarding how long a patient should be in treatment (duration) and how often a patient should be seen within a given period of time (frequency) is influenced by so many different factors that no one variable can be used as a focus. The patient's diagnosis, motivation, expectations, and financial and environmental situation, as well as the therapeutic goals, setting, format, and technique, will all affect how long a patient should be treated and how often (Table 4.1).

In addition, the decision regarding duration and frequency is more subject to change than other decisions the consultant must make. Although the setting, format, and technique may be and often are altered as treatment evolves, the issue of duration and frequency is even less fixed, more fluid. In the course of most treatments, therapist and patient will inevitably reconsider how much longer treatment should and will last.

Because the selection of duration and frequency is codetermined by so many interacting variables and because the issue regarding length of treatment resurfaces at various points of any therapy, we are going to depart somewhat from the structure of previous chapters. Rather than present a case and then discuss the issues involved, we will inter-

TABLE 4-1

Relationship of Co-variables to Duration of Treatment

Co-variable	Factors Affecting Length of Treatment	
	Factors Increasing Duration	Factors Decreasing Duration
Diagnosis	Chronic disorder (e.g., schizophrenia, personality disorder)	Acute disorder (e.g., adjustment reaction)
Premorbid Functioning	Poor	Good
Treatment Goals	Ambitious (e.g., comprehensive character reconstruction)	Limited (e.g., relief of acute symptom, or focused conflict)
Motivation	Wants enduring relationship	Wants brief contact
Patient's Expectations	Takes a long time to change	Brief contact will accomplish the job
Therapist's Expectations	Multiple targets of change	A few focal areas of change
Acute Precipitating Stress	Less likely present	More likely present
Availability of Resources (e.g., patient time and money; clinician availability)	Extensive	Relatively limited
Geography	Easily accessible therapist	Inaccessible treatment
Life Cycle	25–50 years old	Children, adolescents and elderly
Technique	Exploratory (e.g., psychoanalysis)	Directive (e.g., educative consultation)
Setting	Maintenance (e.g., chronic state hospital)	Reparative (e.g., crisis intervention program)
Format	Heterogeneous group, psychoanalysis	Family and marital therapy, behavior therapy

weave a case presentation with a discussion of how the decisions regarding duration and frequency were made first at the beginning of treatment and then at other crucial phases along the way. After this longitudinal case presentation, we will review the available research regarding duration and frequency to see whether scientific studies support the decisions made in this particular situation.

THE CASE OF THE BRUSQUE BUSINESSMAN

When Mr. H. phones for an appointment, he is terse and to the point. He arranges a date and time, then hangs up without even a goodbye.

The first session begins in the same brusque manner. Mr. H. is a successful management consultant in his mid-forties, a short and burly no-nonsense sort of fellow who has come only at his wife's urging. He is driving her crazy because of his constant fretting over a "business divorce" ending a partnership of almost 20 years. As the date of the dissolution of the firm approaches, his resentment toward his partner has increased despite reassuring statements from both Mr. H.'s lawyer and his accountant that the terms are quite equitable, perhaps even advantageous. Mr. H. and his partner are now barely speaking to one another, though Mr. H. has endless bitter conversations in his mind or with his wife about who did what to whom and when and why and on and on into the night.

After 15 minutes of patiently listening to Mr. H.'s spiteful and barbed account of events, the consultant interrupts to suggest that in addition to this resentment toward the partner, Mr. H. might also be feeling some sadness about the breakup. Mr. H. accepts this remark without challenge. Somewhat shamefacedly, he acknowledges that he has indeed been feeling down in the dumps. Particularly at night, when unable to sleep, he stares into the darkness and becomes fearful that he will not succeed on his own. He feels especially shattered because all six of the firm's employees chose to join the partner rather than stay with Mr. H. One after another, each privately told Mr. H. that the partner was easier to work for because he was less demanding and critical. Worried that he will also lose his old clients and never be able to attract new ones, Mr. H. for the first time in his life begins to question his abilities. He is so unsure of himself that he has trouble getting out of bed and dragging himself to the office. He wants help fast — some advice about how to manage his affairs. Without it, he is convinced that he faces professional and personal disaster that would leave him with no reason to live.

The consultant responds by stating the obvious: that Mr. H. has a depression characterized by insomnia, agitation, ruminations, lowered self-esteem, suicidal ideas, and feelings of helplessness and hopelessness. Mr. H. willingly accepts the consultant's remarks but then replies, "Okay, if that's what I've got, what do I do tomorrow that I didn't do today?" When asked to elaborate on his expectations of treatment, Mr. H. makes clear that he was expecting to tell the doctor the problem and be told what to do about it, much in the way he himself advises corporations in trouble. The consultant chooses to pursue this analogy for his own purposes and states that, given the complexities of the problem, an "extended consultation of several sessions" will be required to place the current difficulties in perspective and suggest management decisions including the possible necessity of medication.

As the first session comes to a close, Mr. H. expresses his irritation over not being able to solve the problems more quickly, but he correctly observes that his chronic impatience is the very thing for which he has been so criticized in the past. The consultant spends the remaining few minutes making sure that no serious and imminent problems have been ignored, such as Mr. H.'s suicidal potential or tendencies to act impulsively in some other destructive way. An appointment is then arranged for the following week.

The first encounter with Mr. H. has already raised important issues regarding duration and frequency of treatment, namely, the length of individual sessions, the spacing of appointments, and the ambiguous, open-ended arrangement for an "extended consultation of several sessions" rather than a fixed treatment plan. We will consider each of these issues now before proceeding further with the case of Mr. H.

Mr. H.'s first session lasted just short of an hour. The consultant had purposely scheduled Mr. H. at the end of the day so that the length of the first appointment could be extended depending on what the new and unfamiliar situation required, and also so that time would not be "lost" if the patient canceled at the last moment (as not infrequently happens in such situations). As it turned out, a lengthy initial evaluation did not appear indicated and the conventional 50-minute session felt about right. The reasoning and research supporting this conventional "hour" are not very convincing. For logistical and personal reasons, Freud saw his analytic patients on the hour with very little time for a breather and note-taking in between appointments (Jones, 1953). Even those whose practice is not psychoanalytic have been influenced by this precedent. Primarily for convenience and financial reasons, many therapists have shortened the session to 45 or 50 minutes and see patients "back to back" with no time in between. The application of psychotherapy in clinical and general hospital settings has encouraged a more flexible approach toward session duration. Castelnuovo-Tedesco (1965) has suggested the value of the "20-minute hour" in conducting supportive psychotherapy. For many patients and situations, the standard hour may be far too long for comfort and anything but cost-effective.

Proponents of crisis intervention have stressed the need to tailor the length of sessions to fit the individual's requirements at the time. Some authors have suggested "marathon" sessions to wear down defenses and defensiveness on the unproven assumption that months or even years of treatment can be compressed into a relatively short period of time. At present, the most effective and efficient length for an individual session is not known and until studied systematically, the consultant must rely on convention, clinical judgment, financial factors, personal style, characteristics of the patient, and type of treatment to determine the length of an individual session.

In regard to Mr. H., the consultant believed that a 50-minute session for both the consultative and therapeutic phases of treatment presented a sufficient time for current problems to be explored and related to the patient's past and to his relationship with the therapist. He also believed that a shorter time would have only increased Mr. H.'s tendency to be abrupt and frenetic rather than thoughtful and reflective, that more prolonged sessions would have produced more material than could be assimilated profitably, and that the consultant-therapist's concentration and responsiveness would have diminished significantly if the sessions were extended, increasing the risk of countertransference mistakes. Even taking into account these various factors, the consultant was well aware that the decision about the length of sessions was determined more by tradition, intuition, and convenience than by well-substantiated evidence.

Along with determining the length of an individual session, the consultant had to decide how far apart the sessions should be. Patients often erroneously assume that the frequency of appointments is a direct reflection upon the seriousness of their problem, whereas in fact the frequency is more often related to the kind of treatment and therapist preference rather than to the severity of the psychopathology. A patient with a relatively mild character problem may be seen five times a week in psychoanalysis, whereas a marginally functioning patient with schizophrenia may be seen only once every other month for adjustment of psychotropic medication. In Mr. H.'s case, the consultant believed that by scheduling the next appointment for the same time the following week, he was not just taking advantage of a mutually convenient time, but also implicitly giving a message to Mr. H. that a substantial interval between sessions for contemplation might be helpful and that despite

Mr. H.'s exaggerated fears and impetuous nature, nothing disastrous was likely to happen if the depression was not relieved at once. We will return to this important issue concerning the frequency of sessions when we discuss the kind of treatment which was chosen for Mr. H. at the end of the consultative period.

In addition to the decisions about length of sessions and frequency of visits, the first appointment with Mr. H. also introduced another issue regarding time: At what point in the consultation is a decision to be made about the type, frequency, and duration of treatment? Many, perhaps most, patients assume that treatment begins the moment they walk through the door. Consequently, they may feel disappointed and devalue the encounter if the expected therapeutic interventions are not offered promptly at the end of the first consultative session and instead "nothing happens," whereas from the consultant's point of view, the problem was being carefully evaluated and something substantial was indeed happening. Of course, every interview with a patient has the potential for being therapeutic, but it is often wise to separate clearly the consultation process from the beginning of treatment. On occasion the type of treatment – setting, format, technique, frequency, etc. – can be decided after only one or two visits, such as when a despondent patient will be treated individually as an outpatient with antidepressants. More often, some time is required to assess all the factors that must be considered in choosing a treatment, as was the case with Mr. H. In his case, the consultant separated the consultative process from the treatment per se by stating, "After meeting a few times to evaluate your problems, we can discuss if treatment is necessary and, if so, what kind of treatment is advisable and with whom." This comment also leaves open the possibility that the consultant might not be the person who will be administering the treatment for whatever reason – financial, logistical, limited expertise in the chosen method, or some incompatibility between patient and consultant that would make a therapeutic alliance difficult to form for either of them. (In Chapter 9, we will discuss in more detail the consultative interview for determining the best treatment, and in Chapter 7, we will discuss those situations where no treatment is the best recommendation.)

Mr. H. arrives for the second session appearing just as impatient as when he left the week before. The anguish over his dissolving business and professional future has not abated; he found the first visit to be "unprofitable," and he would now like one of those new nerve pills he's been reading so much about. In the absence of more severe depression, endogenous features, or suicidal risk, the consultant suggests postponing this decision about medication until "the current problems can be placed in some perspective." Mr. H. responds to the consultant's cautious and reflective manner by volunteering that he likes the way the doctor has a mind of his own; then he laughingly yet genuinely adds that he was relieved when he was not "locked up" after the first visit but simply given another appointment for the following week ("I told my wife I must not be *that* crazy").

When asked what else stood out in his mind after the first session, Mr. H. replies that he thought about how the resentment toward his partner was indeed covering over a sadness about losing his fellow employees who were "as close to friends as I ever had." Prompted by only a few open-ended questions, Mr. H. then goes on to depict his lonely and bitter life. He was raised in a somber Catholic home. His father was an aloof and sullen man, who dominated the family from afar with the threat of explosive tantrums and harsh criticism. Mr. H.'s mother assumed a martyred stance, seeking solace with daily retreats to the church for prayers. She encouraged her son to work hard so that he could find rewards not in this world, but in the next.

To his own dismay, Mr. H. "inherited the worst of both" — the oppressed and pessimistic attitude of his mother and the critical and irritable outbursts of his father. With his chin on his chest and the weight of the world on his shoulders, Mr. H. plowed head down through his schooling, using "discipline, drive, and determination" to keep him on the road to success. Fun and friends were not part of his life. Small talk was a waste of time and more intimate conversations made him uncomfortable. Hobbies and sports — woodworking, coin collecting, golf, bridge — were seen as tasks that had to be perfected; ultimately, each was discarded for being either too frustrating or too trivial. In recent years, leisure time had become an intolerable idea, to the point where Mr. H. would plan to have a business journal or his briefcase with him at all times. He would intentionally avoid taking a window seat on the commuter train home so that he would not be tempted to waste potentially valuable time by enjoying the scenery: "I was put in this world to work."

Partly as a result of his unwavering determination and his willingness to confront corporate executives frankly, if not tactfully, he has become an immensely successful corporate consultant: "Most of the smoothies in the big board rooms are all grease but no moving parts. I work to make business work. Simple as that." His wife is a fragile though kind woman whom he suspects married him for security and not love; and, as for his two teenage daughters, he considers them a "distraction." When they were young, he was able to experience love for them only when they were asleep or away at camp, and he now looks forward to the day when they will be off to college. He realizes that he is acting like his father did, but when they are around he simply feels "numb."

Mr. H. leaves the second session without impetuously demanding that the consultant "do something," and he begins the next session where he left off, continuing to describe an oppressed and oppressive existence characterized by the ruthless demands he places on himself and others. His life would probably have been totally unbearable to himself and those around him were it not for his richly evocative, scathingly sarcastic, but ultimately delightful wit, which he sprinkles engagingly throughout his converation as he devalues himself and others (for example, he refers to himself at one point as "a chronic postnatal drip").

Midway through this third session, after a particularly poignant account of being ten years old and locked out of the home by his father, Mr. H. abruptly interrupts the evolving closeness with the consultant, dismisses the moving story as "irrelevant," and demands to know, "When is the real therapy going to start around here?" The consultant first points out how Mr. H. has once again covered over his sadness by being cold and demanding, but he also responds to the question and suggests that they begin to consider what therapy and duration would be most helpful.

What duration and frequency would be most advisable for Mr. H.? The information gathered in the consultation indicates that he meets criteria for an Axis I diagnosis of Adjustment Disorder with Depressed Mood and for Dysthymic Disorder. His Axis II diagnosis is a compulsive personality (and perhaps he could also be labeled Other Personality Disorder — Masochistic). He has no significant medical problem and, therefore, no diagnosis on Axis III. His Axis IV rating of recent stressors would be a 4 in that he is confronted with the moderate stressors of his business breaking up in mid-life and of his employees deserting him. His Axis V rating of the highest level of functioning in the past year is a 4 or fair, since his functioning at work has been somewhat impaired by the personality factors that led to the firm's breakup and his social and family relationships are also impaired by his irritability and isolation.

With our current knowledge of differential therapeutics, these diagnostic considerations do not in themselves indicate either how frequently Mr. H. should be seen or for how long a period of time. At least five reasonable possibilities exist regarding the duration and frequency of his treatment:

1) *a brief and intensive treatment* of several sessions compressed within a month or less (such as crisis intervention);
2) *a brief, less intensive treatment* of one session per week without an established date for termination (such as focal therapy);
3) *a brief and less intensive treatment with definitely established date of termination* (such as time-limited therapy);
4) *an extended, unintensive, and open-ended treatment of once every week* or so for several months or years (such as supportive psychotherapy);
5) *an extended, intensive, and open-ended treatment of two to five times per week* for at least two years (such as psychoanalysis or exploratory psychotherapy).

Although these five possibilities have overlapping boundaries and cannot in actual practice be sharply demarcated, for the purpose of exposition we will summarize separately the background, rationale, advantages, and disadvantages of each approach before describing what the consultant recommended for Mr. H. and what subsequently happened.

BRIEF, INTENSIVE THERAPY (CRISIS INTERVENTION)

We stated at the beginning of this chapter that the choice of duration and frequency of treatment was unavoidably interwoven with other choices the consultant must make, such as selecting the setting, format, and technique. A discussion of crisis intervention for Mr. H. illustrates this point, for choosing this brief and intensive treatment involves more than considering time factors (as indicated in part by our having already discussed crisis intervention in Chapter 1).

Lindemann (1944) pioneered the development of crisis intervention 40 years ago, when studying the responses of those who survived the devastating Coconut Grove fire. He noted that some were able to get over the trauma within roughly six weeks, whereas others were not able to work through their profound grief and to resolve the crisis adaptively. This failure continued to impede their lives. Twenty years later, Caplan (1964), noting the observations of Lindemann and others, developed techniques to support and mobilize all of the patient's available internal and external resources within a compressed period of time. The aim was not only to prevent damage from an inadequately resolved crisis, but also to foster maturation, change, and growth with the acquisition of more adaptive coping skills that emerged as a result of resolving the crisis successfully (Ewing, 1978). Of note, and often noted, is the fact that the Chinese have no word for "crisis" and instead combine the symbols for "danger" and "opportunity"; crisis intervention can be viewed as an elaboration of this concept.

In regard to Mr. H., crisis intervention – an intense, timely, goal-directed treatment lasting less than a month – certainly seems to match the patient's impetuous style. It would, therefore, be likely to meet with his approval and initial willingness to participate and possibly also serve as a role-induction into an extended and less intensive treatment should this later seem necessary after the immediate crisis has been resolved. The breakup of his business is a major and recent precipitating stress which provides a clear focus for intervention, and the patient's depression is severe enough to require urgent attention; the question is whether this attention needs to be so intense.

A disadvantage of crisis intervention for Mr. H. is that a compressed treatment may only perpetuate rather than correct his excessive impatience and his need to view every personal and professional problem as something that should have already been taken care of yesterday because it can't wait until tomorrow. The consultant has not indicated that Mr. H.'s depression is so severe that maximum support and structure are necessary nor that a more reflective, less intensive treatment runs the risk of professional disaster, psychotic decompensation, or suicide. In addition, a crisis-oriented treatment might focus too exclusively on the immediate stress – the business divorce – and an opportunity would be lost to modify other less pressing but nonetheless very important problems for Mr. H., such as his harshly critical view of himself and of others and the effects of this harshness on his self-esteem and on his relationships with his colleagues, friends, wife, and children.

BRIEF THERAPY

What constitutes a "brief" therapy varies from author to author and from model to model. Malan (1963) considers brief "focal" therapy to have an upper limit of about 40 sessions. Others have written about six session brief therapies (Bellak and Small, 1978), and some have noted the therapeutic effect of just one session (Bloom, 1981; Malan, Heath, Bacal, and Balfour, 1975). In the absence of a clear definition, for this discussion about Mr. H. we will consider brief therapy to mean five to 40 weekly or twice weekly sessions spanning one month to one year.

Just as there is no consensus about what makes a treatment "brief," the techniques, formats, and settings of the brief psychotherapies differ as well. In fact, brief therapies are currently as diversified as the longer treatments and include techniques that are derived from the psychodynamic, behavioral, cognitive, abreactive, task-oriented, problem-solving, interpersonal, strategic, biofeedback, hypnosis, marital, family, and sex therapies. Despite this diversity, common features can be found. All the brief therapies focus attention more or less exclusively on one issue, such as a stressful event, or a specific symptom, or a demarcated dynamic conflict. Influenced by the purposeful restriction of time, the therapist and patient engage quickly, mutually determine what problem is most important, and focus on that area with an explicit or implicit recognition that decisions will need to be made with incomplete data and that the goals of treatment will be limited.

With the growth of publications on brief therapy and with the increasing social pressures for psychiatric treatment to be more cost-effective, widely available, and practical, there is a tendency to view brief therapy as a recent phenomenon. Actually, as Gurman (1981) points out, most therapies have always been brief in private practice (Koss, 1979), as well as in psychiatric clinics (Butcher and Koss, 1978). Across the country, in fact, the average number of visits for patients seen in mental health clinics is six. What is new and exciting is that the duration of treatment is now often being limited by explicit design and the implications of this for treatment technique are being investigated systematically.

The rationale for brief therapy depends upon the theoretical model. Some approaches fit quite naturally into a relatively short time period: problem-solving brief therapy (Bellak and Small, 1978; Haley, 1976; Rabkin, 1977); behavioral brief therapies (Lazarus, 1973; Lewinsohn, Biglan, and Zeiss, 1976; Wilson, 1981); cognitive brief therapies (Beck and Greenberg, 1979); and marital brief therapies (Kessler and Glick, 1979; Kingston and Bentovim, 1981; Weiss and Jacobson, 1981). In contrast to these approaches, the development of brief psychodynamic therapies has a more complicated history. Freud's early work involved active interventions within a relatively brief period of time. With the increased interest in transference, resistance, and character analysis, together with the increasing power over therapy traditions exerted by the emerging psychoanalytic institutes, psychoanalytic treatments became longer and therapists became increasingly passive. The developing emphasis on regression, the overdetermination of symptoms, and the necessity for working through the transference neurosis were additional factors that fostered a sense of "timelessness" for psychoanalytic therapies.

Ferenczi (Ferenczi and Rank, 1925) was one of the first to shorten the length of psychoanalysis by "active therapy," during which he would give advice and encouragement and prohibit patients from certain activities. When eventually he went so far as to hug, kiss, and fondle his patients, Ferenczi was severely chastised by Freud. This episode perhaps placed in bad repute all of the more active and briefer treatments that were later developed (even though Freud himself in 1914 placed a time limit in the case of the wolf man [1955c]). Otto Rank was interested in the separation anxiety related to birth trauma and imposed a nine-month time limit for the gestation and completion of treatment. This method took advantage of the established date of termination in order to focus on problems related to separation. Although Rank's etiologic theories are now considered oversimplified and too categorical, *The Development of Psychoanalysis,* published in 1925 by Ferenczi and Rank, anticipates many of the techniques and concepts of modern focal therapy.

About 20 years later, Alexander and French (1946) continued these earlier efforts to shorten and intensify treatment. The most well known (and criticized) of their recommendations was the control and manipulation of the transference relationship to provide a "corrective emotional experience." Following this lead, Balint, his student Malan, and their colleagues at the Tavistock Clinic in London formed a research group and used sophisticated statistical methods to study focal therapy (Malan, 1963, 1976). Malan spelled out his selection criteria and demonstrated that a good therapeutic outcome was correlated with interpretations that linked the present transference distortions to the early experience of parental figures. This work is similar to that done in the United States by Sifneos (1972) and Mann (1973) and in Canada by Davanloo (1978). Sifneos restricts focal therapy to somewhat healthier patients with Oedipal problems and tends to use more directive and cognitive approaches. Mann emphasizes that separation-individuation problems are present in all patients and that a time-limited treatment is therefore an especially apt paradigm to explore such problems. Davanloo and Malan are far more flexible in their selection criteria and techniques. Despite these differences, the distinguishing technical device for most dynamic psychotherapies is the interpretation of unconscious wishes, fears, and defenses in order to clarify and resolve a narrowly-defined intrapsychic conflict that may be responsible for a number of seemingly diverse symptoms and behaviors. Along with relieving symptoms, focal therapy also attempts to promote character change, at least insofar as the undesirable personality traits are an expression of the focal psychodynamic conflict that has been explored.

In considering "focal therapy" for Mr. H., the consultant must decide whether a psychodynamic approach in an individual therapy is the best choice; for this particular treatment, the decision about time is inseparably linked with the decisions about technique and format. As we have already indicated, some treatments (such as behavioral, cognitive, problem-solving and family therapies) are more or less inherently brief, whereas the dynamic therapies are inclined to be more extended unless a conscious attempt is made to limit their duration. There are many good reasons for suggesting a nondynamic therapy for Mr. H. (e.g., a cognitive, behavioral, or problem-solving therapy) or for suggesting a format other than individual (such as group or marital) therapy; but for purposes of this chapter on duration and frequency, we will confine ourselves to the issues of time and intensity. We will discuss the advantages and disadvantages for Mr. H. of participating in a brief rather than an extended, psychodynamic treatment. Other selection decision points will not be addressed.

As with crisis intervention, the brief therapies appeal to Mr. H.'s style and his wish (perhaps need) to have things specific, focused, and structured. Given his impatience and his intolerance of uncertainty, Mr. H. might reject from the start any treatment that was ambiguous and of potentially long duration. Although Mr. H. by nature tends to be stimulus bound and to experience life minute by minute, arrangements for meeting once or twice a week might help him to establish a more reflective attitude and to accept more patiently the unavoidable delays and frustrations of life. By leaving the termination date open, the therapist maintains the option of reassessing along the way the extent to which Mr. H. has improved and become able to participate in the treatment. The length of therapy can then be adjusted accordingly on the basis of the latest data rather than relying on what may have been a premature decision at the time of consultation, one that could not include within its data base information about Mr. H.'s treatment response. Different patients get better and learn from treatment at different rates and each individual's rate of progress is hard to predict in advance. Many studies indicate that the patient's response to the beginning of treatment is the best predictor of ultimate outcome. Additionally, the indications and goals of treatment might change along the way. A more extended treatment is likely to be necessary to deal with Mr. H.'s chronic characterological problems and absence of loving relationships in his life, if he decides that these are his goals and that he wants more than symptom relief. By leaving the date of termination indefinite, a longer-term psychoanalytic or supportive therapy could evolve, if this seems necessary or desirable, without Mr. H. feeling defeated because he did not succeed in living up to a predetermined and definite deadline.

The main disadvantage of a brief treatment for Mr. H. is that the focus and goals might remain too limited. For example, even after there is improvement in his acute depression and worry about work, his long-standing oppressive view of himself and others might remain in its smoldering state; thus, an opportunity for greater change and a more enjoyable and loving life would be lost as the therapy is abruptly dismissed because the "job" is done. As will be discussed below, character change can occur as an outcome of focal therapy, but this is likely to be more circumscribed than is the case in longer-term, psychodynamic treatments.

TIME-LIMITED THERAPY

Time-limited therapy, as developed and described by James Mann (1973), is one type of brief, dynamic psychotherapy. The date of termination is established from the start of the treatment in order to highlight the themes of separation-individuation, as this relates to the patient's chief complaint and character structure. This maneuver confronts directly the problems encountered by all patients when ending treatment. Termination is a time when patients characteristically are likely to become upset, sad, disappointed, angry, and to complain about what hasn't been done. The patient may find new problems or have exacerbations of old ones in a conscious or unconscious attempt to hold on to the therapeutic relationships and avoid having to get on with life "alone." Although time-limited therapy is a specific approach to separation problems, the emphasis upon stating the date of termination at the beginning of treatment also has other implications which can be illustrated by going back to Mr. H.'s situation.

One advantage for Mr. H. of determining what date will be the end of treatment at its very outset is that the therapist is less likely to become a direct substitute for the lost business partner. This reduces the temptation, in both patient and therapist, either to extend treatment indefinitely or to cut it off abruptly rather than deal with Mr. H.'s powerful reactions to once again losing a supportive figure. A fixed termination date precludes such possible collusion between patient and therapist, the experience of separation and loss and its exploration are enhanced by the presence of vividly relevant transference material.

The main disadvantage of limiting the duration of treatment from the start is that the consultative process can never really predict for sure at what rate Mr. H. will improve and whether the goals of treatment will become more limited or more ambitious as treatment proceeds. Possibly Mr. H.'s immediate despair is making the retrospective account of his life more bleak than in fact has been the case. When his mood lifts, it may become clear that what initially appeared to be severe "trait" problems were, in fact, colored black by his depressive "state" and are actually relatively minor and tolerable. If this should prove to be the case, perhaps a very brief treatment of only a few more sessions is necessary and indicated. But it seems equally possible that when his depression improves, Mr. H.'s chronic characterological problems will appear to be far more important than the breakup of his business, which may have been only an incidental ticket of admission into treatment. If this turns out to be the case, a premature time limit for treatment could be a disservice for Mr. H.

EXTENDED, NONINTENSIVE, OPEN-ENDED TREATMENT
(SUPPORTIVE PSYCHOTHERAPY)

In striking contrast to brief therapies, extended supportive psychiatric treatments do not have clearly defined goals or techniques. These treatments depend more on the therapist's clinical judgment, interpersonal skills, and personality than on a prearranged and theoretically sanctioned set of treatment techniques. In part because of this lack of defined technique, extended supportive treatments are sometimes viewed pejoratively: that patients are either too healthy to need such treatments and are using them as an unnecessary "crutch"; or that patients are so sick that they need treatment for the rest of their lives. Training programs tend to underemphasize teaching in this area and many practitioners do not realize that supportive treatment may require the highest skill and is inherently interesting. It is easier to make direct interpretations about intrapsychic or interpersonal conflicts than to use one's understanding to inform behavior within the therapeutic alliance. Supportive treatments establish a therapist-patient relationship that comes closest to the valued traditional relationship offered by physicians, priests, and advisors who are sought by those in need for varying intervals, and often for many years, to lend an ear and give advice as the situation requires.

For Mr. H., an extended treatment might provide the caring and close relationship he has been unable to sustain elsewhere in his life. Using the support from this ongoing relationship and from various therapeutic interventions intended to strengthen those of his defenses that are most adaptive, Mr. H. in time might be able to develop and maintain similar relationships outside of the therapeutic situation. As different problems arise in his life — professional crises, marital stress, confrontations with the children — an extended treatment would provide the flexibility to approach them with whatever frequency and techniques were required at the time. Supportive treatments can be very flexible and may be delivered in packages as variable as a few sessions within one week to a lifetime relationship.

A distinct disadvantage of an open-ended and unintensive treatment is that Mr. H. might reject such a suggestion as being an impractical waste of time. Even if accepted, the therapy might never become sufficiently intensive to catalyze change; the problems would continue to simmer, never boil, and little of substance might transpire. In addition, the constant availability of help might conceivably impede Mr. H.'s autonomous growth and reduce his acceptance of life's inevitable losses and disappointments. Therapy can sometimes indeed become a "crutch" while a potentially healthy leg becomes weak and wasted. These concerns do not seem particularly worrisome in regard to Mr. H. who has a much more severe problem in establishing intimacy than in achieving autonomy.

EXTENDED, INTENSIVE, OPEN-ENDED TREATMENT (PSYCHOANALYSIS OR EXPLORATORY PSYCHOTHERAPY)

Treatments which are extended, intensive, and open-ended are often delivered in an individual format using psychodynamic techniques. The large commitment of time is necessary for the patient to develop a deeply emotional relationship with the therapist and to recall and to reexperience in regard to him (or her) the repressed wishes, fears, fantasies, attitudes, and conflicts that originated in childhood and that continue to influence current behavior. The therapist interprets how the patient is distorting the current relationships, both within and outside treatment, in terms of past significant relationships. Sessions must be relatively frequent to allow for transference regression and so that a "crust" of resistance and forgetting does not again settle over the recalled, anxiety-laden material. The duration is long because considerable time is generally required for the patient gradually, and often painfully, to develop powerful transference feelings toward the therapist, and then to analyze and correct misperceptions and character traits in order to find a more suitable way of resolving infantile conflicts. In general, the more ambitious and global the treatment goals, the more the duration and frequency are increased. Explicitly or implicitly, setting a time limitation for treatment, even if this is framed in terms of years, might provide the patient with a mode of resistance and prevent a full transference regression, exploration, and working through of important material.

Without being aware of it, the patient might be inclined to avoid certain issues when such a premature closure is in view.

An extended, intensive, and open-ended exploratory psychotherapy might be recommended for Mr. H. if his presenting depression is seen less as an isolated problem and more as the inevitable consequence of many serious characterological difficulties spanning his entire life. Such a treatment might also be indicated if a focal, circumscribed uncovering appraisal is not deemed possible because Mr. H. does not meet the rather stringent selection criteria for focal therapy. To focus on the current crisis, to relieve his depression, and to go no further might sacrifice an opportunity to use this "ticket of admission" and attempt to modify the chronic oppressive way he treats both himself and others.

The major disadvantages of such a recommendation are that his motivation and capacity for such a commitment at this time are questionable and that an extensive (and expensive) treatment may be ill-advised until a more limited therapy is first tried. This can serve as a trial of treatment and induction to treatment, should further work seem necessary. Moreover, intensive exploratory treatments can sometimes worsen acute symptoms—for instance, Mr. H. might become more ruminative and self-incriminatory during the uncovering inquiry. Given his despair and professional crisis, Mr. H. might require more structure, support, hope, and encouragement than an extended exploratory treatment customarily provides, at least at its outset.

After considering the many possibilities of different treatment durations and frequencies, the consultant and Mr. H. decided upon focal therapy. In choosing a recommended frequency, the decision was made on the grounds that Mr. H. had already begun to accept and adjust to the weekly sessions during the consultative process. Despite his characteristic impatience, he had not placed demands upon the consultant to be seen more frequently and he had been able to reflect upon the discussed material during the interval rather than simply dismissing it after a couple of days. In terms of the duration, the consultant believed that Mr. H. met many of the selection criteria for focal therapy and that the prospect of a more prolonged treatment would probably not be accepted at this point by Mr. H. The consultant was reluctant to set a definite date for termination (time-limited therapy) because of more than usual doubts about how well Mr. H.'s chronic characterological problems would respond to a short treatment. The consultant wanted to leave open the option to extend the treatment if Mr. H. became motivated to work out more extensive characterological problems that were not resolved during the focal therapy.

In this case, because the consultant had an adequate expertise in focal therapy and because an acceptable rapport had developed between the patient and the consultant, the consultant became the therapist and a referral was not necessary. The suggestion was made that they meet "once a week over the next few months" to learn why Mr. H. consistently made such strict and unreasonable demands on himself and on others, all of which inevitably led to disappointment, despair, and strife. He accepted the recommended duration, frequency, and focus of treatment; gradually over the next 14 sessions (four months) his depression lifted, as previously automatic and unconscious defenses were explored.

Because the emphasis of this chapter is on the selection of duration and frequency, we will not elaborate on all the themes and interventions which ensued during Mr. H.'s focal therapy. Some aspects are worth mentioning, however, because they relate directly to the management of time as a therapeutic technique. For instance, Mr. H. at first responded quite favorably to the suggestion that the treatment have a specific focus (i.e., Mr. H.'s critical attitude toward himself and others) and an approximate time limit of a few months rather than, as he put it, "letting it drag on for years and years while we talk about everything and nothing." The pressure to get the therapeutic work done "now" was a close fit for Mr. H.'s natural inclination toward action, and gave an immediacy and urgency to the transference and to the therapist's interventions. The notion that treatment would soon be ending prevented Mr. H. from simply rationalizing and saying, "Yes, these are the kinds of problems I someday will have to work out." His behavior in the treatment revealed to Mr. H. that his brusque superiority defended against strong fears of being rejected by others and was meant to hide his longings for acceptance. Mr. H. realized that despite his discomfort, he was, in fact, able to extend kindness and affection to others. Concomitantly, he also became much kinder and more forgiving of himself. He gradually came to realize that he did not inevitably have to behave in the same harshly critical fashion he had experienced in his father.

TERMINATION

After five months of weekly meetings (18 sessions), the therapist wondered whether to bring up the issue of termination or whether it would be useful to extend the treatment's goals and duration. The therapist had long previously announced a planned three-week vacation, which was scheduled to begin the next week. Surprisingly (or not so surprisingly), Mr. H. had not mentioned anything at all about this pending event or about termination. The therapist, appreciating how Mr. H.'s presenting depression had been in part a reaction to a "separation" from another "partner," wondered how he was reacting to this vacation and to the possibility that treatment might be nearing its end. Therefore, shortly after the beginning of the next session, the therapist repeated the dates of his holiday. At first, Mr. H. just reacted by thanking the therapist for "reminding me." Although he did not appear upset, he immediately went on to talk about how one of his secretaries was out sick, an important employee was taking maternity leave, his wife was going to visit her mother, and his older daughter was being a real "pain" getting ready to go to college in the fall and was not doing her chores at home. The therapist pointed out that all of Mr. H.'s thoughts were about being deserted by those whom he needed, and that perhaps he had more feelings related to the therapist's being away than he had at first known or acknowledged. The interpretation was vigorously denied. Mr. H. claimed that actually he was looking forward to having some more time to do his work and that, furthermore, this might be an excellent and opportune time to stop treatment altogether. Mr. H. was feeling "as well as anyone has any right to expect."

With the time of the session drawing to a close, the therapist suggested to Mr. H. that the decision whether to stop or continue treatment was too important to make on the spur of the moment and that the two of them could give the decision more thought and discuss it further when the therapist returned. Mr. H. accepted the suggestions in a rather business-like, perfunctory manner, and the session ended.

Let us look at the two main options confronting the therapist and Mr. H. Should treatment be terminated now that the goals of the brief dynamic therapy have been reached, or should a long-term exploratory treatment be initiated? By now, the reader should be aware that we believe there are no easy or categorical or right answers to these questions. Much depends on the balancing of a variety of factors – goals, motivations, dissatisfaction with current functioning, resources, diagnosis, severity of impairment, as well as the phrase that connotes both our wisdom and ignorance, namely, "clinical judgment." Nevertheless, we have by now obtained a large amount of information about Mr. H. and, on the basis of these data, we can discuss the possible advantages and disadvantages of either stopping or extending his treatment.

In favor of continuing treatment, Mr. H. has made substantial gains in his brief therapy. He has become aware of those specific aspects of his behavior that are most off-putting, has some idea of their origin, and has more ability to control them. Rather than to experience himself as a basically "bad" and "unlikable" person, he can now act in a way that attracts rather than repels others. He realizes that the rejection he suffered from his employees does not mean that he is, as he feared, "a thoroughgoing son-of-a-bitch now and forevermore." Partially because of this understanding, his depression has lifted and he has achieved substantial business success as the principal of his own firm. In addition, as a result of explorations in therapy, he has been able to trace his maladaptive perfectionism to early experiences with a father and mother who could never be pleased by their son or seemingly by anything else. To terminate treatment at what might be a premature juncture and sacrifice the potential for further gains might sell short Mr. H.'s potential for even more dramatic change. His longstanding inability to relax, have fun, be close to his wife, and enjoy his daughters and friends might persist in crippling him needlessly for the rest of his life.

But there are also disadvantages for extending Mr. H.'s treatment. His therapy may have become a surrogate source of support and gratification, a kind of amulet to ward off hardship. Any delay in terminating may put off rather than work through the inevitable pain of separation and "divorce," the very problems with which Mr. H. presented. Extending treatment might also foster a magical dependency on the therapy and therapist. Mr. H.'s confidence and autonomy would be diminished if inwardly he believes that the only reason he has done so well during the crisis is his weekly contact with the therapist and that if he ends treatment, he will not be capable of functioning on his own. Paradoxically, extending treatment might prevent Mr. H. from making further improvements. Rather than confronting issues directly and immediately, some patients become locked into treatment by assuming an attitude of, "I'm still working on that problem," or worse, "I haven't gotten to that point in my treatment yet," or even worse, "So long as I'm in treatment, I don't have to worry about that." In Chapter 7, we will discuss further how certain patients sometimes use treatment as a way of not changing until some mythical "tomorrow" — a tomorrow that sadly enough often never comes. Another disadvantage for extending Mr. H.'s treatment relates specifically to his narcissistic-obsessive-masochistic dynamics: He is liable to continue therapy as a way of becoming "perfect" like his overly idealized "perfect" therapist, or unconsciously to conceive of sessions as a punishment, another form of fire and brimstone offering penance for his inherent badness.

In addition to these disadvantages for continuing therapy, there are a number of possible advantages that come with stopping. Mr. H.'s acute symptoms have remitted and treatment is no longer vital. He has functioned more or less successfully in the past, and has no guarantees that his imbedded character problems will change much more with longer-term therapy. Mr. H. may be given an added boost of reassurance if he no longer views himself as a "psychiatric patient." Often the gains that are made in brief treatment catalyze further change. The benefits of treatment may be amplified in a positive feedback loop establishing what has been called a virtuous (as opposed to vicious) circle (Wender, 1971). For example, a more tolerant Mr. H. is likely to elicit more positive responses from those around him which is likely to make him even more tolerant of himself and others which is likely to elicit even more positive responses from others and so on. Brief treatment may reverse vicious cycles and establish benign cycles with the benefits continuing long after treatment has ended. Moreover, the decision to end treatment need not be irreversible—if more treatment seems desirable later on, he can always return. Often it may be more efficient to offer a patient a lifetime of several brief treatments each around a particular life or developmental crisis, with easy return to and termination from treatment each time, rather than one prolonged therapy.

Yet, there are a number of definite disadvantages for stopping treatment at this time. Termination, particularly if abrupt, may serve to confirm Mr. H.'s pessimistic view of the human condition: Nobody, including the therapist, ever really comes through in the long run; a caring relationship can never be sustained; and one must work hard to seek rewards in the next world, but not in this one. Stopping now might repeat rather than resolve Mr. H.'s tendency to play "hit and run" and to avoid the anxiety experienced in all intimate relationships. Rather than learning new attitudes and behaviors, he may regard the treatment as yet another confirmation of his previous ways of perceiving and doing things.

Having considered some of the pros and cons for either continuing or stopping Mr. H.'s treatment, we must add that many patients enter, continue, or terminate therapy with an admixture of complicated reasons, some of which are quite reasonable and most of which are unconsciously determined, magical, and consonant with character pathology. If given an opportunity over time to explore these reasons, many, perhaps most, patients learn that they embarked on the right treatment, but for the wrong reason.

One final note: To prevent our discussion from being redundant and convoluted, we have at this point discussed only the issue of duration and not frequency. We realize that the therapist also had to consider, if treatment continued, whether the frequency should be made more or less intense. As it turned out, the decision about frequency was intrinsically interwoven with the decision about what technique would be implemented if treatment continued.

After considering the advantages and disadvantages of either extending or ending Mr. H.'s treatment, the therapist and patient in this case chose to continue. The weekly focal therapy was changed into a twice weekly, open-ended exploratory psychotherapy. The goals of treatment were changed as well: The aim would be not simply to reduce Mr. H.'s depression by modifying the harsh view he had held of himself and others, but also to explore and change more general characterological difficulties, such as his inability to enjoy himself and to share an intimate, loving relationship with his wife and daughters. If the format had been different from the start (for example, marital therapy) or if the approach had been different (for example, behavioral or cognitive therapy) or if a date of termination had been predetermined (time-limited therapy), the therapist might have been less inclined to extend the treatment and enlarge the goals. Psychodynamic therapies may be inherently more difficult to terminate, in part because the goals are more difficult to define and to limit. The dynamic focal therapy of 20 sessions had inducted the patient into what seemed to be a profitable exploratory process which neither the therapist nor patient wished to end just yet because both felt that further gains might be made.

As intended, this change in the duration and frequency had a direct effect on the process of Mr. H.'s treatment. The brief focal therapy had dealt primarily with Mr. H.'s critical attitude toward himself and others which had led to the business divorce and his reactive depression. Psychodynamic material from his past (such as the punitive attitude of Mr. H.'s father) was used to understand the current crisis (for example, the way Mr. H. dealt with his "family" of employees) but this understanding was mostly cognitive and was not connected to the transference by interpretation. Now, partially as a result of the increased frequency of sessions and the extended duration, the therapy became more emotional and reflective and consequently more repressed memories were recovered, and more transferential distortions became manifest and accessible to interpretation. Both the therapist and the patient felt less pressure to resolve an immediate specific problem with directive and interpretive techniques. Instead, the aim was to use uncovering, exploratory methods to understand Mr. H.'s behavior in a more general and comprehensive fashion.

To keep the focus of this chapter on the issue of time, we will not elaborate on the multifaceted and intricate working through of Mr. H.'s problems which ensued over the 18 months of exploratory psychotherapy. The following example, however, does illustrate how the intensity and extension of treatment helped make Mr. H. aware of certain ego-syntonic character problems and how this awareness could then be used for constructive change.

Quite typically, Mr. H. would leave work for his session at the last possible moment, rush frantically through traffic, arrive exactly at the moment of his appointment, and obsequiously apologize for being late (which, in fact, he rarely was). Then, as he entered the office, he would politely ask if it were "all right" if he took off his coat. During the focal treatment, the therapist had tried in vain to show Mr. H. how his fear of being late and his oversolicitous attitude were signs of the harsh way he treated himself and the way he feared he would be treated by others if he did not anticipate and submit to their strict and unreasonable demands. Such comments fell on deaf ears. Mr. H. would simply rationalize that "the three Ds" – discipline, drive and determination – were necessary if one were to stay ahead of the game.

But then, after four months of exploratory psychotherapy, as Mr. H. became more involved with the therapist in an uncovering inquiry, he "had time" to mention toward the end of one session a "funny dream": He dreamt that the therapist had recommended that the patient "buy a handgun to keep over (sic) his pillow for protection before it was too late." Mr. H.'s associations to the dream ("living under the gun"), along with his recalling early memories (the frightening discovery of the gun his father kept by the bedside), helped convince Mr. H. how he was terrorized by his own conscience and by the projection of that terror onto others, including in this case the therapist. Before very long, his own violent impulses were discussed for the first time in the treatment. Much more could be said about this dream and its further impact on the therapy, but the point here is that, at least in the case of Mr. H., the change in duration and frequency appeared to be instrumental in bringing such material to the fore and making it accessible for interpretation.

NEGOTIATION AND COMPLIANCE

A discussion of the duration and frequency of treatment would be incomplete without considering the issue of negotiation and compliance. After all, the therapist is not the only one who determines how long a treatment will last; whether or not the patient agrees with the recommendation is crucial. At one point in Mr. H.'s treatment, he stopped coming for a period of seven weeks, partly as a bitter response to the therapist's week-long vacation and partly because a negative, paternal transference had become unbearably intense. Fortunately, the therapeutic alliance was strong enough to weather this transferential storm and a productive treatment continued.

Just as a premature termination may be a severe form of resistance, an overextended treatment may also be a form of resistance if both patient and therapist are covertly colluding with each other to avoid the inevitable loss and pain accompanying separation. With Mr. H., after almost two years of therapy the major goals of treatment had been achieved: His profound depression had not returned; his business partnership had dissolved much less bitterly and disastrously than he had feared; he was able to hire a new staff, keep most of his old clients and even to find new ones with an ease that bewildered him and confounded his excessively pessimistic predictions; he was able to relax and enjoy himself, both with his wife and alone; and, although his relationship with his daughters remained distant and stilted, he came to terms with the irreversible loss which had resulted from his not being more loving toward them. He looked forward to doing better with his grandchildren in the years to come.

Believing that treatment had now reached the point where Mr. H. was using it primarily to seek some goal of ultimate perfection, the therapist introduced the idea of termination. Mr. H. at first responded with only a mild anxiety, but during the next few sessions the thought of termination evoked near panic and despair, quite similar to the symptoms which had originally brought him to treatment. This time around, however, Mr. H. was able to use the gains he had made in treatment to withstand the loss and to grieve rather than collapse over "another divorce." The concluding sessions dealt with the distinction between his "treatment goals," which had been met, and his "life goals," many of which he would still have to strive for (Ticho, 1972). Mr. H. would have to come to terms with what was reasonable to expect from himself and others. The Christmas and Easter cards sent to the therapist during the next few years indicated that the gains of treatment withstood the test of time and, in fact, were deepened and extended after termination.

RESEARCH ON FREQUENCY AND TEMPORAL FACTORS IN PSYCHOTHERAPY

In our review of the research regarding time factors in psychotherapy, we will start by discussing those studies which investigated frequency of sessions and then turn to the literature comparing brief and long-term treatments. We will conclude this section by summarizing studies that show how different techniques and formats influence both frequency and duration.

Frequency

Results on this question have been mixed. Orlinsky and Howard (1978) did an excellent review of the research attempting to measure how treatment outcome is affected by the frequency of sessions. After carefully examining 16 different studies, they concluded that in general *no harm came from more intensive therapies and that some studies documented real advantages if the patient were seen more than once a week.* Graham (1958) found that neurotic adults such as Mr. H. did significantly better if seen twice a week as opposed to once a week, and Imber, Frank, Nash, Stone and Gliedman (1957) and Frank, Gliedman, Imber, Stone, and Nash (1959) found weekly individual or group therapy superior to seeing patients for half an hour every two weeks.

However, other studies have not supported this positive relationship between frequency and outcome. For example, Lorr and colleagues (Lorr, McNair, Michaux, and Raskin, 1962) studied a large population of V.A. clinic patients after four and eight months of treatment and found that improvement was not related to frequency of sessions. Similarly, when Kernberg and his group (Kernberg, Bernstein, Coyne, Appelbaum, Horwitz, and Voth, 1972) at the Menninger Clinic compared psychoanalytically-oriented psychotherapy with full psychoanalysis, they could find no significant relationship between outcome and session frequency – a conclusion that has also been reached by at least six other studies performed in widely varying settings and with diverse patient populations (Heilbrunn, 1966; Heinicke, 1969; Kaufman, Frank, Freind, Heims, and Weiss, 1962; Rosenbaum, Friedlander, and Kaplan, 1956; Van Slambrouck, 1973; Zirkle, 1961). A point worth noting is that at least one study found an increased number of sessions to be harmful in certain situations. Graham (1958) discovered that adult psychotic outpatients did less well if seen twice rather than once a week, supporting the clinical impression that severely disturbed patients may have difficulty with intense therapy relationships.

In summary, the available research does not absolutely substantiate the decisions made regarding the treatment of Mr. H., but the existing evidence is compatible with his being seen once a week until his depression improved and then increasing the frequency of sessions when the goals changed to working out more chronic characterological problems.

Brief Versus Long-term Therapy

Current research strongly favors brief therapy. *Most comparative studies fail to demonstrate a significant advantage of longer treatments.* Three different reviews of the research literature in this area have independently arrived at the same conclusion. Using the "box score" method, Luborsky and his co-workers (Luborsky, Singer, and Luborsky, 1975) looked at eight studies comparing brief with long-term therapies. In two studies brief therapy was better, in five studies no difference could be found, and in only one study was longer treatment more beneficial. When Butcher and Koss (1978) and Smith, Glass, and Miller (1980) did their own reviews of research studies involving duration, they too concluded that, in general, brief therapies are just as effective as longer treatments.

The conclusions reached by these three systematic reviews should, however, be approached with considerable caution. A closer look at the individual studies reveals how methods of measuring outcome tend to favor the initial impact of brief treatments (Henry and Shlien, 1958; Pascal and Zax, 1956; Reid and Schyne, 1969; Shlien, 1957; Shlien, Mosak, and Dreikurs, 1962). For example, Muench (1965) found that both time-limited individual therapy and short-term group therapy provided more improvement than long-term therapy, but he measured outcome with the Rotter Test of Internal-External Control and Mazlow's Security-Insecurity Inventory. Many therapists might question whether such tests validly assess those aspects of patient behavior that are most relevant to change in psychotherapy and whether these measures in effect serve to bias outcome results so as to favor briefer treatments. There are other limitations in many other studies comparing brief with longer treatments: 1) it is not always clear whether the brevity is planned or reflects dropping out; 2) severity of impairment is often uncontrolled; and 3) brief treatments are favored by regression to the mean (patients are seen initially at their worst and are bound to improve) and by using measurements of symptom relief rather than of character change. For instance, if Mr. H. were in a study measuring only relief of depression, he would have appeared to have done so superbly well in brief therapy that no advantage could have been documented from extending his treatment.

Total Amount of Psychotherapy

The research comparing brief versus longer treatments must be distinguished from research assessing the total amount of psychotherapy. This subtle distinction is important because brief treatments, whatever their orientation, tend to be more active, directive, and focused on specific problems; therefore, the comparison of brief and longer treatments may be more a comparison of different techniques than of different time schedules per se.

With this in mind, Orlinsky and Howard (1978) did an exhaustive review of 33 studies that related the therapeutic benefit to the total number of sessions. In 20 of these, there was a positive relationship between the amount of psychotherapy and the outcome; in seven there was no significant relationship; and in six the relationship was curvilinear.

Orlinsky and Howard also located 22 studies that dealt with the total time spent in treatment (as distinguished from the total number of sessions). Twelve such studies, a little over one-half, reported a positive relationship between outcome and duration; nine found no significant relationship; and the remaining study by Muench (1965) actually found a negative relationship between these variables.

After closely evaluating all these studies, Orlinsky and Howard concluded that *the total number of sessions is generally correlated with more positive outcome and, to a somewhat lesser extent, the total duration of treatment also significantly correlates with greater therapeutic benefits.* This conclusion would have supported the therapist's decision to extend Mr. H.'s brief therapy in hopes of achieving greater gains. However, before becoming too content with this conclusion, we must mention that Smith et al. (1980) in their meta-analysis could find no simple relationship between the duration and effect of therapy. They noted that peak therapeutic effect occurred somewhere between the first and seventh session – although it must be remembered that this result was obtained mostly in studies of behavioral therapy and may not generalize to other modalities. If one were to quantify the rate of change with Mr. H., the greatest incremental improvement probably did occur within the first two months of his treatment (four to eight sessions), yet this does not mean that extending the duration was of little additional value.

Open-ended Versus Time-limited Therapy

From the sparse research to date, few data support definitive reasons for assigning particular kinds of patients to specific brief therapy formats, such as open-ended as opposed to time-limited brief treatments. But there are tantalizing leads that the clinician must use with caution. For instance, the impressive clinical experiments of Malan (1963, 1976) suggest that certain constellations of patients' motivation and capacity to focus are predictive of success in brief focal dynamic psychotherapy. Patients with high motivation and low focality of conflict did well in therapy but often required longer treatments than those for whom there was high focality. Patients with low motivation for change did poorly, regardless of duration. The particular constellations that were obtained in a given therapy could be predicted between the fifth and eighth sessions. In addition, Sloane, Staples, Cristol, Yorkston, and Whipple (1975) found that individuals with acting-out behavior may do better in brief behavioral psychotherapy rather than insight-oriented psychotherapy.

No patient variables have yet been found to indicate whether a patient should or should not be given a time limit for therapy in advance. Though some brief therapists believe setting such a limit is in itself an important therapeutic technique (Mann, 1973), Butcher and Koss (1978) point out that current research evidence does not substantiate such a claim. For example, Shlien, Mosak, and Dreikurs (1962) compared time-limited psychotherapy with unlimited psychotherapy and found similar results. In the case of Mr. H., therefore, we must rely mainly on the consultant's judgment and patient's preference and not on available research to support the decision to keep the brief therapy open-ended.

Duration of Treatment as a Function of Therapeutic Modality

As we implied at the beginning of this chapter when describing the relationship of temporal factors with other treatment variables, the two-year duration of Mr. H.'s therapy may have been very largely determined by the consultant's selection of an outpatient setting with an individual format and an exploratory technique. To illustrate this point, we will summarize the literature indicating that had a marital or family therapy been chosen, Mr. H.'s treatment would probably have been relatively brief, and had a behavioral approach been used, his treatment would most likely not have lasted two years (though, of course, the results might have been quite different as well).

The data suggest that the format of marital or family therapy is associated with treatments of brief duration. Gurman (1981) found that the average marital therapy lasted just over 17 sessions. In a later review of marital and family therapy outcome studies, Gurman and Kniskern (1978) found that 70% of the cases had a length of less than 20 sessions.

This relatively brief duration of marital or family therapy does not appear to be significantly altered by the approaches used: Framo, a dynamically-oriented family therapist, reported that the average treatment in his own private practice lasted about 15 sessions (1981); behavioral marriage therapists such as Stuart (1980), Weiss (1975), and Jacobson and Margolin (1979) all limit treatment to under 12 sessions; and the strategic therapists of the Mental Research Institute report similar lengths of treatment (Weakland, Fisch, Watzlawick, and Bodin, 1974). Because the evidence overwhelmingly suggests that almost all marital or family treatments are brief, Gurman (1981) has provocatively suggested that the term "brief marital treatment" is redundant.

Wilson (1981) did a superb review of the relationship between time factors and the various kinds of behavioral therapy. He concluded that most often behavioral therapy is focused and brief, lasting from ten to 25 sessions. As might have been predicted, he found that the duration of behavioral therapy depended upon: 1) the motivation of the patient; 2) the ability of the patient to practice behavioral techniques in between sessions; 3) the patient's social and family support systems; and, of course, 4) the nature of the presenting problems. Complex and multifaceted problems required a "broad spectrum" behavioral approach of longer duration, whereas specific phobias (such as fear of heights and closed spaces) treated with in vivo exposure responded on the average within ten to 12 sessions.

This correlation between specificity of the problem and brevity of behavioral treatment appears elsewhere in the literature. For instance, addictive problems such as alcoholism have been treated effectively in behavioral therapy programs lasting around 17 sessions (Sobell and Sobell, 1978); specific sexual dysfunctions, such as premature ejaculation or vaginismus, have been treated in behavioral programs varying from six to 15 weekly sessions – a departure from the intensive two-week treatment introduced by Masters and Johnson (1970). But, as Kaplan has described (1979), when the sexual problem becomes less specific and more diffuse (such as a diminished sexual desire), longer and more complicated treatments are necessary. In the same way, severe obsessive-compulsive disorders, if focused around specific themes, have been successfully treated in three weeks with 15 one-hour sessions of relaxation training (Hodgson, Rachman, and Marks, 1972); but, when dealing with a more ego-syntonic and generalized obsessive character (such as with Mr. H.), the behavioral treatment can become quite extended. One cannot, therefore, conclude that all behavioral treatments are brief. For instance, during the first four years that the Institute of Behavioral Therapy in New York City was in operation, the average length of treatment was 50 weekly one-hour sessions (Fishman and Lubetkin, 1980).

When we return to Mr. H.'s depression (the initial problem confronting the consultant), we find that effective behavioral and cognitive approaches described in the literature do not differ substantially from brief dynamic therapies in terms of frequency and duration. Rush, Beck, Kovacs, and Hollon (1977) treated depressed outpatients with a type of cognitive behavioral therapy that lasted on the average 11 weeks (see also Chapter 3). Lewinsohn (Lewinsohn and Arconad, 1981) has developed a brief treatment of depression based on a social learning approach. As part of the initial contact with the patient, he set a time limit ranging from four weeks to three months, which typically involved 12 sessions. Such a treatment might have been quite appropriate for Mr. H., especially since the program is based on the belief that depression arises from the loss of social reinforcement due to inadequate social skills. Treatment techniques include rehearsing skills to enhance social reinforcement. A 12-session interpersonal psychotherapy has also been developed by Klerman and Weissman (1982). Rehm (1981) has developed a behavioral program which also might have been suitable for Mr. H. His model emphasizes that depression is a result of faulty self-monitoring, self-evaluation, and self-reinforcement. Treatment is offered in a group format and is time-limited varying from six to 12 weekly sessions of 90 minutes' duration. Likewise, McLean (1981) describes a treatment package designed to reverse deficits in the areas of interpersonal communication and social interaction—problems for Mr. H. This treatment is also usually brief with once-a-week sessions tapered at the seventh or eighth week to every other week, and with the last treatment scheduled for a month later. McLean further suggests that reactive depressions can be treated in this time frame but, if the depression is an inherent part of one's lifestyle, monthly review sessions may be necessary for another six months.

As Wilson points out (1981), this practice of extending the duration of treatment in order to address more characterological problems is not at all unusual. For instance, half the patients in the "time-limited 13 sessions" behavioral cell of Sloane's study (Sloane et al., 1975) requested and received additional therapy during the next year. The average was an additional ten sessions, but some patients received much more. It seems that even with the behavioral therapies, it is not unusual and is becoming more common to start treatment by attacking a focal problem and then to proceed by adding appropriate subsequent "booster sessions" to deal with other problems. Thus, the treatment of Mr. H.'s depression might well have been relatively prolonged even if a behavioral and not a psychodynamic approach had been selected.

SUMMARY

We conclude our review of the research regarding duration and frequency of treatment with the same cautions with which we began this chapter. Our current knowledge about time factors in psychotherapy is very limited and confounded by the many co-variables influencing how intense and how long any treatment should be. Nevertheless, this discussion of Mr. H. might help remind all of us that decisions about frequency and duration must be made throughout any treatment and cannot simply be deferred because they are too difficult or complex. Further research will, no doubt, heighten this awareness and document that the handling of duration and frequency can have a profound effect on the quality and quantity of therapeutic results.

CHAPTER 5

The Choice of Somatic Treatment

In every psychiatric evaluation, one must decide whether or not to recommend a psychotropic medication as part of the overall treatment plan. There are times when the choice is easy and straightforward, i.e., some clinical situations very clearly require that medication be prescribed; other situations seem equally certain to improve without such action. Often, however, the decision whether or not to use medication is much more uncertain, controversial, and/or greatly influenced by local or individual habit or taste. If the clinician, in collaboration with the patient, has decided that medication is indicated, the next series of questions is perhaps even more difficult — which class of medication, which specific drug, what dose, and for how long?

This book can neither avoid these interesting questions entirely, nor come close to providing anything that approaches adequate answers to them. Given the great value of psychotropic medications in the treatment of many disorders, it has now become impossible for the mental health clinician, of whatever discipline, to make informed treatment recommendations without having a fairly wide knowledge about the indications and effects of the various available drugs. We would be remiss in writing about the psychiatric treatment selection were we not to emphasize the importance of this decision point and to devote at least some attention to the choices and problems involved. On the other hand, the topic is so large in scope, and so complicated in detail, that textbook length is required to cover it in any really meaningful way. Fortunately, a number of excellent texts are already available and we recommend them to readers who want more than the brief overview that we can provide here (Appleton and Davis, 1980; Baldessarini, 1977; Kalinowsky, Hippins, and Klein, 1982; Klein, Gittelman, Quitkin, and Rifkin, 1980;

Reid, 1983; Usdin, Davis, Glassman, Greenblatt, Perel, and Shader, 1981).

We will begin this chapter with an historical background and discussion of trends in the area of psychotropic medication. Next, we will provide certain general observations about factors that influence the selection of medications and increase the likelihood of patient cooperation in their management. Finally, we will outline briefly the indications for the major classes of psychotropic medication and provide a sketch of their modes of action and side effects. Electroconvulsive therapy will be discussed in the same fashion. The next chapter will pursue in some detail the important question of when psychotropic drugs and psychotherapy are best delivered in combination.

HISTORICAL PERSPECTIVE

The prescription of medication (and other somatic therapies) for the treatment and prevention of emotional disorders is a practice that extends far back through the history, and indeed the prehistory, of the human race. The "medicine" man, whether he practiced as a shaman in a primitive tribe, as an alchemist in medieval Europe, or as a physician in Egypt, Greece, Rome, Moorish Spain, or in colonial America (cf., Benjamin Rush), had very definite ideas about and faith in somatic treatments, which were prescribed for a wide variety of physical and emotional disorders. Furthermore, the results obtained must have been convincing to healer and patient alike, despite the fact that very few of the substances in use could have conferred any active pharmacological benefit.

This intriguing paradox of good outcome resulting from pharmacologically nonsensical treatment has usually been labeled the "placebo" effect. There has been very little understanding about what actually causes the placebo effect even though it has been the essential ingredient (along with natural healing) in most of the "cures" accomplished by physicians, until the quite recent acquisition of active pharmacologic agents (Shapiro and Morris, 1978). Modern, double-blind, randomized studies have confirmed repeatedly that the placebo effect is quite powerful (e.g., accounting for responses rates of 30%–40% in depressed patients). Moreover, there are exciting recent studies that have associated the placebo effect with definitive physiological changes (e.g., in endorphin levels and immuno-competence), which suggest the happy thought that there are biochemical correlates to hope and expectation. The historical evidence seems to confirm that the wrong medicine (or inert medicine) given the right way (with hope, cultural sanction, and/or magic) by the right person (doctor, healer, priest, shaman, or psychotherapist) often works wonders for a variety of emotional and physical disorders. Of course, the right medicine does even better.

Early psychobiologists also had at their command some few, active psychotropic medications (e.g., alcohol, hallucinogens, antihistamines, anticholinergics, narcotics, and bromides). Unfortunately, these substances were so nonspecific in their action and so fraught with complications that they were more frequently harmful than helpful. The treatment very often turned out to be worse than the disease.

In the early 1950s, there was a dramatic psychobiological revolution sparked by the development of a number of specific and quite potent psychotropic medications. Within a few years, and with an almost casual serendipity, it was noted that several different classes of medication had dramatic effects on the specific target symptoms of psychosis, depression, mania, and anxiety. The way in which these discoveries were made is interesting and will surprise anyone who expects clinical science to progress in slow and predictable steps. The application of lithium to bipolar disorders is an illustrative case in point. Lithium had been used for generations in the treatment of gout, because lithium-urate is very soluble. In the form of its bromide salt, lithium had also seen some action as a sedative in the 19th century. During the late 1940s, Cade was investigating the metabolism of uric acid and happened to notice in passing that lithium had a sedating effect on his experimental animals. Cade's was an alert and prepared mind and he soon tried lithium with manic patients with amazingly gratifying results.

The psychotropic effects of the phenothiazines were also stumbled upon serendipitously. This family of compounds had been synthesized by the French chemical industry in the latter part of the 19th century during the development of the aniline dyes. In the 1930s, promethazine was found to have antihistaminic and sedative (but not antipsychotic) properties. Chlorpromazine, the pioneer psychotropic in this family, was initially introduced in 1951 as a preanesthetic sedative for surgery. Only later was it tried as an antipsychotic with astounding success. Similarly, the monoamine oxidase inhibitors were tried to treat depression only after it was noted that isoniazid caused euphoria and activation, as side effects of its use in the treatment of tuberculosis. Rounding out the discoveries of the 1950s was the realization that tricyclic compounds, like imipramine, had antidepressant effects. This was also a surprise. The tricyclics were originally categorized as antipsychotics because they are structurally similar to the phenothiazines and have many similar side effects. The tricyclics were ineffective in this regard but did induce mood elevation, an effect that was noted (as were the others we have described) almost in passing.

The introduction of a whole modern medicine cabinet full of effective psychotropic drugs has had an enormous effect on psychiatric practice and theory. The biological model of behavior and psychopathology became the frontier of new research in psychiatry. The availability of active treatments created an urgent need to improve diagnostic reliability and predictability in order to establish which syndromes responded best to which medication. This led psychiatric diagnosis out of the wilderness of confusion and neglect in which it had languished for the previous half century, and it was no accident that the comprehensive and systematic *Diagnostic and Statistical Manual of Mental Disorders III* (APA, 1980) was enormously influential. Furthermore, the availability of active psychotropic drugs provided an opportunity to dissect diagnostic categories pharmacologically by noting differential treatment responses. This has led to an expanding, if still very inconclusive, increase in knowledge about and methods of measuring brain neurotransmitters and receptors.

The clinical impact of psychotropic drugs over the past 30 years has been nothing short of remarkable. Many conditions that were previously refractory to all available treatments are now well controlled and in some cases prevented. The success of psychotropic medications and their popularity is evidenced by the fact that these are now the best-selling of all prescription pharmaceuticals and are used, at least occasionally, by 10% of the population of the United States. If anything, psychotropic medications are probably overprescribed by the general physician and underprescribed by the psychiatrist.

SOME GENERAL PRINCIPLES IN THE SELECTION OF PSYCHOTROPIC DRUGS

Target Symptoms

As we discussed briefly in the introduction, the patient's target symptoms are usually a better guide to treatment selection than is the diagnosis. This issue is worth reiterating here because it applies most particularly to the prescription of psychotropic drugs. Psychiatric syndromes, as defined in DSM-III, are for the most part no more than clinical descriptions of symptoms that have been observed to correlate with one another. When two patients qualify for the same diagnosis, this means only that they have a more or less similar clinical presentation, it does not assure that their conditions have the same etiology, pathogenesis, neurochemistry, or treatment response.

Moreover, there is considerable overlap among the DSM-III syndromes and, unfortunately, many patients fall at the boundaries rather than clearly within one category. It is certainly common enough to have a patient who appears to be some mixture of what we call schizophrenia and what we call affective disorder. Too often, in our experience, this circumstance leads to a passionate and rather futile debate about whether the patient indeed is "really" schizophrenic or "really" affective, as if this arbitrary placement of the boundary patient within one or the other descriptive diagnostic label has some value in the decision about the best course of treatment. It usually does not. We must remember that most psychiatric diagnoses are mental abstractions, thought up for convenience sake by diagnosticians. Most available diagnoses have not been closely linked to cause or treatment and should not be reified or regarded as concrete realities. Target symptoms, on the other hand, are easier to agree upon and more closely related to treatment response — particularly to the responses that are achieved by psychotropic drugs.

Polypharmacy

This issue follows from our previous discussion and will be touched upon again in Chapter 8 on combination of treatments. The long-standing prejudice against polypharmacy (itself a clearly pejorative term) makes sense when two or more drugs within the same family are each prescribed at less than optimal dosages. This concern should not extend routinely in the same way to situations in which drugs of different families are prescribed simultaneously for different clinical indications, or because the combination is more effective or less risky than either drug would be if used alone. Examples of such rational combinations of medications include: antidepressant plus antipsychotic for delusional depression (the combination is much more effective than either drug used alone); antidepressant plus lithium for depression in bipolar disorder (reduces likelihood of inducing mania); antipsychotic plus lithium for manic episode (the former works faster in acute situations); and antidepressant plus antianxiety agent for panic attacks and agoraphobia (the first for panic attacks, the second for expectant anxiety).

Compliance

Any number of studies have demonstrated conclusively that patients, both psychiatric and medical, are really very good at not listening to doctors. There is up to a 50% chance (Blackwell, 1973; Rosenstock, 1975) that a given prescription may never be filled, and even among those that are filled there remains a fair chance that the medicine will be taken in a way that differs substantially from the stated directions. Although patients have many reasons for not complying with medication orders, the only one that need concern us here has to do with the way in which the particular medication has been selected. Patients are much more likely to take a medicine when they understand its action, are given some say in its selection, know its side effects, and have some control over dosage. It is clear that the doctor has expertise, prerogatives, and responsibility in prescribing medication but, even given these considerations, pulling rank on the patient is only rarely effective. It is usually best to negotiate an arrangement that the patient endorses. In most instances, the choice of a medicine regimen requires, at the very least, the informed consent of a knowledgeable patient and sometimes the whole family.

Drug Selection Based on Side Effects

It is of great interest that the pioneer drugs within each class of medication are still actively prescribed and have kept their usefulness in the face of very stiff commercial competition from the many related compounds that have since been developed. In each family of medication, the second, third, and fourth generation contenders have failed to exceed the originals in therapeutic effectiveness, although often they do have a somewhat different profile of side effects. The choice of a specific drug within a family is therefore more often based on a consideration of differential side effects than on any expectation that the different drugs will have differential therapeutic effects. The therapist and patient must decide which of the various side-effect profiles will be most or least desirable for the given circumstance. For example, all else being equal (and the therapeutic effect usually is), a more sedating antidepressant will be used (at bedtime) for a patient with insomnia, while a patient who is sleeping too much will receive an antidepressant that is less sedating.

Past Performance

As in most aspects of life, the track record is usually the best predictor of what will happen next. If a patient has previously responded well to a given medication, one must have a good reason not to select it again for the same symptoms. Conversely, if a patient has failed to respond to adequate doses of a given medication in the past, there is no reason to prove conclusively that it will fail yet again. However, it is wiser to try something else. Furthermore, if the patient happens to have relatives with a similar disorder that has responded (or failed to respond) to a particular drug, this provides a valuable clue as to the patient's most likely pattern of response.

Treatment Trials

The proof of the pudding is often in the eating. For certain patients, especially those frequent ones who are so puzzling that they are labeled "atypical," it may not be at all clear which family of medications and which specific drug are most indicated. It is wise to be empirical and flexible about this question, rather than to feel any great confidence that the correct answer will emerge from endless ratiocination. First, one tries a representative from among the family of medications that seems to be most closely attuned to the leading target symptoms. If the first drug does not work after an adequate trial, then one tries the next most likely choice and so on. It is wise to prepare the patient for the possibility that more than one trial of medication may be necessary before the right regimen is established. This takes some of the mystery out of the procedure, reduces disappointment when any given medication fails, and in the process improves compliance.

FAMILIES OF MEDICATIONS

Tricyclics

The tricyclic antidepressants are probably misnamed insofar as they also seem to be effective for a variety of conditions other than classical depression. These compounds are fairly similar in chemical structure to the phenothiazine family, but they differ in having a seven-membered central ring. All tertiary amine tricyclics are metabolized to the secondary amine form (e.g., imipramine to desipramine). A number of these secondary amines are also marketed under separate trademarks.

A major proposed mechanism of action of the tricyclics involves their ability to block the reuptake of the neurotransmitters, norepinephrine and serotonin, at the presynaptic nerve ending. It may be important that certain tricyclics (especially the secondary amines) preferentially block reuptake of norepinephrine, while others operate more on the serotonin system. There has been some hope that different subtypes of depression would be characterized by specific neurotransmitter deficits. Thus far, however, the specific matching of depressive subtype, neurotransmitter deficit, and most indicated tricyclic has not been confirmed. Moreover, the tricyclics also have many other central nervous system actions (e.g., on receptors), and the exact mechanism of beneficial therapeutic effect awaits much further research investigation.

At this point, the selection of any one particular drug from all of the possible tricyclic medications is based mostly on the decision about which profile of side effects will be most or least desirable in the particular situation. For example, amitriptyline is the most sedating tricyclic and thus may be especially indicated for patients with agitated depression and insomnia. On the other hand, amitriptyline is also the most anticholinergic of the tricyclics and should be avoided when these side effects (constipation, urinary retention, visual blurring, sweating, dry mouth, or drowsiness) are most undesirable. The secondary amines have less tendency to cause postural hypotension and they are more useful for patients with cardiovascular problems.

A major limitation in the prescription of tricyclic medications is that they can be lethal when ingested in even relatively small overdoses — often as little as one week's supply. In most instances, they also require two or more weeks to attain therapeutic effectiveness. For these reasons, seriously suicidal patients must receive the medication in a structured inpatient hospital setting.

The clearest indication for tricyclic medication is for moderate to severe unipolar major depression with melancholia. Tricyclics also are effective for depression occurring in bipolar patients, but often lithium is a useful adjunct to avoid the risks of provoking manic episodes and of reducing cycle length. It is not yet established whether tricyclics are effective for chronic depression, although some early data suggest that they may be indicated at least when vegetative symptoms are present. Tricyclic medication has been very useful in eliminating panic attacks in patients with panic disorder, whether or not they also have accompanying agoraphobia. However, tricyclics seem not to be useful for panic consequent to specific simple phobias or for the expectant anxiety that is often present in patients who have experienced panic disorder. Tricyclics have been useful in the treatment of enuresis. There are also preliminary unpublished reports that they may be helpful in some patients with obsessive-compulsive and eating disorders.

Newer generation antidepressants (e.g., trazodone, amoxapine, mapratoline) with chemical structures that differ appreciably from the tricyclics have recently been marketed. By and large, these medications seem to have an effectiveness and range of indications similar to the

tricyclics and they also work as either serotonin or norepinephrine reuptake inhibitors. They claim interest mainly because of reported reduced side effects (particularly cardiovascular) and possible faster onset
of action.

Monoamine Oxidase (MAO) Inhibitors

As described by their family name, these medications irreversibly tie
up the enzyme, monoamine oxidase, and in the process increase the
synaptic availability of its substrates, most importantly norepinephrine
and serotonin. Since the MAO inhibitors also have many other central
nervous system effects, their precise method of therapeutic action remains to be elucidated. Therapeutic effect usually correlates with fairly
complete MAO inhibition, but some potent MAO inhibitors are not good
antidepressants.

Although the MAO inhibitors were the first antidepressants to be
discovered, they have had something of a checkered career and their
current indications remain controversial. Until fairly recently, the MAO
inhibitors had fallen into considerable disrepute and neglect, especially in the United States, because they seemed to be less effective than
tricyclics for severe depressions and to be potentially much more
dangerous and difficult to use.

Let us take up the latter issue first. The MAO inhibitors, on their
own and without consideration for interaction effects, have a profile of
side effects that is no worse than that of other potent psychotropic
drugs. The special caution that has surrounded their use has to do with
their potentially devastating interactions with certain foods, drinks, and
other drugs. Because of depletion of available monoamine oxidase (and
perhaps also through other less well established mechanisms), a patient
who is taking MAO inhibitors may have a serious hypertensive crisis
in response to the ingestion of tyramine or other aromatic amines. Unfortunately, tyramine is a natural and fairly widely distributed by-
product of bacterial fermentation and is present in many very tasty
foods and appealing wines. The MAO diet restricts the intake of aged
cheeses, chocolates, nuts, beans, citrus fruits, chopped liver, coffee, tea,
beer, wine, and many other expendable but otherwise very desirable com-
estibles. The patient must also avoid drugs containing sympathomimetic
agents (including nosedrops). Treatment selection dilemmas arise because these restrictions are least likely to be followed faithfully by those
very patients (e.g., atypical depressives, borderlines) for whom the MAO
inhibitors may be most indicated. Moreover, like the tricyclics, the MAO
inhibitors can be fatal in relatively small overdoses. In prescribing them,

one gives the potentially suicidal and impulsive patient two ready means for self-harm — the choice of overdosing on pills or on blue cheese.

Now, we can return to the efficacy question. The early systematic studies of the MAO inhibitors fairly consistently found them to be considerably less effective than tricyclics or ECT in severe endogenous depressions. In the United States, the MAO inhibitors were barely used at all until recently, because clinicians assumed them to be less effective and more dangerous than the tricyclics or ECT. In Great Britain, on the other hand, the MAO inhibitors continued to receive study and use both alone and in combination with tricyclics (a potentially risky combination that requires special expertise). The MAO picture began changing in the early 1970s. Studies using larger doses of the MAO inhibitors revealed them to be much more effective for depression (even serious, endogenous depression) than had previously been determined. It seems likely that much of the early pessimism about efficacy may have resulted from inadequate dose ranging. Moreover, in actual practice these drugs are much less dangerous than one might expect. They are associated with a rather low rate of fatalities, not exceeding that of available alternatives. The MAO family is now enjoying a strong comeback of interest in the United States and is receiving very active research attention. One particularly promising development has been the isolation of two specific types of MAO inhibitor (the A and B forms). There are some early indications that the specific MAO B inhibitor, deprenyl, may have good antidepressant efficacy but without the accompanying risk of the "cheese" or tyramine effect (Mann, Frances, and Kaplan, 1982).

The indications for the MAO inhibitors remain extremely controversial. Some studies (and clinical lore) suggest that this family is particularly effective in "atypical" or "neurotic" depressions and is less effective in the more severe, endogenous depressions. Although "atypicality" has been poorly and very variously defined, MAO inhibitors might be prescribed preferentially for those patients whose depression is also associated with prominent phobias or anxiety, or with reverse vegetative symptoms (i.e., increased rather than decreased sleep or appetite), and/or with other neurotic symptoms. MAO inhibitors would be a less likely first choice for patients with classical and severe endogenous depression, but might be prescribed for such patients who had failed to respond to tricyclic antidepressants. The MAO inhibitors have also been suggested as preferentially effective for patients whose depression is atypical and associated with marked rejection sensitivity and reactivity (i.e., the ability to rebound in response to pleasurable environmental stimuli).

This division of antidepressant labor, i.e., tricyclics and ECT for severe, endogenous depression and MAO inhibitors for milder, atypical anxious depression would be welcome indeed. Unfortunately, more recent attempts at replication have been inconsistent and often fail to support it. In a number of recent studies, both families of antidepressant medication turn out to be equivalently effective, and specific differential indications for MAO inhibitors and tricyclics have not emerged (Rowan, Paykell, and Parker, 1981; Ravaris, Robinson, and Ives, 1980). Since other studies do still find matches of clinical picture and specific drug, the whole picture remains cloudy. MAO inhibitors have been found to be equivalent to tricyclics in the prevention of panic attacks (Sheehan, Ballenger, and Jacobson, 1981), and may have antianxiety action as well.

Electroconvulsive Therapy (ECT)

ECT seems to inspire an almost primitive shudder of dread in the general public, so much so that a county in California voted recently to outlaw its delivery. This stigma probably arises from a variety of causes: the lurid ways in which shock treatments have been depicted in the movies; ECT's association with the unappealing words "fits," "convulsion," and "shock"; the ancient mystique attached to individuals undergoing seizures; and, most practically, the injuries that occurred in the early days when ECT was delivered without benefit of anesthesia or muscle relaxation. Perhaps, also, it is unnerving that a treatment seemingly so lacking in clear rationale is so very effective. Although it has been shown the ECT acts in various ways on brain neurotransmitters, receptors, and electrolytes, its specific mode of effect is still unknown. In fact, some investigators believe that the key to understanding the etiology of depression is the understanding of how ECT works, since it is specifically effective in this disorder.

Whatever its mechanisms, the effectiveness of ECT in depression is unquestionable. Consistently, in study after study, ECT has been shown to be considerably more effective than any of the available antidepressants. This is particularly true in the treatment of delusional depression for which antidepressants or antipsychotics alone do not work at all well, and ECT is more effective than the second best choice – antidepressants plus antipsychotics in combination. ECT may also be the treatment of choice (and at times is lifesaving) in patients with serious suicidal ideation, severe agitation, insomnia, retardation, or life threatening weight loss. Other somatic treatments often require a much longer lead time for the onset of action and are less likely to be effective.

ECT is often the best second treatment for seriously depressed patients who have already failed to respond to an adequate trial of antidepressant medication. ECT has only one absolute contraindication (increased intracranial pressure) and is the safest form of treatment for patients at higher risk from antidepressants (e.g., those who have cardiovascular problems, the elderly, the pregnant). ECT may also be indicated in situations which require rapid and severe remission: for example, a businessman who must get back to work quickly or risk losing his job.

ECT also works quite well in slowing down patients in manic storm, is often effective in catatonic patients, and sometimes works in patients with atypical psychoses who have not responded to other treatments. ECT, usually provided in a longer series of 15–20 treatments, has been used as a treatment of last resort for schizophrenic patients who have been refractory to repeated trials of antipsychotics.

Thus far, we have suggested that ECT has many real virtues and an almost equal number of imagined dangers. What then are its real limitations, complications, and risks? The major limitation of ECT is that its results are not always long-lasting; not infrequently, relapses occur unless the patient is placed on continuation antidepressants or maintenance ECT (which has not really received sufficient systematic study). Antidepressants are often chosen in preference to ECT in order to discover the medication to which a patient is most responsive – information that is of value both for prophylaxis and for possible subsequent relapses. Antidepressants are somewhat cheaper and easier to prescribe on an inpatient basis and are much more convenient for outpatients.

Memory loss is the most frequent troubling complication of ECT, particularly in elderly patients. Many studies suggest that this difficulty is reduced by the use of unilateral ECT applied to the nondominant hemisphere, although the advantages of this procedure remain controversial. There are some risks associated with the use of anesthesia and neuromuscular blockade, but these are only slight and acceptable, especially if an anesthetist is present during the treatments.

In summary, ECT has received quite a bum rap. It is the most effective and perhaps the most specific treatment for severe acute depressive disorders. It is especially indicated for delusional depression, for emergencies, and for patients at high risk for medical complications of antidepressants. It is relatively safe. Prejudices die hard, but it is time that ECT be recognized and not stigmatized. It certainly should not be outlawed.

Lithium

It is quite remarkable that the unassuming salts of lithium, a very uncomplicated and abundantly distributed element, should have such dramatic effects in the acute and prophylactic treatment of bipolar disorder. Lithium is the lightest member of the sodium family of elements and is readily absorbed after oral administration. It tends to distribute equally throughout the total body water space, having neither the intracellular preference of potassium, nor the extracellular preference of sodium. Equilibration between blood and brain occurs within 24 hours after oral administration and plasma lithium levels can be monitored conveniently. It has not yet been clearly established just how lithium works. Its most characteristic action may involve intracellular and extracellular neuronal electrolyte concentrations and the workings of the sodium pump, but lithium also has an impact on synaptic concentrations of neuroleptics and on receptor activity.

The major indication of lithium – to stabilize mood – is among the most well established and specific in psychiatry. Lithium is effective in the treatment of acute manic episodes (although neuroleptics are also often necessary at the outset), and in prophylaxis against bipolar cycling; it may also be effective in the treatment of the depressive phase of bipolar disorder. There is still controversy about its acute and prophylactic effects in unipolar depression. Moreover, lithium may have nonspecific sedating properties and may be effective in some activated schizophrenic and violent patients. Although its use in patients with cyclothymic and emotionally unstable personality disorder is not well established, this indication feels intuitively and clinically right. Lithium may help potentiate antidepressant effects in patients previously not responding to tricyclics.

Lithium is a potentially dangerous medication with serious toxicities if it is not prescribed and monitored carefully. Because acutely manic and hypomanic patients are notoriously poor compliers, they must generally begin treatment within the structure of an inpatient setting. Lithium must be given cautiously to patients who are suicidal, psychotic, suffering from poor judgment, likely to have medical complications, or who are subject to fluid and electrolyte imbalance (e.g., severe weight loss or marathon running).

Antipsychotic Agents

These consist of a large variety of substances derived from the phenothiazine, butyrophenone, thioxanthene, dibenzoxazepine, and indolone families. These compounds are quite effective in the treatment of psychotic symptoms and have a number of fortunate characteristics. They are not addictive, are remarkably nonlethal even in large overdosages, and demonstrate no tolerance for beneficial antipsychotic effects, although they do have tolerance for anticholinergic and other side effects. Unfortunately, however, patients often do not like taking them because of their side effects, and compliance is a problem.

The antipsychotic agents are powerful dopamine antagonists and work at various sites on the central nervous system (CNS). Their specific antipsychotic effect may be mediated by their ability to block dopamine neurotransmission in the limbic forebrain. Their parkinsonian side effects may result from dopamine blockade in the basal ganglion. Hypothalamic effects may be responsible for their characteristic neuroendocrine alternations (increased release of prolactin from the pituitary and decreased growth hormone). The antipsychotics also have many other CNS effects and, as with all the psychotropic agents, their exact mechanism of action remains unclear.

The question of how best to select from among the many available antipsychotics in a given clinical situation is usually answered in just the same way that we suggested previously for the antidepressant medications. Although they vary very widely in potency (i.e., effect per milligram), all of the available antipsychotics are essentially equivalent in their therapeutic efficacy, provided that adequate doses of each are used. The choice among antipsychotics will therefore be determined by matching the patient's needs, tastes, and dreads with the individual drug's profile of sometimes desirable (i.e., sedation), but usually undesirable, side effects.

The side effect profiles of the antipsychotics vary much more than their therapeutic efficacy. The high potency antipsychotics tend to be less sedating and to have fewer anticholinergic and cardiovascular side effects (this makes them especially useful in older patients), but they are much more likely to affect the extrapyramidal motor system and to cause acute dystonia, akathisia, and parkinsonism (which happens to occur most frequently in younger male patients). The selection of a particular drug takes into account how a given patient is likely to tolerate its most characteristic side effects. Careful matching is a crucial step in increasing the likelihood of patient compliance which is a special problem both because the agents have unpleasant side effects and because they are prescribed to an unusually difficult and demanding patient group. The clinician must obtain a careful history of the patient's prior experiences with, reactions to, and fantasies about these medications in order to pick the one with the greatest chance of current success. One striking example of the importance of matching side effects is the effect of thioridazine in slowing male ejaculation. This may make it the antipsychotic of choice in a schizophrenic patient who also has premature ejaculation, but may make it the worst possible choice in another patient who is preoccupied with potency and the ability to ejaculate.

Unfortunately, the most distressing complication of the antipsychotic medications, tardive dyskinesia, seems equally likely to occur with all of the compounds under discussion and therefore does not serve as a criterion for choosing from amongst them. Although often advertised by drug companies for use in low doses as tranquilizers in nonpsychotic patients, the antipsychotics are not really very effective as antianxiety agents. The risk of tardive dyskinesia is very rarely worth taking for the alleviation of anxiety unless the patient is also psychotic. Exceptions to this caveat are situations in which the antianxiety agents are even more likely to be risky, e.g., in the elderly patient with organic brain syndrome or in the addiction-prone.

The antipsychotic agents are not specific for any one psychiatric diagnosis. They work well in ameliorating psychotic symptoms associated with schizophrenic, manic, depressive, organic, and drug-induced disorders. They work particularly well for patients whose psychotic symptoms are florid, acute, and accompanied by anxiety and agitation. They work much less well in schizophrenic patients who are chronically impaired and characterized by many so-called negative symptoms, e.g., poverty of thought and lack of affect and volition.

Antianxiety Drugs

A large number of fairly diverse substances might qualify for classification under this general and somewhat vaguely defined heading. Anxiety is such a ubiquitous, unavoidable, and unpleasant aspect of the human experience that many remedies have been devised for its alleviation. These have enjoyed a very considerable popularity and wide distribution, and have achieved an almost sacred role in many societies. Unfortunately, however, antianxiety agents are often a very mixed blessing. They are generally burdened by the undesirable characteristics of tolerance and withdrawal and tend to induce physiological and psychological dependence. Problems of abuse and addiction limit their clinical usefulness and greatly impact upon treatment decisions concerning when to prescribe them.

The most venerable, widely used and abused, and perhaps the most effective and also most dangerous of the antianxiety agents is that old standby, alcohol. Dionysus was raised to the status of demigod for his patronage of wine, thereby setting a precedent that many others have attempted to emulate with only indifferent success. Derivatives of naturally occurring narcotic agents also have an impressive history as tranquilizers and have also caused their share of problems.

During the 19th century, bromide salts were immensely popular and often combined with alcohol in patent remedies designed to cure all kinds of ailments. Around the turn of the century, the emerging chemical industry began to synthesize agents like paraldehyde and chloral hydrate, which had a range of action (and addictive potential) similar to that of alcohol. The next great wonder drugs were those of the barbiturate family. These became the standard sedative/hypnotics until their high addictive potential, withdrawal syndrome, and lethality in overdosage became clear. The never-ending search for a nonaddictive antianxiety agent led to the synthesis and testing in the late 1950s of the propanolol family of muscle relaxant and sedative drugs, the best known of which is meprobamate. These have had a remarkable popularity despite very high addiction potential, high lethality, with serious withdrawal complications.

The current leading antianxiety agents are the benzodiazepines. These were first synthesized in the 1930s but their antianxiety effects were realized only with the introduction in 1960 of chlordiazepoxide (Librium), followed soon after by diazepam (Valium). Later flurazepam (Dalmane), the best of the hypnotic drugs, was introduced. These medications made the pharmaceutical industry's wildest sales and revenue dreams come true and far surpassed in volume of prescription any other family of compounds. This kind of popularity is the most telling reflection that these substances work and in a way that is immediately recognizable and gratifying to the patient. The compliance problem encountered in the use of the antianxiety agents is very different from those discussed for the antidepressants and antipsychotics. For these latter drugs the issue is usually the patient's refusal to take the pills because he feels no benefit and/or dislikes the side effects. In sharp contrast, patients are usually all too eager to take antianxiety agents. If they fail to comply, it is usually by taking more than have been prescribed. The great virtue of these agents is that they are so immediately and tangibly effective; in some ways, this (and their addictive potential) is also their great vice and danger. Patients often come to feel that they cannot live without the antianxiety agent, are inhibited in learning other ways of coping, and lose opportunities for extinguishing their sensitivity to anxiety.

All of the various antianxiety agents cause degrees of CNS depression that is roughly proportional to dosage: i.e., anxiolysis in low dosages; sedation and then hypnosis in higher dosage; and, finally, coma, respiratory depression, and death in progressively higher overdosage. The benzodiazepines are superior to their predecessors in their improved therapeutic index. They induce less sedation for a given antianxiety effect, less tendency to addiction, and have lower lethality on overdosage. There is much cross-tolerance among antianxiety agents and many of them have anticonvulsant and muscle relaxant properties.

The antianxiety agents are only rarely of any use in severe psychiatric disorders. They generally do not have antipsychotic, antidepressant, or antipanic properties and find their major indication in the treatment of relatively mild and acute anxiety syndromes. Their tendency to produce tolerance and addiction, as well as frequent incidence of abuse, suggests that for most patients these agents should be used in a specific and temporary manner to assist emergency coping. Antianxiety agents are also prescribed to encourage patients to attempt activities that might otherwise be avoided because of expectant anxiety. Often, just having the medication handy is magic enough to get an otherwise stalemated patient back on the move. PRN dosage is useful for such purposes.

The major dilemma in the prescription of these medications is that the patients who most want and seem to need them are also those most likely to abuse them and to use them in combination with alcohol in a particularly devastating combination. Before prescribing antianxiety agents, a careful history of previous addictions is crucial. Other means of controlling anxiety and stress (e.g., psychotherapy, relaxation exercises, biofeedback) are indicated in preference to antianxiety agents for longer-term prophylaxis and for patients with high addiction potential. These medications are also used commonly in alcohol detoxification and for stress management in a variety of medical conditions (e.g., hypertension). They must be prescribed with great care in the elderly and in those with brain pathology, because CNS depression may exacerbate or unmask any tendency toward confusion, delirium, and other organic mental syndromes.

SUMMARY

Effective medications now exist for the treatment of depression, bipolar mood swings, panic disorder, psychosis, and acute episodes of anxiety. These have dramatically changed the delivery of mental health services in ways that are too familiar to require extensive discussion here. Psychotropic medication has become an area of very active and exciting research. Although the psychiatrist is ultimately responsible for prescribing medication, all clinicians must keep abreast of new developments and be knowledgeable about the indications, side effects, complications, and limitations of the major families of psychotropic drugs.

In the treatment of severe unipolar depressions, ECT is consistently the most effective but least convenient choice (especially for outpatients and during the continuation phase). It is usually reserved for delusional depressions, for acute emergencies that require fast results, for patients in whom it is a safer alternative to medication, and for those who have failed to respond to other treatments. ECT is probably underutilized because of the unfair and uninformed stigma that has been attached to it.

Tricyclic antidepressants remain the treatment of choice for most moderate to severe endogenous depressions. MAO inhibitors are generally second-line medications for those who have already failed to respond with tricyclics, although they may be the treatment of choice for "atypical depressions." The role of antidepressants in chronic or "characterological" depression remains to be elucidated.

Lithium is the treatment of choice for bipolar disorders although it is often most effective in combination with other medication (with antipsychotics for delusional and agitated patients and with antidepressants for depressed patients).

The tricyclics and MAO inhibitors are equally effective for so-called "spontaneous" panic attacks, i.e., those that are unassociated with specific or simple phobias. This finding has been documented fairly recently (Sheehan et al., 1981) and has not yet had a sufficiently extensive impact on general clinical practice. These medications have little effect on the expectant or generalized anxiety that often accompanies panic disorder. This symptom requires psychotherapeutic intervention (and occasionally the temporary use of antianxiety agents).

The antipsychotic medications are quite effective in the treatment of acute, florid psychotic symptoms arising from a variety of sources. A major problem in their use is poor patient compliance occasioned by their unpleasant side effects and use in a difficult patient population. Close attention to side effects in the selection of a particular drug and its dosage schedule may dramatically reduce relapse ratio by increasing compliance.

The antianxiety aspects are often the victim of their own popularity. These drugs are remarkably effective and patients love to take them. They also have some risk for producing tolerance, withdrawal, abuse, and dependence. Antianxiety drugs should be targeted to specific situations and used for brief durations.

CHAPTER 6

Combination of Treatments

Many of us were trained, and not so very long ago, to be quite skeptical about any use of combined therapies and to regard them as a sure sign of sloppy and inelegant practice. The prescription of a combined drug regimen invited a variety of mocking nicknames like "polypharmacy," "cocktails," "shotguns" and the "kitchen sink." Many clinicians also took the parallel position that psychotherapy and drug therapy were strange bedfellows and mixed poorly. It was, for example, not uncommon for psychotherapists to believe that patients on medication would lose motivation for psychological exploration, whereas psychopharmacologists often seemed to believe that drugs were self-sufficient and superior to psychotherapy. For example, Langs (1973) states,

> The use of drugs can undermine the quest for insight, internal change and ego development. Their use, when not truly indicated, can reflect serious inadequacies and countertransference problems in the therapist which lead him to avoid the struggle with the patient. . . . If a therapist truly believes in the powers of insight and the healthy resolution of conflict, he will seldom find need for medication. . . . There is no substitute for the patient's ego and resources (p. 215).

Meanwhile, the proponents of the various developing schools of psychotherapy tended to maintain the pristine and competitive purity of their technical innovations, rather than attempt to determine how these could best be combined with one another. There have always been a few synthesizers and bridgebuilders (often derided from all sides as "eclectic"), but, for the most part, clinicians who were trained in one form of therapy tended to regard other types with disdain and suspicion. Many clinicians would still consider it highly unorthodox, perhaps even sacrilegious or foolish, to formulate a treatment plan like the one suggested below, which includes both psychodynamic and behavioral techniques, and would be particularly appalled if these approaches were made simultaneously and by different therapists.

The tendency for the different psychotherapies to remain separate was only in part an expression of unreasonable xenophobia or rivalry. During their early development, the different schools understandably wanted to test the implementation and value of their approaches in relative isolation, without having their results confounded and complicated by the intrusion of outside variables. Another concern was that the combining of treatments might divide the patient into a number of syndromes with no appreciation of possibly integrating etiologies or of the person as a working (or malfunctioning) unit. As an extreme and therefore absurd example, a patient with obesity, premature ejaculation, work inhibition, insomnia, and obsessive character problems might be referred in a travesty of combined therapy to a homogeneous group, sex therapist, behavior therapist, psychopharmacotherapist, and psychoanalyst—even though all of the symptoms might be traced to the same set of underlying causes. The resistance to combined therapies arose in part as a way of avoiding a "kitchen sink" approach that could lead to fragmentation of the patient—and of the field itself.

Another reason for the limited discussion in the literature of combined therapies—and the very limited research—is that the area is overwhelmingly complex. The permutations of various possible combinations of settings, formats, techniques, drugs, durations, and frequencies very quickly enter into the millions and most of the alternatives generated in this way are not altogether farfetched.

Despite this complexity, we believe that several interrelated factors make this an opportune time to lessen the tensions between various schools of psychiatric treatment and to reassess the pros and cons of combined treatment.

First, many of the vying psychotherapies have matured. Psychodynamic therapy, behavior therapy, pharmacotherapy, family therapy, group therapy, cognitive therapy, gestalt therapy, brief dynamic therapy, and crisis intervention are representative of treatments that now have a more established identity. Their advocates no longer need fear that characteristic innovations will be lost when combined with other types of treatment.

Second, many treatments have already proved their worth. Having established their efficacy, the various kinds of psychotherapists are less inclined to assume that different techniques are in a horse race. They are more willing to find ways in which their particular approaches can be integrated to complement and augment one another. No one has a monopoly on the understanding or treatment of psychopathology.

A third reason why the time is now ripe for reassessing combined treatments is that we now have evidence that certain combinations have additive and possibly even synergistic effects. The evidence for these effects of combined treatments comes most impressively from psychopharmacotherapy (Smith, Glass, and Miller, 1980). Drug combinations that were once disparagingly called "polypharmacy" are now regarded as well-substantiated and acceptable treatments for certain disorders: the combined use of antidepressants and antipsychotics for psychotic depressions (Brown, Frances, Kocsis, and Mann, 1982); the combination of antidepressants and minor tranquilizers for agoraphobia with panic disorder (Klein, Gittelman, Quitkin, and Rifkin, 1980); and the combination of lithium and antidepressants for bipolar disorders. Moreover, despite previous doubts, recent research also suggests that pharmacotherapy and psychotherapy do mix quite well, are often additively effective, and may each address different target symptoms so that for certain disorders neither treatment alone is really sufficient. When we come to the question of combining different psychotherapies, our impression is that outcome research will someday support emerging clinical opinion that rational combinations are often the treatment of choice. There is no reason to assume, and our experience does not support, that techniques derived from different orientations are necessarily incompatible.

A fourth reason for confronting at this time the issue of combined treatments is that advances in outcome research, such as "dismantling" and "meta-analysis," provide the possibility of mastering the complexities involved. These research innovations will be discussed in Chapter 8.

ADVANTAGES OF COMBINED TREATMENT

1) Treatments delivered in combination may have additive and at times even synergistic effects. The term additive effects describes the situation in which the combined benefits of treatments A and B are equal to the sum of their individual benefits. The term synergistic effects describes the special bonus situation in which the combined benefits of A and B exceed the sum of their individual parts, i.e., the treatments are in some ways potentiating each other.

2) There is evidence that different types of therapy are differentially effective in resolving different types of target symptom, even as these

present themselves simultaneously in a given patient. Certain patients may obtain more comprehensive improvement if different treatment interventions are directed to particular target symptoms, rather than if any one approach is expected to be totally adequate to do the job on all fronts. A fairly well documented example has to do with the treatment of depression. It seems that psychotropic drugs are most effective in reducing affective and vegetative symptoms, while psychotherapy is most effective in improving cognitive symptoms, interpersonal relatedness, and social adjustment. It may have constituted an unrealistic idealization of the various psychotherapies to expect each of them independently and individually to be effective for all of the problems in each of the patients treated with that technique. In somewhat analogous situations in medical practice, an internist would not expect a patient with both hypertension and heart failure to forego digitalis, just because he is also on propanalol.

3) Not infrequently, a needed treatment is impossible to deliver unless another treatment is provided either concurrently or in a preparatory induction phase. A severely depressed or psychotic patient is often inaccessible to psychotherapy unless the otherwise disabling symptoms are first improved or stabilized with psychotropic drugs. The reciprocal situation is equally frequent — the patient improving from his/her depression or psychotic episode is likely to discontinue the medication unless he/she is simultaneously engaged in psychotherapy.

4) Different treatments induce change at different speeds. A patient who requires fast improvement for a specific, urgent problem occasionally may need referral for the amelioration of that one specific problem, even if he is already engaged and doing good work in a longer term, more ambitious treatment aimed at more pervasive character change. Perhaps the most frequent example would be the referral of a patient in long-term exploratory psychotherapy to a more behaviorally oriented therapist for the concurrent, brief, focused treatment of sexual, phobic, anxiety, or psychosomatic disorders. This would be indicated when the symptom is pressing, requires quick resolution, and has thus far resisted interpretation (e.g., a student with test anxiety the week before an important final exam). Although the therapist with training and expertise in both techniques may choose to apply the combination him- or herself, in some instances referral may be, nonetheless, desirable in order to protect the process of transference evolution in the uncovering treatment.

5) For patients who are especially needy and who tend to get excessively attached to one therapist, combined treatment may provide a desirable dilution of what would otherwise be an actualized and unworkably intense transference relationship. Combined treatment can also

provide a backup for vacations and other therapeutic interruptions which are otherwise often devastating for this kind of patient.

6) On a more general level, an acceptance of the possible utility of combined treatments may help to promote clinical innovation, flexibility, and a lessening of tensions among the various schools of psychotherapy. For too long, psychiatry has been fragmented into warring biological, psychological, social systems, and behavioral camps, each acting as if it had a monopoly on the understanding of psychopathology and on the methods for treating it. It is time to stop assuming that treatment techniques are in a horse race and, instead, to find ways in which they can be integrated to complement and augment one another.

DISADVANTAGES OF COMBINED TREATMENT

1) When two treatments are used simultaneously, it is never possible to know for sure just what is working and how. Let us suppose a depressed patient begins psychotherapy and antidepressant medication on the same day and three weeks later shows marked improvement. Is this caused by the psychotherapy, by the drug, by spontaneous remission, or by some combination? How does the therapist decide whether or not to continue the medication for six months? Sequential treatments, if more than one turns out to be necessary, allow for a clearer understanding of what causes patient response and what does not, thus providing a clearer guide for future interventions.

2) It is conceivable that at least some treatments in combination interact negatively with one another, i.e., the benefits of treatments A and B are less than the sum of their parts or, in the more extreme case, less than what either would achieve if given alone.

3) Side effects and complications of combined treatments are probably additive in many instances.

4) When combined treatments are performed by different therapists, and particularly if they occur simultaneously, there is the danger of having too many cooks stirring and ruining the treatment broth. At its worst, combined therapy can become a nightmare. The different therapists may unwittingly compete for the patient's favor, work at cross purposes, or each fail to take responsibility, assuming that the other is, and so on. It may also allow the patient to "split," i.e., to see one therapist as a good guy and the other as a bad guy and to externalize the internal, intrapsychic conflict onto the external, real or imagined battle between therapists. On the other hand, combined therapy may allow some patients to take neither of their treatments very seriously and/or to regard therapy as a social event or an interesting hobby.

5) Combined therapies, especially if done by more than one therapist, may convey to the patient the notion that he or she is especially sick because he or she requires so many different kinds of help.

6) Combined therapies by different therapists may contribute to the patient's dependency on therapy as a way of life. Moreover, some patients use their participation in therapy as proof to themselves and to others that they are doing all they possibly can to change their lives. Therapy in this situation serves as an excuse (and expiation) for avoiding necessary but feared activities.

7) Combined treatments are expensive in time and money for the patient and in resources for the mental health system. This practical limitation leads very quickly to a value and public policy question: Does one patient deserve two treatments if this means that someone else will have to go completely without?

8) The use, or rather misuse, of combined treatment might on a more general level contribute to an excessively compartmentalized target symptom and organ-specific approach to human behavior and psychopathology. The patient might receive multiple treatments instead of the one definitive treatment for the underlying factor most responsible for the surface symptoms. It is certainly true that combined therapy done mindlessly can lead to a sloppy "kitchen sink" level of practice—one that seriously underestimates the integration and connectedness of human nature. It is conceivable that rather than bringing psychiatry together, a hoped-for advantage listed above, an emphasis on combined treatments might encourage even greater fragmentation and subspecialization in the field.

TYPES OF COMBINED TREATMENT

Drug and Drug

The rational use of what has been derisively called "polypharmacy" has been briefly alluded to in the introduction to this chapter and will not be discussed any further now, since it is outside the scope of this book.

Psychotherapy and Drug Delivered Simultaneously

If one allows the broadest definition of psychotherapy—the careful attention to and use of the doctor-patient relationship—it is almost inconceivable that drugs will ever be dispensed completely independent of some form of accompanying psychotherapy. Doctors should not, and in ordinary ethical practice do not, act like vending machines in providing their patients with medications. The way in which the medication treatment is explained and questions are answered greatly influences the extent to which the patient will comply with and benefit from the suggested regimen. It is a rewarding and sobering observation that physicians were regarded, and indeed performed successfully, as healers for many centuries without having in their possession any great store of truly active pharmacologic agents. The power and frequency of the placebo effect—one that depends on patient hope and expectation and a psychotherapeutically healing relationship—has been documented scientifically in many modern studies and is a biologically as well as a psychologically mediated phenomenon. Medication is often powerful, even if it is pharmacologically inert, when it is delivered in a certain way. A physician who attends to the patient's concerns, is able to explain the purpose and risks of a medication in an educative, convincing, and reassuring way, and conveys hope and concern in the offering of help is likely to have a much higher success rate than one who provides medicines without explanation or in a negative manner. In other words, the greater the psychotherapeutic skills (again defined in a broad way) possessed by the prescriber, the more likely it is that the medication will work. Therefore, it would seem that there is no situation in which medication should be given without the accompaniment of at least some education and medical supportive psychotherapy.

The recent research and discussion on the combination of psychotherapy and drug therapy have addressed a somewhat different issue than that reviewed above. In research investigations, the definition of psychotherapy is restricted to a much more specific package of verbal, interactive techniques designed specifically to influence the patient's behavior and psychopathology. Here the question is whether one or another form of psychotherapy, e.g., cognitive, behavioral, interpersonal, psychodynamic, when provided simultaneously with one or another form of drug therapy, has effects that are synergistic, additive, or negatively interacting in the treatment of one or another psychiatric condition. We will return to this question in the section on Research Review.

Delivered Sequentially

There may be certain situations in which the most rational combination of drug and psychotherapy requires that they be given consecutively rather than simultaneously. In the acute phase of some conditions, it may be wise to sequence interventions. A patient with a nonsuicidal, nonendogenous depression or panic attacks of recent onset may be treated first with psychotherapy alone, in order to test whether medication will also be necessary. This is particularly advisable if the side effects of the medication are to be feared in the given clinical situation. On the other hand, there are a few conditions (such as severe acute psychosis or depression) that so remove a patient from participation in a therapeutic alliance that medication is a precondition to meaningful psychotherapy.

Combinations of Psychotherapy Techniques

This important topic has received very little attention in the literature. Given the great variety of specific psychotherapy techniques, it is of great interest to begin learning which mix best with one another and for which conditions and in which situations it is best to have one therapist providing a range of different techniques or to have two or more experts in different particular approaches working separately. Up until now, there has been a proliferation of new schools of psychotherapy, each of which has emphasized the ways in which it is different from what has come before in an attempt to establish itself as a new panacea. In most instances, clinical innovations are a lot less new and different than initially meets the eye and are quite susceptible to synthesis with other established techniques. We have lived through the era of the creative "splitters" promoting new psychotherapeutic techniques, and it is now time for the "lumpers" to shape what is best in the variety of these seemingly disparate techniques into higher order, coherent, flexible, and integrated wholes (Goldfried, 1980).

RESEARCH REVIEW

We are not interested here in reviewing those research investigations that have compared the efficacy of one drug with that of drug combinations. Moreover, there is very little available research on the use of combined psychotherapeutic techniques (this was done only in the mantling-dismantling strategy for studying behavioral techniques — see Chapter 8). Therefore, our research review will focus on the studies performed to compare the results achieved by a combination of psychotherapy and psychotropic drugs, with the results of psychotherapy used alone and the results of drugs used alone.

In his 1971 review of research on this topic, May concluded that for hospitalized psychotic patients there is little difference between drug alone and drug plus psychotherapy. Even in the face of this conclusion, May nonetheless recommends therapeutic management for the psychotic inpatient — work with other members of the family, milieu therapy, and social casework — and he suggests that psychotherapy may be of most help during the outpatient phase, after the current episode has responded to medication treatment. Moreover, May concludes that for neurotic outpatients, drugs generally should be used only when psychotherapy is not available or when its goals cannot be reached without the aid of drugs.

In their review of studies that compare combined treatment versus drugs alone versus psychotherapy alone, Luborsky, Singer, and Luborsky (1975) concluded that the combination of therapy and drugs is clearly superior to either drugs alone or therapy alone.

Hollon and Beck (1978) summarized seven additional studies (Claghorn, Johnstone, Cook, and Itschner, 1974; Lipsedge, Hajioff, Huggins, Napier, Pearce, Pike, and Rich, 1973; Paul, Tobias, and Holly, 1972; Rush, Beck, Kovacs, and Hollon, 1977; Shader, Grinspoon, Ewalt, and Zahn, 1969; Solyon, Heseltine, McClure, Solyon, Ledridge, and Steinberg, 1973; Zitrin, Klein, Lindemann, Tobak, Rock, Kaplan, and Ganz, 1976) that did not appear in the Smith et al. (1980) review (mentioned in detail below), and used many of the other studies that were included in previous reviews. This 1978 review covered research in the following areas: depression, anxiety states and phobias, and schizophrenia.

According to Hollon and Beck (1978), only cognitive therapy among the psychotherapies had a direct effect on the depressive symptomatology, while individual therapy and marital therapy had positive effects on related phenomena, such as marital interaction. The combination of drugs and therapy may have joint but independent effects on different but related phenomena, thus broadening the impact provided by the drugs or therapy for depression, if these were delivered alone.

Three studies reviewed in the treatment of phobias yielded inconclusive data, according to the reviewers. Lipsedge (1973) found no differences in the comparison of combined drug and behavior therapy, behavior therapy and placebo, and drug alone in treatment of agoraphobics. Solyon et al. (1973) found no difference between behavior therapy versus drug plus supportive therapy, but the medication was superior to placebo in conjunction with supportive therapy. Zitrin et al. (1976) found drug plus behavior therapy or drug plus supportive therapy superior to placebo plus behavior therapy for agoraphobia, but not for specific phobic conditions.

In seven studies reviewed on chronic schizophrenic inpatients, the reviewers (Hollon and Beck, 1978) concluded that drug and psychotherapy combinations appeared to add little over drugs alone. However, in two of these studies (Evangelakis, 1961; Honigfeld, Rosenblum, Blumenthal, Lambert, and Roberts, 1965), adjunctive therapy and group therapy did have some impact on such dimensions as time of discharge, irritability, cooperation, and personal neatness. In three of four studies reviewed on acute onset inpatient schizophrenics, drugs alone were superior to psychotherapy and equivalent to drug plus psychotherapy. In the maintenance of schizophrenics, one study (Paul et al., 1972) found positive behavioral changes associated with social skills training. A second study (Hogarty et al., 1973) found that drugs have a significant effect in reducing the need for rehospitalization of schizophrenics, while social role therapy had little to add except possibly in a subsample of the patients.

Smith et al. (1980) have summarized six reviews of studies comparing combinations of therapy and drug versus psychotherapy (pp. 136–140). The reviews summarized and compared included: Luborsky et al., 1975; Uhlenhuth, Lipman, and Covi, 1969; May, 1968, 1971; Gilligan, 1965; and GAP, 1975). The only major review prior to 1980 that is not included is that of Hollon and Beck (1978) which we have mentioned already. In their review of the reviews, Smith et al. aggregate studies and arrive at the following summary: 22 studies showed drug plus psychotherapy superior to psychotherapy alone, while 12 showed the combination equal to psychotherapy. Drug therapy was less effective than the combination in nine studies, while 16 showed them to be equal in effect and only one study showed drug superior to drug plus psychotherapy. Drug alone was more effective than therapy alone in 11 studies, five showed them equal, and, in three, therapy was superior to drug. The obvious problem with such a general overview is that it summarizes somewhat mindlessly across drugs and diagnostic groups, and thus leaves the clinician without guidelines as to precisely when to combine therapy and drugs, when to go more with one or the other.

In their own meta-analysis (to be discussed in more detail in Chapter 8), Smith et al. (1980) used all known studies in which drug therapy was compared to drug plus therapy. In contrast with many prior reviews that required certain specifications before a study would be included in the review, Smith et al. included studies without requirements for proper drug dose level, patient diagnosis, duration of treatment, homogeneity of patient subsample, and so forth. This strategy was used to avoid selectivity and bias in the resulting review and conclusions, but it does leave the results wide open to dispute. The relevant Smith et al. findings may be summarized as follows:

1) The separate effect size for psychotherapy alone (.31) is essentially the same as that for drug therapy alone (.42).
2) The interactive effect of drugs and therapy is virtually nil: .02. Their effects are therefore essentially additive.
3) The effect sizes went in order of decreasing magnitude from anti-anxiety drugs to antipsychotic drugs to antidepressant drugs. This may have to do with the high level of placebo response in depressed patients.
4) The effect sizes for drugs only in schizophrenics (.495) and depressives (.367) are less than for the combination of drugs and therapy for schizophrenics (.802) and depressives (.460).

Smith and colleagues conclude that even in the serious illnesses, therapy is nearly as effective as drug therapy. When provided together, the combination produced essentially the same net effect as the sum of their separate effects, thus giving no evidence for synergistic or negatively interacting effects. As we will discuss in considerable detail in the next chapter, the major limitation of the Smith, Glass, and Miller review lies not with their method of meta-analysis, but rather with the data that are aggregated. Much of the available outcome research has been weak in design and inadequate in the definition of patient groups, treatments, and measures. Smith and her associates believe that their overall review is more robust than are the individual studies forming its data base. However, caution is indicated until the method of meta-analysis is applied to better outcome data.

Specific Research Studies

While the aggregation of studies is extremely important in making generalizations, it is only by considering the results of individual investigations that one can make statements about specific drug and therapy combinations for specific diagnoses and target symptoms. We will review several relevant, well-done, and influential studies that examine the efficacy of psychotherapy in combination with chemotherapy in the treatment of schizophrenic, depressive, and anxiety disorders.

The New Haven-Boston collaborative depression project

The New Haven-Boston Collaborative Depression Project, conducted by Klerman and associates (Klerman, Dimascio, and Weissman, 1974), provides interesting data on the differential effects of drug treatment and psychotherapy in outpatients who are depressed and nonpsychotic.

The subjects were 150 moderately depressed women between the ages of 29 and 60. Patients who had a depression of at least two weeks' duration that reached a total rating of 7 or more on the Raskin Depression Scale were admitted to the acute treatment phase of the study and received amitriptyline. Those who showed at least a 50% improvement on the Raskin Depression Scale at the end of four-to-six-weeks of the medication treatment were assigned randomly to an experimental maintenance treatment design – to receive either weekly psychotherapy (high contact) with a psychiatric social worker or monthly brief interviews (low contact) for assessment and drug prescription with a psychiatrist. Both the psychotherapy group and the low contact group continued to receive amitriptyline for two or more months and then were further randomized as to drug. One-third of the psychotherapy patients received amitriptyline, one-third were withdrawn double-blind onto placebo, and one-third were withdrawn overtly onto no medication. An equal distribution was also made for the low contact group. Treatment continued in this way for a further six months.

The high contact psychotherapy was done by a social worker in a minimum of one session per week. The therapy is described as supportive with a focus on current problems, maladaptive interpersonal patterns, and the achievement of better levels of adaptation. Multiple outcome measures were used throughout the eight months. Clinical relapse was defined as return to depressive symptoms at the level of 7 or more on the Raskin Depression Scale. Symptoms were measured by self-report and psychiatrist rating, and social adjustment was assessed.

In summary, the results indicated a differential effect for drug therapy and psychotherapy. Compared to placebo medication and no medication, amitriptyline significantly reduced relapse rate and prevented a return of depressive symptomatology, but it had no greater effect on social adjustment. In contrast, psychotherapy did not prevent relapse or symptom return but did significantly increase social adjustment ratings in those patients who completed the eight-month trial of therapy and did not relapse. The psychotherapy significantly improved work performance and marital and family communication and decreased interpersonal arguments, resentment, subjective feelings of stress, and anxious dissatisfaction.

What differential therapeutic guidelines can be drawn from this study? The authors argue that this investigation supports the utilization of psychotherapy (supportive) for six to eight months for the enhancement of social adjustment of a recovered, depressed (moderate) female outpatient. The efficacy of this psychotherapy, however, is contingent on the patient remaining symptomatically well, either by psychopharmacology or natural remission. The appropriate goal of the psychotherapy is increased social adjustment and not the prevention of relapse or depressive symptoms. Amitriptyline is the appropriate treatment if the goal is prevention of relapse; such treatment reduces the relapse rate by around 50%.

Thus, the following guidelines are useful: 1) Maintenance treatment of moderate depression in those who initially respond to chemotherapy is best handled with continued chemotherapy. Supportive psychotherapy has little if any impact on this course; 2) those ambulatory, depressed patients with problems in social relationships and work adjustment could be assigned to supportive psychotherapy, if the goal is improvement in such areas. Many, probably most, patients will require both.

One comes away from the Klerman study still wondering about the extent to which there is any direct connection between faulty interpersonal adjustment and mild to moderate depression. The psychotherapy performed on this group of depressed patients was not very specific and could just as well have been done on a nondepressed group of patients with faulty social and work adjustment. It may well be that the psychotherapy produces results most specific to the areas on which it is focused. Beck and his colleagues in a study to be discussed next have developed a cognitive therapy that is more focused on variables related to depression and therefore may possibly be more potent in directly treating depression than was the psychotherapy used by the Klerman group. In fact, there is now under way a large, multicentered collaborative study, investigating this question, as well as studying the interaction of each form of psychotherapy with antidepressant medication.

Cognitive therapy vs. chemotherapy in the treatment of depression

Rush, Beck, Kovacs, and Hollon (1977) compared cognitive psychotherapy as contrasted to imipramine in the treatment of unipolar, depressed outpatients. Thirty-nine percent of the sample had been depressed for more than one year and more than 75% of the group complained of suicidal ideation. The patients were at least moderately depressed as defined by a score of 20 or more on the Hamilton Rating Scale for Depression and exhibited a depressive syndrome according to the Feighner criteria. Patients were excluded if they had a history of schizophrenia, alcoholism, drug addiction, bipolar disorder, organic brain syndrome, hallucinations or delusions, or poor response to a previous adequate trial of tricyclic medication.

Self-rating and clinical rating scales of symptomatology and standardized personality inventories were used as outcome measures. The treatment modalities were well specified. Cognitive therapy is described by Beck as a verbal and behavioral technique to assist the patient in learning to recognize his negative thoughts and distorted cognitions, their relationship to his mood, and to substitute more reality-oriented interpretations for his negative cognitions. The therapy was given for a maximum of 20 50-minute sessions. Pharmacotherapy involved once-a-week 20-minute sessions for a maximum of 12 treatment visits. These visits involved evaluation of the medications, as well as global supportive therapy. Imipramine was administered flexibly to obtain optimum clinical response.

The results indicated that in both treatment modalities the patients exhibited a statistically significant reduction in depressive symptomatology and a significant reduction in the level of anxiety. Independent ratings suggested that cognitive therapy produced significantly more improvement in depression scores than did pharmacotherapy. Fifteen of 18 cognitive therapy patients were judged to exhibit marked improvement or complete remission of symptoms, whereas only five of 14 psychopharmacological therapy patients did so. There was no significant difference in favor of one treatment over the other in anxiety reduction. Follow-up ratings indicated that the cognitive therapy group had significantly lower depression scores at three months, but that there was no significant difference at six months. Eight of the 22 patients assigned to pharmacotherapy discontinued treatment as compared to only one out of 19 in cognitive therapy – a statistically significant difference.

The findings of this study are at variance with the usual results of comparisons of pharmacotherapy with psychotherapy, and it will be interesting to learn if they hold up in the currently ongoing replication mentioned above. It is especially important to learn if there are possible additive or synergistic effects of the combination of cognitive therapy and pharmacotherapy both for acute depressive episodes and in prophylactic treatment. This study raised the exciting possibility that specific treatment packages composed of focused verbal and behavioral techniques can be effectively employed for the treatment of specific target symptoms.

Combined treatment of schizophrenia

May, Tuma, and colleagues (May, 1968; May and Tuma, 1965; May, Tuma, and Dixon, 1976) carried out an impressive and well-controlled investigation comparing the results of treatment of hospitalized schizophrenics receiving psychotherapy, psychotherapy plus neuroleptics, neuroleptics alone, electroconvulsive therapy, and standard hospital care. The therapists were inexperienced but supervised by experienced psychoanalysts. The therapy techniques emphasized ego support, definition of reality, confronting the patient about his or her conception of reality, and clarification of reality distortions. Treatment consisted on an average of one to two weekly sessions of one hour for one year or until the patient was discharged from the hospital. Following discharge, patients were followed for up to five years and assessed on a wide array of outcome measures, including the global rating, Camarillo Assessment Scale, behavioral ratings by nursing staff, ratings on idiosyncratic symptoms, and tally of subsequent days of hospitalization. The results indicated the clear superiority of antipsychotic drugs. Drug therapy was superior to psychotherapy, and psychotherapy was no more effective than the low contact therapy given to the control group. Drugs plus psychotherapy were only slightly better than the drugs alone. ECT treatment was intermediately effective.

This study has received great publicity and is outstanding for many of its design qualities including length of treatment, length of follow-up, and wide array of outcome measures. However, it can be criticized for having utilized inexperienced therapists, who were doing psychotherapy on schizophrenics who were not selected on the basis of suitability for psychotherapy. Indeed, in this regard, the heterogeneity of any group of schizophrenic patients is quite impressive and well-known to anyone who has worked clinically with such a population.

The community treatment of schizophrenic patients

In contrast to the studies done by May on the inpatient treatment of schizophrenia, Goldstein and his colleagues (Goldstein, Rodnick, Evans, May, and Steinberg, 1978) have done an impressive series of studies on the community treatment of schizophrenics following hospitalization. These studies are extremely relevant and clinically applicable in an era in which the schizophrenics are hospitalized for only brief periods of time and community placement and aftercare become a necessary and serious mental health issue. Goldstein et al. point out that the thrust of their investigation was not to ask whether psychotherapy is effective in helping the schizophrenic patient to reconstitute from psychosis but, rather, whether psychotherapies alone or combined with chemotherapy play a significant role in community adjustment once the patient's recompensation has been effected. The schizophrenic patients in this study were consecutive first and second inpatient admissions, released to the community after an average of 14 days of hospitalization. Upon admission to the hospital, patients were randomly assigned to either a high or low dose of fluphenazine and were kept on this dosage throughout the study. In addition, patients were randomly assigned to either crisis-oriented family therapy or no family therapy. The crisis-oriented therapy had the objective of helping the family to come to terms with the fact that a member had a psychosis, to identify possible precipitating stresses, and to plan family life in order to reduce these stresses in the future. The results suggest that both medication and family therapy play a significant role in decreasing relapses, and that the combination was particularly effective. The high dose plus therapy group had not a single relapse during the study period, while the low dose plus no therapy group had a 50% relapse rate.

Of special interest with regard to interaction effects were the therapists' ratings of the extent to which patients and families had reached the goals of family treatment. Results suggested that when a patient manifested hostility, suspicion, and uncooperativeness at discharge, high doses of phenothiazines were necessary to achieve family therapy goals. For patients below the median level of hostility at discharge, family therapy goals were more likely attained by patients assigned to the low dose condition.

CLINICAL GUIDELINES FOR COMBINATIONS OF TREATMENT

1) Medication should never be prescribed outside of a therapeutic relationship and is thus always a part of a combined treatment. The only question concerns the nature of the psychotherapeutic relationship that will most enhance medication compliance and overall treatment effect.

2) As research and clinical practice clarify the nature of specific treatment effects on specific problems, there will be increasing use of rationally planned combinations. A balance must be struck to avoid the extremes of providing a confusing and redundant plethora of treatments to each patient versus insisting that one global treatment will be a panacea.

3) It seems likely that the most effective therapies are those that flexibly and smoothly combine attention to psychodynamic, behavioral, cognitive, and social systems issues and techniques. Different treatments may be applied concurrently or sequentially, by different or the same therapist, and may be defined as separate entities or be delivered in a seamless fashion.

4) Combinations are most indicated for what Beutler (1983) has called "complex" problems. Perhaps the most frequent example is when the patient's treatment has short-term, circumscribed, and perhaps urgent goals, in addition to more ambitious, long-term goals (e.g., sex therapy for premature ejaculation, psychoanalysis for resolution of compulsive personality traits).

5) In our experience, certain combinations are particularly likely to be recommended:

(a) medication plus psychotherapy for the treatment of major affective and anxiety disorders;
(b) medication plus psychosocial and educative interventions for schizophrenia;
(c) behavioral plus psychodynamic interventions for anxiety, sexual, and personality disorders;
(d) individual and group therapies;
(e) family/marital and individual therapies (particularly in this sequence, although at times concurrently).

6) There is little research or experience on the contraindications for various combinations. One controversial possibility is that behavior therapy and psychotropic medication may not mix well in the treatment of anxiety disorders or depression, because the patient may attribute positive changes to the medication which would undercut the reinforcement of newly tried, anti-symptomatic behaviors.

7) Combinations of treatment have to be highly individualized not only to the needs, tastes, and enabling factors of the patient, but also to the resources of the system. Marginal utility and cost effectiveness may be an issue in allocating scarce therapeutic resources.

We have chosen to avoid any detailed discussion of a very interesting and important question, but one that is forbiddingly complicated. In what way do specific settings, formats, techniques, durations, intensities and medications covary with one another? Which combinations are particularly common and well-matched (e.g., a likely recommendation might be: setting/outpatient; format/individual; duration/brief; technique/behavioral therapy; frequency/once a week; without medication), and which are absurd and nonexistent (e.g., inpatient, group, psychoanalysis, done briefly in conjunction with chlorpromazine treatment).

Covariation of the various elements in the treatment plan is often crucial but is quite an individual matter about which it is hard to generalize. With certain borderline patients, for example, the use of psychodynamic techniques requires that the setting be quite structured (inpatient or day hospital) and an outpatient setting will imply that a more directive treatment is necessary, even though we generally do not closely associate inpatient settings and psychodynamic techniques as the most natural of matches. The process of linking choices along the steps of the decision tree makes the most demands on the art of treatment planning and is the researcher's nightmare.

SUMMARY

Combinations of various forms of psychiatric treatment are often more effective than any one of the components delivered alone. As treatments become more specific and targeted to particular types of patient problem, rational combinations emerge that are tailored to the individual's array of symptoms. The additive effects of psychotherapy and psychotropic medication have generally been established for a variety of psychiatric disorders. The combination of different psychotherapeutic techniques remains a topic of controversy and uncertainty. Clinical innovators naturally espouse the use of their techniques in relatively pure form, often for all types of problems. Experience suggests, however, that a flexible and creative weaving together of techniques derived from the various orientations provides maximum therapeutic effectiveness. This is a difficult, but necessary, arena for future research.

CHAPTER 7

No Treatment as the Recommendation of Choice

Now that we have considered methods of selecting a therapeutic setting, format, technique, frequency and duration, and have also described somatic treatment and ways of combining different kinds of treatment, we are better prepared to discuss what may be the most difficult of decisions for the consultant, a choice that is in fact all too often totally overlooked: Is psychiatric treatment advisable at all or would no treatment be the preferred recommendation?

This decision is frequently deferred, avoided, or left in the hands of the patient. In our own clinic, despite our interest in this topic and teaching on it, a recent survey of 500 consecutive evaluations revealed only four occasions when no treatment was recommended by the consultant. In discussing this matter with our staff and trainees, we found that on many more occasions the thought that treatment might not work had indeed occurred to them, but most consultants nonetheless preferred to recommend a treatment and to rely on the later judgment of either the therapist or the patient to terminate it, if the risks came to outweigh potential benefits. In our survey, 52 of the 500 patients did, in fact, refuse to continue evaluation or to accept the consultant's recommended treatment, indicating that patients were approximately ten times more prepared to initiate no treatment than were their consultants to offer it. We do not know how many other patients in this sample actually followed through with the proposed treatment in spite of the fact that they would have been better served without it — that is the very issue to be addressed in this chapter.

We will begin our discussion by examining the understandable reluctance of consultants to suggest to the patient that no treatment is the recommendation of choice. We will then describe some of the problems that may occur if the consultant does not overcome this reluctance and instead automatically recommends treatment to all who request it. The remainder of the chapter will provide clinical examples to illustrate some of the relative indications for recommending no treatment (these indications are outlined in Table 7-1). Unfortunately, the research regarding no treatment is so limited that we cannot present a separate section devoted to this area, but we will comment on whatever research is available and, in our concluding remarks, we will consider the methodological and ethical problems inherent in any investigation of no treatment.

RELUCTANCE TO RECOMMEND NO TREATMENT

One reason a consultant may be reluctant to consider no treatment is that the patients who are the most likely to qualify for this recommendation are often the most unfortunate and needy of people. In the main, these are not reasonably happy individuals for whom therapy would be an unnecessary extravagance; on the contrary, many of them are leading miserable lives, desperately want relief from their suffering, and may well continue to do poorly if left to their own devices. The consultant understandably wants to provide these patients with the help they seek and seemingly need, and is hesitant to turn them away without knowing for sure how they will fare on their own.

The consultant may also be reluctant to acknowledge the limitations and the risks of psychiatric treatment. The findings of outcome research demonstrate psychotherapy to be, on the average, significantly more effective than no treatment. Nonetheless, psychotherapy probably is analogous to any potent medicine: It may on occasion not only fail, but also induce its own particular brand of side effects, adverse reactions, dependency, and overdosage. The consultant is not necessarily rejecting the patient when he recommends no treatment, but rather is rejecting the erroneous assumption that "even if treatment may not help, it can't hurt."

Moreover, in his concern about a particular patient's problems, the consultant may lose sight of his responsibilities to the community at large. When the resources of the mental health system and of third-party payments are expended on any given patient, this necessarily limits their availability for someone else — someone who is perhaps more in need or more likely to benefit. Despite the immense difficulty and uncertainty of predicting in advance the outcome of a patient's treatment, the consultant has some obligation to make such an attempt. Although we hope to remind the consultant that every treatment requires a calculation of its risk/benefit and cost/benefit ratios, we are not advocating pessimism or austerity; rather, we are intending in some rough way to define psychotherapy's realistic limits and boundaries.

RISKS OF DEFERRING RECOMMENDATION OF NO TREATMENT

As pointed out above, consultants often routinely recommend treatment, even when this choice seems questionable, and defer the decision to forgo treatment to the therapist or the patient. Such a deferment is usually based on a belief that the therapist, after observing how the patient has responded to the early stages of a trial of treatment, will be in a better position to recommend no further treatment. This belief is often well-founded, but at times it serves as a rationalization for passing the buck. Once therapy is formally begun and both the patient and the therapist have together made a substantial commitment, their relationship gathers a momentum of its own (fraught with transference meanings) regardless of how well or poorly it is working. An investment of time, money, fantasies, feelings, and concern has been made, and both parties usually find it easier to continue their involvement with one another than to cut their losses, limit their goals, and acknowledge that no treatment might have been and might still be a preferred choice. Once the patient has developed strong transference feelings toward the therapist, a recommendation of no treatment will be understood and responded to within this frame of transference reference. The recommendation of no treatment can often be heard and accepted in a much more realistic way when it is made by a consultant who is not yet invested with the same degree of feeling or fantasy and who is more likely to be regarded as a disinterested expert without his own ax to grind.

Deferring the recommendation of no treatment has a number of inherent risks. If there is a lack of improvement or worsening of the patient's condition, the therapist may attribute this to some failure in the patient, rather than to the unsuitability of the therapy. Attempts are made to interpret the patient's "resistance" or to confront the patient's "lack of motivation." When these maneuvers prove futile, the inclination is then to change some aspect of the treatment – setting, format, technique, intensity – rather than to consider no treatment as the best option. When the patient still "fails to respond," the heated but stalemated therapeutic situation may ferment frustration and bitterness in both parties. The therapeutic climate beomes even more unsettling if the patient has actually gotten worse during the course of treatment.

Feeling at least partly responsible for this deterioration, the therapist may attempt to overcome his or her guilt with increased therapeutic zeal and the recommendation of no treatment becomes an even more untenable possibility. It is common to hope that more of the same will at some future point turn things around, even in face of impressive evidence to the contrary.

During peer reviews of cases in which the patient has remained unchanged or gotten worse, we have found that once therapists can disentangle themselves from the immediate pressures of the treatment, they often acknowledge (with hindsight) that perhaps no treatment might have been a better choice from the start. Not surprisingly, therapists are less able to make such an acknowledgment if the patient has improved. Many find it hard to admit that, despite the patient's improvement, the risks or liabilities of treatment might have been greater than its benefits. For those patients whose symptoms might have remitted spontaneously or who might have been able to use the help of relatives and friends rather than a therapist to achieve similar gains, dependency on treatment may have deprived them of a sense of mastery and autonomy and instead reinforced a false sense of helplessness when future crises occur.

RELATIVE INDICATIONS FOR NO TREATMENT

Having considered the reluctance of consultants to recommend no treatment and having mentioned some potential risks if the decision is deferred, we are now ready to examine what specific factors favor such a recommendation. The consultant is faced with the difficult task of predicting the future, that is, making an informed guess about what is most likely to happen if the patient receives one or another treatment or goes without. In Chapter 9 we will elaborate on the kinds of data, interviewing techniques, and procedures which can be helpful in this attempt. For now, we will concentrate on the more specific considerations regarding the recommendation of no treatment. For purposes of conceptualization, we have subdivided the relative indications for no treatment into three categories of treatment outcome: Treatment should be avoided because it may be 1) harmful and cause a negative response, 2) useless and lead to no response, or 3) unnecessary in a patient headed already for a spontaneous remission (see Table 7-1). After describing the patients and relevant research in each of these categories, we will discuss a fourth category in which the recommendation of no treatment is made as a specific therapeutic maneuver and not just to avoid the risks and costs of therapy.

TABLE 7-1
Relative Indications for No Treatment

Patients at Risk for Negative Response	Patients at Risk for No Response	Patients Likely to Have Spontaneous Improvement	Recommendations of No Treatment as a Therapeutic Intervention
Patients prone to severe negative therapeutic reactions, such as severe masochistic, narcissistic, and oppositional patients. Possible exception: – brief, unambitious treatment if need immense and unavoidable	Antisocial or criminal behavior. Possible exceptions: – coexisting treatable psychiatric disorder. – no evasion of legal responsibility by becoming psychiatric patient	Healthy patients in crisis. Possible exceptions: – history of pathological response to similar crisis – presence of pathological symptoms or mourning process – avoidance of crisis, mourning or developmental tasks – nontechnical help (friend, family, church, etc.) unavailable or has not worked	Oppositional patients refusing treatment
Borderline patients with a history of treatment failures. Possible exceptions: – circumscribed problem amenable to brief treatment – life immediately endangered or absolutely intolerable – opportunity and resources for the first time to obtain expert treatment	Patients with malingering or factitious illness. Possible exceptions: – malingering result of treatable psychiatric disorder	Healthy patients with minor chronic problems. Possible exception: – training purposes	To support adaptive defenses
Patients who enter treatment primarily to support a lawsuit or to justify a claim for compensation or disability. Possible exceptions: – coexisting treatable psychiatric disorder. – chronic invalidism so severe that therapeutic support is necessary	The iatrogenically infantilized patient. Possible exceptions: – severe refractory impairment requiring continuous maintenance therapy – history of suicide attempts, decompensation, and deterioration when patient out of treatment – long-term medication regimen		Advisable delay in starting treatment
	Poorly motivated patients without incapacitating symptoms		

1) Patients at Risk for Negative Response

Patients prone to immutable negative therapeutic reactions

"Negative therapeutic reaction" is a technical term originally introduced by Freud (1955d) to describe patients who pradoxically became worse in response to a correct interpretation at a time when they seemed most likely to achieve a beneficial result from the treatment. This intriguing, but frustrating, phenomenon has since been observed and elaborated by numerous authors (e.g., Sandler, Holder, and Dave, 1973); two major explanations have been offered:

1) In masochistic patients, the negative therapeutic reaction represents a need to remain sick or even to become worse as a form of punishment; this punishment is necessary either to assuage an abiding sense of guilt or to maintain a relationship with an ambivalently perceived and punishing love object (represented now by the therapist);
2) In narcissistic and oppositional patients, the negative therapeutic reactions represent a wish to defeat the therapist and to prevent him or her from being helpful, useful, or important; the patient is able in this way to remain autonomous, distant, and superior.

The terms *negative therapeutic reaction* and *negative therapeutic outcome* have often been confused or used interchangeably, but it is useful to keep their definitions distinct. The term *negative therapeutic reaction* does not describe those treatments that have a negative outcome because of faulty technique or poor patient-therapist match, because the wrong treatment was chosen, or because the natural course of the patient's condition is downhill. The term applies instead to those therapeutic situations in which the patient's self-defeating character traits work tenaciously to subvert and sabotage progress just when substantial gains are liable to be made. Although the concept has been most extensively described by psychoanalysts, characteristics within the patient probably comprise at least to some extent the otherwise unaccountable failures experienced in any form of treatment. This may even be true for strategic therapists, like Haley (1963), who cleverly and paradoxically attempt to short-circuit negative therapeutic reactions by becoming even more negative than the oppositional patient. The therapist might state, "I agree that this problem is hopeless. If anything, you are underestimating the difficulties." It is hoped that the oppositional patient will be forced to do well in order to defeat the therapist. It is our impression that this maneuver is unsuccessful (and potentially dangerous) when the negative therapeutic reaction is motivated by guilt rather than oppositionalism.

The extent of damage done during a negative therapeutic reaction varies greatly. In some patients it amounts to no more than the average expected resistance to treatment and becomes a useful, often a central, arena for investigation into self-defeating patterns of behavior. In other patients, the need to be punished or to defeat the therapist is so strong that treatment remains a futile endeavor throughout. At the far end of this spectrum, the negative therapeutic reaction can be life-threating. The case of Ms. C. illustrates this potential.

THE CASE OF THE SELF-DESTRUCTIVE SUICIDE

Ms. C.'s life was filled with tragedy. Her mother died during her childbirth. Her father remarried two months later but shortly thereafter he left home in the throes of a drunken binge and never returned. Ms. C. was left to be raised by the young, abandoned bride. Although the "wicked stepmother" displaced her bitterness about being deserted onto the hated and physically abused child, she also sought solace from her loneliness by clinging to Ms. C. Before this ambivalent relationship could be at all resolved, the stepmother contracted tuberculosis. Throughout grade school Ms. C. ushered her stepmother through a prolonged, debilitating illness. This ended in a nightmarish, fatal bout of hemoptysis that allegedly occurred on the very day that Ms. C. had her first menstrual period.

Ms. C. was then bounced from one foster home to another. Finally, she experienced a series of rapes by a foster father and took to the streets to begin a career of prostitution and pushing drugs. At the age of 16, following her fourth arrest, she was referred by the court for psychiatric treatment. Ms. C. was all but "adopted" by a young female social worker who met with the patient daily, telephoned her during weekends, and offered a maximum of support and guidance in helping Ms. C. obtain a job as a filing clerk. This well-meaning therapist was totally unprepared for what followed when she mentioned with some admiration and pride that Ms. C. was doing so well and seemed to have turned the corner. The patient quickly sabotaged all the gains that had been made. She went to work drunk, became abusive, and lost her job. She then began to miss her appointments and was out of touch for three weeks until the therapist was awakened at home early one morning by a telephone call from Ms. C., who had been arrested for shoplifting in a liquor store.

Disappointed and frustrated, the social worker countered her guilt over being angry at the patient by becoming even more solicitous and caring. It was not until Ms. C. superficially cut her wrist that her therapist began to feel out of her depth. When Ms. C. was hospitalized for this suicidal gesture, the social worker felt safe in telling her that treatment would now have to stop since it seemed to be causing more harm than good. Probably in reaction to this, Ms. C.'s hospitalization was particularly stormy and characterized by temper tantrums and multiple suicide attempts before she could finally be discharged to a day hospital, four months later.

Although the experience of the therapist and the particulars of the therapy could perhaps explain Ms. C.'s negative response to treatment in this one instance, the same pattern was to be repeated again and again during the next several years with other therapists of different persuasions, disciplines, expertise, style, and techniques. A hostile dependent relationship would evolve quickly and then inevitably result in a suicide attempt whenever the patient began to improve or whenever an actual or symbolic separation was in sight. This same pattern occurred also with her numerous lovers, who at first would find her immensely appealing and attractive, take her underwing, and then become enmeshed in a clinging, destructive relationship from which they could not disentangle gracefully. Attempts to interpret the patient's guilt over the death of her mother, her rage at her father and stepmother, her identification with lost objects, and her need to self-destruct in order to defeat and cling to therapists and lovers were to no avail. Such correct and timely interpretations would usually be followed by negative reactions.

At the age of 34, after being abandoned by yet one more lover, Ms. C. mailed a long and moving poem to her original therapist describing a baby bleeding to death while the umbilical cord was in the process of being slashed. On the date of the postmark, Ms. C. was found dead in a pool of blood in a public bathroom where she had repeatedly stabbed herself in the belly.

Most often, negative therapeutic reactions are far more subtle and less destructive than the one that ended Ms. C.'s life. Although we do not know how her course might have evolved without any psychiatric intervention, we cannot assume blithely that the treatment did no harm. Her story emphasizes that for patients who have demonstrated a devastating proneness to negative therapeutic reactions in their previous treatments, additional treatment should probably be offered only if the need is very great and unavoidable. Even if unavoidable, treatment should in most instances be brief and unambitious so that there is little opportunity for the patient to defeat therapeutic optimism or punish him/herself for being given or for taking too much.

Borderline patients with a history of treatment failures

The borderline personality disorder constitutes a syndrome that is variously defined by a growing, if very vague and unsystematic, literature. The most consistent deficits are affective, behavioral, and interpersonal instability and a fragile sense of self. The more severely afflicted patients have a tendency to become at least briefly psychotic in times of stress and to lead chaotic lives punctuated by stormy and unsatisfying relationships. The relative refractoriness of borderline patients to treatment has often been noted, as has their poor tolerance of the ambiguities, temptations, and frustrations of the transference situation (Kernberg, Bernstein, Coyne, Appelbaum, Horwitz, and Voth, 1972). They are prone to actualize their transference fantasies rather than to investigate them and often they do this in the most self-destructive and provocative manner. In extreme cases, this actualization takes on a delusional intensity and becomes a "transference psychosis."

The following case illustrates how psychiatric treatment, particularly those kinds that are intense and dyadic, must be regarded as a high risk procedure for at least some people with borderline personality disorders.

THE CASE OF THE TRANSFERENCE STORMS

Ms. R. began her career as a psychiatric patient when, as a college junior, she was accepted as a training case by a psychoanalytic institute. A bright, articulate, and attractive woman, she complained at that time of "jealousy" and "a hypercritical attitude" toward herself and others. The induction into analysis went smoothly enough and session after session she produced engaging and insightful tales of her urban Jewish life and proclaimed herself a "female Portnoy." After two years of analysis, she had entered a graduate psychology program and begun a sexually intimate relationship with a medical student.

Ms. R.'s life and analysis were proceeding so well that her analyst was completely unprepared for the chaotic events that occurred during his August vacation. Ms. R. had been uncharacteristically promiscuous during his absence, had become pregnant, and was now considering marriage to the medical student's divorced father. She described her analyst's interpretations of this acting-out as "obvious" and "pedantic." Her frenetic behavior outside the analysis diminished but only because she became inordinately preoccupied with the analyst's opinion of her. She could not decide when to do the laundry or what to cook for dinner without first pondering how the analyst would judge such a decision. These ruminations became paralyzing and as a result, she could not date, socialize, or attend classes. Furthermore, despite her analyst's urgings, she could not decide whether or not to have an abortion because she believed the analyst might not really mean what he was recommending. In brief, by the final week of her pregnancy, Ms. R.'s life consisted only of attending her daily sessions and for the rest of the day sitting alone in her studio apartment thinking about her analyst and writing intellectualized journals about her psychodynamics. Her parents had disowned her, her friends were ostracized, and her analyst felt powerless to influence events even when he introduced more structuring and directive techniques. Ms. R.'s destructive downhill course continued to gather momentum. Finally, she became flagrantly bizarre in her thoughts and behavior two days after the delivery of a stillborn son and she was transferred to a psychiatric hospital.

The staff on the inpatient ward was highly critical of Ms. R.'s psychoanalyst and blamed him for causing the patient's decline. Her new therapist, a female psychiatry resident, used neuroleptics and supportive interventions to usher Ms. R. out of her brief psychosis and, after four weeks, out of the hospital. Ms. R. went on to obtain her master's degree in psychology, worked part-time as a waitress, and resumed dating. Soon, however she became involved in a lesbian relationship with her new boyfriend's pubescent sister. She announced to her new therapist, and then inappropriately to everyone else, that she was a confirmed lesbian. When the young girl's parents discovered the homosexual affair, they exposed and humiliated Ms. R. in a manner that contributed to another profound depression, serious suicide attempt, and rehospitalization. She refused to continue with her female therapist and held her responsible for her homosexual affair.

The same pattern of therapy repeated itself again and again. A honeymoon period of mutual admiration shared by patient and therapist would be followed by a series of successes, an unexpressed intense transference involvement, unpredicted self-destructive acts, and eventually a profound crash. Changes in setting, format, technique, and intensity made no difference, nor did trials of phenothiazines, antidepressants, or lithium modify the pattern. After ten years of different treatments and during Ms. R.'s fifth psychiatric hospitalization, a consulting psychiatrist suggested a trial of no treatment. The reasons for this recommendation were carefully explained to the patient, namely, that treatment seemed more to complicate her life than to help her and that she would be wise to make do as best she could on her own. Ms. R. agreed. Two-and-a-half years later, by a coincidental follow-up, the consulting psychiatrist learned that Ms. R. had been working steadily and reliably as a secretary for a lawyer.

The case of Ms. R. indicates how repeated treatment may increase rather than sort out the chaos in such a patient's life. Our evaluation service is frequently visited by borderline patients who are seeking relief from treatments that have failed or are failing; and not infrequently we find ourselves similarly stalemated in our own work with such patients. Certainly some borderline patients are able to use supportive or exploratory therapies in a constructive manner, but our experience strongly suggests that the current methods of community care for a subgroup of borderline patients often causes more havoc than cure.

There is an urgent need for well-designed studies to compare the outcome of borderline patients who have been randomized to various treatment modalities and also to no treatment at all. As a first attempt, the Menninger (Kernberg et al., 1972) study examined the results in a handful of therapies with such patients. The findings were that an intense, expressive therapy was superior to a supportive one, and that the therapist's skill was much more important in promoting the successful treatment of borderline than of healthier patients. The serious methodological problems of this study and the few patients from which the conclusions were generalized have been noted by us (Perry, Frances, Klar, and Clarkin, in press) and by others (Malan, 1973; May, 1973; McNair, 1976). We should be aware that, although borderline patients may be leading miserable lives and often are crying out for treatment, psychotherapy for this subgroup of patients has distinct limitations and serious risks. Although, the case of Ms. R. does not provide systematic evidence, it offers support and courage to the consultant who recommends no treatment as a preferred alternative for borderline patients who have had repeated treatment failures and dangerous transference actualizations. We include a separate section later on in the chapter, in which we specify four exceptions when therapy might be advisable for a borderline patient.

Patients who enter treatment to support a lawsuit or to justify a claim for compensation or disability

When faced with patients in the above situations, the consultant must try to distinguish primary from secondary gain. The terms have often been used ambiguously and incorrectly. Primary gain is the reduction of intrapsychic conflict achieved by the symptoms and results from the operation of unconscious defense mechanisms. Secondary gain represents the benefits which come to the individual secondarily and which reinforce the intrapsychic resolution. The following vignette illustrates these two phenomena.

THE CASE OF THE DIZZY LONGSHOREMAN

Mr. M., a robust longshoreman, had worked in shipyards since his youth and had always been praised by his employers for his zeal and fearlessness in tackling the most difficult assignments. At the age of 32 he was temporarily knocked unconscious as a result of a co-worker's error and, although he had no signs of serious injury, he was hospitalized for a brief period of observation. In part because he was an appealing fellow with colorful stories of the docks, Mr. M. was chosen by the medical students for a psychiatric teaching conference regarding reactions of patients to medical illness.

During the first half of the interview Mr. M. spun out his entertaining tales of the waterfront, but during the second half he felt "slightly dizzy" as he revealed to the psychiatrist that his father had been an alcoholic and was often physically violent to his mother and the children. A few hours after the interview, the medical students were feeling concerned (and perhaps guilty) about subjecting this admired patient to the clinical conference. Several students returned to the patient's bedside to comfort and reassure Mr. M., but their reassurance had just the opposite effect from what they intended: Mr. M. again began to feel increasingly dizzy, worried about irreversible brain damage from the trauma, and convinced that he would not be able to return to work. The more the concerned medical students spoke with Mr. M. about his fears and problems in the present and in the past, the more dizzy and upset he became. He told his wife that there must be something seriously wrong with him since the doctors were constantly in attendance around his bedside.

Over the next week of Mr. M.'s hospitalization, the attending physician tried in vain to tell Mr. M. that no neurological reason for his dizziness could be found. Mr. M. refused to leave the hospital until he had "a better answer and more care." A psychiatrist was called. This psychiatrist (not the one who had interviewed Mr. M. initially) suspected that the patient's dizziness was a conversion reaction stemming from the anxiety stirred up by remembering and recounting upsetting events in the patient's past. It could also have resulted from hyperventilation. The primary gain reflected in his dizziness was the intrapsychic resolution of the conflict over his violent anger toward the co-worker who was responsible for his injury and toward his father, and the reciprocal fear that he would be subjected to further violent attacks. The secondary gain included his ability to avoid the waterfront and to engage the interest and admiration of the medical students and of other hospital staff. The consulting psychiatrist recommended that the patient be discharged with routine follow-up care and that psychiatric support not be provided at this time. He suggested that the physician state unequivocally that the patient could and should return to work, that he did not require compensation, and in fact would be harmed by it. This recommendation was not accepted by the treating physician, who instead referred the patient to the psychiatrist who had done the initial interview with the students. After this referral, Mr. M. agreed to leave the hospital, but after four months of psychiatric treatment, he still had not returned to work. Only when the attending physician finally refused to sign the disability forms any longer and the patient could no longer afford psychiatric treatment did Mr. M. eventually return to the waterfront.

As the case of Mr. M. points out, the possible psychiatric and material benefits to be derived from treatment must be balanced against the danger that psychiatric treatment inadvertently will encourage chronic invalidism. If the patient has a treatable psychiatric disorder, then the risk of increasing secondary gain may be worth taking. In addition, some patients are already so disabled by secondary gain that, paradoxically, they may require psychiatric treatment in order to be weaned off gradually from the benefits that have accrued from illness; and in extreme cases, some patients have become so dependent upon secondary gain that they require the support and gratification of psychiatric treatment in an ongoing way. These exceptions do not, however, contradict the general principle that no treatment should be considered as a recommendation for those patients who are consciously or unconsciously seeking further reinforcement of their secondary gain.

Research regarding negative response

Little information is available on the specific patient attributes that predict a negative response to psychiatric treatment. Uncontrolled studies suggest that severely disturbed patients may deteriorate in some exploratory individual and group therapies (Aronson and Weintraub, 1968; Fairweather, Simon, Gebhard, Weingarten, Holland, Sanders, Stone, and Reahl, 1960; Kernberg et al., 1972; Weber, Elinson, and Moss, 1965). However, conceivably these same patients might have benefited from other forms of treatment and they do not necessarily constitute a group for whom no treatment would have been the preferred recommendation. Strupp and his associates (Strupp, Fox, and Lessler, 1969) were interested in the negative responses to psychotherapy and conducted a survey of experienced therapists whose opinion it was that negative responses are related to some of the personality factors we have already mentioned (borderline and masochistic), to the patient's low ego strength and motivation, and to lack of skill in the therapist.

The most extensive review of negative responses was done by Bergin and Lambert (1978), who summarize data from 40 reports of negative outcome from psychotherapy. In the nine best studies, the occurrence of negative responses ranged from 3% to 28%, but the value of these findings was compromised by considerable limitations in the research designs. Some studies did not distinguish a negative response from a nonresponse (Cartwright and Vogel, 1960); other studies assumed a negative response only on the basis of differential variance in treatment outcome (Carkhuff and Truax, 1965; Mink and Isaksen, 1959); and two studies could not distinguish which negative responses were the result of psychotherapy and which were due to other interventions (Powers and Witmer, 1951; Fairweather et al., 1960). These inconclusive reports suggest that researchers must make greater efforts to measure negative results and the factors that predict them.

2) Patients at Risk for No Response

Antisocial or criminal behavior

The legal system, as well as the individual offender, is often quite happy to have a legal charge converted into a psychiatric problem. This happens in various ways. The apprehending police officer usually has wide personal discretion in deciding whether a given lawbreaker should be brought to jail and booked or instead be taken to a psychiatric facility and admitted. Even if the offender is taken to jail, he may still be labeled a psychiatric patient if he appears unable to participate in his defense, if he is declared incompetent to stand trial, or if he makes a suicide attempt. And even if the offender is not remanded to a psychiatric hospital and does eventually go to trial, the court may determine that he is not responsible for his acts and can recommend psychiatric observation and treatment. Finally, the court may find that the individual is responsible and guilty but permit the penalties to be suspended if the offender agrees to pursue psychiatric treatment. The role of psychiatric patient is thus a frequent alternative to assuming criminal responsibility.

Mental health professionals must be wary of colluding with the legal system too readily and encouraging this potentially disastrous conversion from criminal offender to psychiatric patient. Because of our belief in unconscious processes and psychic determinism, we may as a group be too prone to regard antisocial behavior as the result of forces beyond the individual's willed control and therefore be too eager to try to treat and change criminal offenders. This spreading of the treatment umbrella is sometimes undertaken despite compelling evidence that most offenders do not have treatable psychiatric disorders (Liss and Frances, 1975). We may do a disservice to society, the legal system, the offenders, and ourselves if we are too willing to treat problems for which no effective treatment is available. The case of Mr. V. illustrates this point.

THE CASE OF THE UNACCOUNTABLE ACCOUNTANT

Mr. V. claimed that he left his Ivy League college during his junior year because of "administrative hassles," but the truth was that he was forced to leave when the school uncovered his clever way of cheating during exams. To avoid the draft and Vietnam, Mr. V. joined the Marines and used his father's political clout to assure a desirable assignment in the States as a general's assistant. Mr. V.'s charm, wit, and intelligence impressed the general and led to exceptionally rapid promotions; but when Mr. V. was caught black-marketing the general's personal supplies, he barely escaped a court martial before being granted a general administrative discharge. Mr. V. embellished his military career to make it look far more distinguished than it actually was and forged letters of recommendation in order to be readmitted to college. He studied accounting and was graduated.

Mr. V. had joked with friends that "you can marry more money in a minute than you can make in a lifetime" and he managed to marry the daughter of a wealthy corporate executive. He settled comfortably into a leisurely life of late breakfasts, long lunches with clients, and afternoon squash games at the University Club. After ten years of marriage, numerous casual affairs, a wife whom he largely ignored, and two children he "adored" but hardly knew, Mr. V. was completely unprepared for the events to follow. His wife and one child were killed in a car accident and his father-in-law (never much of an admirer of Mr. V.) established a trust for the remaining grandchild, but cut off all other support. Mr. V. was now forced to earn a living.

Four years later Mr. V. was indicted for embezzlement and attempts to defraud a small accounting firm. While the matter was sluggishly making its way through the courts, he consulted a psychiatrist because he was "depressed." After 18 months of conducting weekly psychotherapy, the therapist was subpoenaed to appear in court by Mr. V.'s lawyer, who argued convincingly to the jury that Mr. V.'s "depression" after the loss of his wife had caused the crime—after all, Mr. V. had sought extensive psychiatric treatment. Whereas the psychiatrist had hoped eventually to treat Mr. V.'s psychopathic tendencies, he had unwittingly given them support. Whether Mr. V. could have been more amenable to treatment if convicted of his crimes cannot be known.

Having observed many cases similar to that of Mr. V., we believe that when evaluating patients who have manifested antisocial behavior, the consultant should determine to what extent a treatable psychiatric disorder (such as psychosis or organic mental syndrome) is present. If this is not the case, a legal or correctional disposition is usually more appropriate than psychiatric treatment. If the person will not evade legal responsibility by becoming a patient or if the therapy can be provided within the auspices of the legal system, then the consultant can be somewhat less cautious in recommending treatment.

Patients with malingering or factitious illness

The essential feature of malingering is the voluntary production and presentation of false or grossly exaggerated physical or psychological symptoms. The symptoms are produced in pursuit of a goal that is obviously recognizable. Malingering may be used to avoid work, to get out of military service, to obtain financial compensation, to avoid criminal prosecution, or to obtain drugs. Factitious disorders are also voluntary and may mimic physical or psychological symptoms, but they have a compulsive quality and are done more for psychological reasons than for obvious material gain. An example would be the nurse who ingests anticoagulants in order to produce hematuria and to be cared for in a hospital. Although malingering and factitious illness are motivated by different factors (material vs. psychological gain), they share the aspects of conscious deception and a generally poor response to psychiatric treatment. For these reasons, they have been combined here for purposes of discussion.

As noted, the criterion that distinguishes malingering and factitious disorder from other diagnostic categories is the conscious intent to deceive. (Conscious and unconscious motivations are on a continuum and the consultant must use inference, judgment, and corroborative evidence in deciding the extent to which the patient is aware of the deception.) Suspicion of malingering should be aroused if the patient has an antisocial personality disorder, does not cooperate with the diagnostic evaluation and prescribed treatment, shows a marked discrepancy between the objective findings and the claimed distress or disability, or presents in a medical-legal context, e.g., is referred by an attorney representing the client after an accident. Whenever malingering or factitious disorders are suspected, the consultant must exclude other diagnostic possibilities. These include: 1) conversion symptoms (the unconscious assumption of disability for primary gain); 2) a delusional system (the false belief in the existence of disease); 3) somatic preoccupations (as occur, for example, in hypochondriacal and depressed patients); and 4) actual physical or psychiatric disease beyond the detection of current technology.

After excluding other diagnostic possibilities, the consultant's next task is to determine if the malingering or factitious disorder is primary or secondary to a treatable condition. In the former situation, no treatment is often the preferred recommendation; in the latter, suitable treatment for the primary condition is indicated. The case of Mrs. K. illustrates how deception, even though conscious and intentional, may be the result of treatable underlying emotional problems. In this context, treatment is indicated.

THE CASE OF FEIGNED FEVER

A psychiatric consultation was requested for Mrs. K., a 46-year-old woman admitted to the neurology service with a low-grade fever and complaints of memory lapses. She had been hospitalized twice during the preceding three months, once complaining of chest pains and shortness of breath and once complaining of fever. On neither admission was any abnormality discovered on physical examination or after extensive laboratory investigations. During the second admission, a nurse had discovered her holding a thermometer under running hot water. This behavior was not challenged at the time, but Mrs. K. did remain afebrile throughout the remainder of the hospitalization.

During the consultation, the psychiatrist was able to elicit Mrs. K.'s unhappy life history. She was pregnant at the time of her marriage 24 years earlier. Her son from that pregnancy was diagnosed in early childhood as having systemic lupus erythematosus, and demands for his medical care created severe strains in her marriage. Her disabled son eventually required maintenance institutionalization and her second child, a daughter, also had SLE and had died of complications five years previously. Of note, the symptoms prompting the daughter's terminal hospitalization had been chest pain and shortness of breath.

The son's deterioration, the daughter's death, the husband's alcoholism, and Mrs. K.'s despair all further weakened the marriage. At the time of the consultation, Mrs. K. was separated from her husband and filing for divorce. She openly admitted that the three hospitalizations would be used in court by her attorney as evidence to substantiate her demand for a large financial settlement so that future medical expenses would be covered. But Mrs. K. appeared to be less concerned about her own welfare and more concerned for her third child, a daughter whose life was being made miserable by her mother's physical complaints and despondency – and indeed Mrs. K.'s depression was evident throughout the consultation. She sat downcast and teary-eyed, reported a weight loss of 20 pounds over the past three months and a history of early morning awakenings. She had felt so despondent at one point that she asked her son to remove a can of gasoline from her garage so that she would not be tempted to immolate herself.

The consultant concluded that Mrs. K. was malingering, had consciously created a "fever" by manipulating the thermometer readings, and was hoping to use her illness to acquire a larger divorce settlement. Whether or not she was also willfully feigning her other symptoms – memory lapses, chest pains, shortness of breath – could only be inferred, and different examiners formed different opinions; but no one doubted that she was suffering from a major affective illness. Accordingly, Mrs. K. was treated with therapeutic doses of a tricyclic antidepressant to which she responded with improved sleep, appetite, and mood, and with a decrease in the intensity of her somatic complaints.

As her depression lifted, she was able to work psychotherapeutically. She came to realize that on the one hand she was furious at the disruption caused by her late daughter's illness and on the other hand, she was tremendously guilty over such hostile feelings. Her illness had allowed her to identify with her daughter, share her suffering, punish herself for such hostile thoughts, and at the same time make life difficult for her surviving daughter, a displacement of her still-unvented rage. With this acquired understanding and with the support of the therapist she was able to settle her divorce without using her hospitalization or physical symptoms to substantiate her claim.

Unfortunately, malingering is usually not secondary to an underlying treatable condition and only rarely does it have the favorable outcome shown with Mrs. K. More often psychiatric interventions tend to be futile, enormously wasteful of professional time, and sometimes make a bad situation even worse. Dr. X. illustrates this point.

THE CASE OF THE DECEITFUL DENTIST

Dr. X. was 37 years old when he first became involved with mental health professionals. At that time he was a retired dentist, allegedly having already made a small fortune as an art collector and entrepreneur. He was referred to a psychiatrist by his neurologist who had been evaluating Dr. X. for pain in the neck and slight weakness and numbness of the fingers following a whiplash car injury. Dr. X. accepted the referral because he had been "a little depressed" since the accident but, in fact, the actual reason for the referral was that the neurologist suspected Dr. X. was malingering to obtain a large insurance settlement. After an extensive evaluation, the psychiatrist could find no evidence for a significant depression and informed both the patient and the neurologist that psychiatric treatment was not indicated at this time. The psychiatrist also told the neurologist that malingering was a definite possibility but, under the circumstances of a time-limited consultation, this possibility could not be confirmed. The patient, feeling humiliated by the referral and misunderstood by the psychiatrist, sought another opinion from another psychotherapist who, as it turned out, had been recommended by the patient's attorney. Dr. X. was then treated in weekly psychotherapy for the next six months for "depression."

Three years later when Dr. X.'s claim finally came to trial, the insurance company's attorney subpoenaed both the neurologist and the original psychiatrist and, when asked under oath, they both testified they had suspected Dr. X. was malingering. Probably because of this testimony, Dr. X received a relatively small settlement. He decided not only to appeal his case, but also to sue both the neurologist and the psychiatrist for negligence. In addition, while the various cases were being pinballed through the courts, Dr. X. allegedly again became "depressed" as a result of his suffering. Finally, after superficially scratching his wrist in a suicidal gesture, he was treated by another therapist for six months with psychotherapy and small doses of antidepressant medication. An additional complicating legal matter arose when the very first psychiatrist (the one now being sued) learned from a psychiatric colleague that Dr. X. had in fact never been a legally licensed dentist and had stopped his practice years ago when the threat of this exposure grew likely. On several social occasions, the sued psychiatrist had inadvertently divulged this information when discussing the ordeal. When Dr. X. learned of this disclosure, he added a libel suit to the others already in progress. Although not all of the cases have been resolved, Dr. X. has already received one settlement in the negligence suit based mainly on the testimony of the two therapists who had treated Dr. X. for several months because of his alleged depressions.

The case of Dr. X. reminds us that patients with malingering may not respond to psychiatric treatment and also may deceitfully use psychiatric as well as physical symptoms to obtain compensation. Providing psychotherapy reinforces this deceit and may increase the eventual financial reward. We therefore recommend that if malingering is not secondary to a treatable underlying psychiatric condition and if the malingering has not responded to past psychiatric interventions, then the consultant's responsibility is to suggest to the patient in a non-punitive way that further medical and psychiatric procedures are not worth the inherent risks. If the malingering patient has been seen in the general hospital, the consultant's recommendation of no treatment can be complemented by helping the staff deal with the rage and helplessness provoked by such patients.

The iatrogenically infantilized patient

Many authors have emphasized that the essence of any successful therapy is to enhance a patient's capacity for self-control, competence, and mastery. There are many instances, however, in which the therapy situation can itself become more of a threat than a potential benefit to the individual's long-range autonomy. This possibility is occasionally clear even in a person who has never had therapy, but more often the risk of needlessly infantilizing a patient by offering more treatment is based on the patient's persistent clinging to previous therapies despite the fact that these have resulted in repeatedly poor responses. Mrs. N. is such a patient.

THE CASE OF THE DEPENDENT DIVORCEE

Although Mrs. N., a tall, attractive but stark 40-year-old woman, has a commanding presence, she has, in fact, never really been on her own. She went immediately from college graduation into a June wedding. When the marriage ended with a childless divorce three years later, Mrs. N. took some of her alimony settlement and entered psychiatric treatment. She has never left.

When seen in consultation, she began by handing the interviewer a three-page, single-spaced typewritten list of her problems, presenting in exquisite detail every conceivable depressive symptom, phobia, obsessive rumination, and compulsive ritual. She then told her story as though totally bored: "I've done it 30 times before." She described her life and her therapy (the two were by now quite inseparable) as unrelieved suffering and a waste. She had "been through" 16 years of consecutive treatments, including "a traditional therapist, a lay and a Jungian analyst, a behavior therapist, two groups, one brief hospitalization, and every available psychotropic medication." Typically, each treatment would bog down, she would attack the therapist for not being more helpful, and a series of implicit or explicit mutual recriminations would follow. She would then leave in a huff, move to another treatment with great expectations, but inevitably feel disappointed. Treatment with her last therapist had ended after a futile battle: The therapist had insisted that she was "self-destructive," while she kept insisting that his "insight orientation" was failing to address her symptoms. (In the past, she had also resented her therapist for the contrary reason that he had focused on symptoms and ignored her self-destructiveness.) Fortunately, in spite of her problems, she had managed to support herself adequately over the years and had dated occasionally.

The consultant, unimpressed by Mrs. N.'s need for lifetime support, thought it remotely possible that she could accept no treatment as "a new approach to her problems." She left the interview intrigued and even hopeful about the prospect, but the consultant learned from a colleague three months later that Mrs. N. was once again in "supportive psychotherapy" because of an "unsettling" experience at a post-est group session.

Mrs. N. exemplifies a group of psychiatric patients who have a history of extensive and varying treatments without any sustained improvement. These patients attach themselves to the mental health system as if they were barnacles on a ship, and treatment becomes for them the crucial (or, at least, interesting) part of their lives, rather than a means to living better in the future without treatment. They may use treatment as a "holding pattern," thereby never making any commitments or taking any concrete action in their lives until they have worked through the problem. When this avoidance takes its toll and life's opportunities pass them by, these iatrogenically dependent patients then blame their problems, their failures, and their poverty on the many psychiatric treatments that have failed them.

When assessing patients who have become chronically dependent on treatment, the consultant should determine if the patient is so impaired that he in fact does require continuous, perhaps lifetime, maintenance therapy. A history of serious suicide attempts, of decompensation, or of deterioration when the patient is out of treatment would be relative indications. If these are not present, the consultant might suggest a brief and limited crisis intervention to help wean the patient from treatment. Many times, however, the chronically dependent patient might well survive without any intervention and should be encouraged to take at least a temporary vacation from his or her routine of treatment as a way of life. In our experience, some patients manage to respond to this suggestion and the option is recommended all too infrequently.

Poorly motivated patients without incapacitating symptoms

Motivation for treatment is always ambivalent and complex. Even the most highly motivated of patients has powerful reasons for not changing and will necessarily present at least unconscious resistances to treatment. Conversely, the least motivated patient who rejects consciously and outwardly every kind of therapeutic endeavor is often pleading inwardly, and perhaps unconsciously, that such efforts continue. In Chapter 9 on the consultative interview, we will discuss how to predict motivation for treatment and to encourage its growth. For now, we are interested in reminding the consultant that treatment should not be imposed routinely on those who have relatively mild problems and relatively little motivation to change. This reminder would seem unnecessary were it not for the enormous dropout rates reported by most outpatient clinics and the possibility that because of a widely shared tendency toward therapeutic perfectionism and missionary zeal, psychiatric treatment is repeatedly offered to those who simply don't want it very much and don't greatly need it. The case of Mr. O. illustrates this point.

THE CASE OF THE QUIET TAILOR

Mr. O. was satisfied with his life, but after five years of marriage and two children, Mrs. O. was not. She had become increasingly dissatisfied with Mr. O.'s quiet, unassuming manner and his lack of professional success (he owned and operated a small tailor shop). Mrs. O. particularly resented the way Mr. O. would sit at home every night methodically studying North American birds while listening to classical music on the old floor radio. On social occasions, which were rare, he participated little and let his wife lead the conversation about her many interests. Mr. O. was affectionate toward his children, though not much involved with their daily lives. They accepted their father for what he was and was not, but Mrs. O. wanted and expected much more.

At the age of 28, out of kindness to his wife – and so that she would stop harping at him – Mr. O. agreed to see a psychiatrist. Twenty months of twice weekly exploratory individual psychotherapy accomplished nothing except increasing the wife's resentment toward Mr. O. for "refusing to change." Mrs. O. considered divorce, but because of the children and financial pressures, decided to wait it out. When the children were in their teens, she returned to school and obtained a degree in social work. This again fueled her ambition for the potential gains of psychotherapy. At her prodding, Mr. O. attended encounter groups, week-end marathons, family therapy sessions, and, at one point, even took low dosages of antidepressant medications.

Therapy for Mr. O. produced no change and not even any particular interest in changing. Finally, during a marital session (the last), the therapist acknowledged that Mr. O. would probably remain about the same the rest of his life and that the therapeutic task was for Mrs. O. either to accept him for what he was or to leave. She decided to stay with him and they lived more or less unhappily ever after.

Many patients have crippling or potentially lethal problems and deserve every attempt to increase their motivation for and/or to reduce their resistance to treatment, particularly when there is an effective treatment available; but, as the case of Mr. O. points out, therapeutic optimism should not be confused with perfectionism and no treatment as the recommendation may be better than trying to sell psychotherapy to someone who is simply not interested.

Research regarding nonresponders

After a biased review of the literature, many years ago Eysenck (1952; 1960; 1966) concluded that psychotherapy was ineffective, or at least those who had been in psychotherapy could not be distinguished from those who had not. This provocative claim, though almost completely misguided, did have the virtue of stimulating many further studies and reviews of these studies. The most systematic, statistical review of 475 outcome studies using meta-analysis has demonstrated psychotherapy to be, on the average, definitely more effective than no treatment (Smith, Glass, and Miller, 1980). The rate of various positive responses to the many kinds of psychotherapy and psychotropic medications tends to cluster at roughly 60% to 70%. This means that about one-third of patients either do not respond measurably to treatment or get worse. We emphasize that they do not *measurably* improve because some patients, designated as either nonresponders or negative responders, may have benefited from treatment but not in ways that were being measured in the particular study. Moreover, they might have deteriorated further had treatment not been offered.

Even if psychotherapy turns out to be even more helpful than outcome studies have already determined it to be, clinicians would agree that some patients show no change in treatment. This lack of apparent, positive results can be divided into the following three distinct hypothetical categories: 1) patients who would have gotten worse except for the beneficial effects of treatment and are able to maintain the status quo only because of treatment (these are really veiled positive responders); 2) patients who are untouched by treatment and continue to follow the natural course of their disorder (these are the true nonresponders); and 3) patients who would have gotten better except for the noxious effects of treatment and are held in a stalemate because of it (these are actually veiled negative responders). One of the many tasks confronting the consultant is to judge which patients are liable to fall into the second or third groups and to steer them away from treatment. As of now, no studies have satisfactorily delineated what characteristics of the patient, therapist, or therapy could reliably predict a nonresponse. We must therefore rely on the patient's past experiences and the clinician's judgment, which we hope will be enhanced by the tentative suggestions and case histories presented above and also by the discussions of other cases and research throughout this book.

3) Patients Likely to Have Spontaneous Improvement

Psychologically healthy patients in crisis

Not every individual in crisis needs psychiatric treatment. This obvious statement would not be necessary except that recent changes in our society have made it difficult for mental health professionals to delineate their specific areas of expertise. The Western industrialized world has evolved in such a way as to weaken many of the traditional supports and amenities. The extended family, the small town, the lifetime job, the stable marriage, the church, and the family doctor are now less available for help and comfort during crises. As these social supports have declined, mental health workers have multiplied both in numbers and range of responsibility to the point where they are sometimes regarded – and even regard themselves – as modern-day philosophers, wise men, healers, priests, erstwhile Mr. Fix-its, social reformers, and correction officers.

Many problems in this world are not caused by specific individual or family psychopathology, but are inherent in the ultimate imperfectibility of man and the social systems he has constructed. Before psychiatry assumes a leading role in changing society and solacing its victims, we mental health professionals should explore and then acknowledge our collective limitations. Some reconsideration and retreat from professional grandiosity has occurred in recent years. More realistic boundaries for our endeavors are being established – but the lines are not always easy to draw. Should every married couple see a therapist before breaking up – just as in the old days they might have gone to a clergyman or family elder or perhaps have continued to bear each other in silence? What about the child who is truant or doing poorly in school? The teenager who becomes pregnant or smokes pot or gets in trouble with the law? The recently bereaved widow? Or the man who is distraught after losing a job, or having a heart attack, or being told he has cancer?

Whether these people in crisis should receive psychiatric treatment is often a question left unresolved or determined by individual tastes and habits. When asked to help in such decisions, the consultant must decide where each situation falls on the continuum that has, at one pole, patients suffering due to psychopathology (an area of our competence) and, at the other pole, those whose suffering is due to the miseries of everyday life (an area over which we have no control and often can provide only limited expertise). The case of Mr. Q. illustrates how hard this determination can be.

THE CASE OF THE REJECTED GROOM

Mr. Q., a 22-year-old senior, sought psychiatric treatment because he had grown increasingly worried and depressed over the past few weeks ever since his parents told him that they would abide by their refusal to attend his forthcoming wedding. Their stated reason was that Mr. Q. was "too young," but the real objection was the girl's faith and the planned religious ceremony.

Mr. Q. pleaded and struggled to reach some compromise. When his parents remained adamant, he became more despondent, cried alone at night over the difficulties, and found it hard to concentrate in preparation for his final exams. He began to doubt his abilities and wondered if he were not in fact "too young," if he could neither separate from his parents nor deal with them more adequately.

The consultation helped clarify Mr. Q.'s feelings, options, and ways of handling his parents during past crises. A well-integrated and likeable young man, he would have made a fine treatment case either alone or with his family. On the other hand, he had already managed an appropriate separation from his family and had no enduring psychiatric symptoms. On this basis, the consultant recommended that no further treatment was required at this time. This reassured Mr. Q., who called back three months later to inform the consultant that he was now married—and, at the last minute, he had successfully persuaded his parents to attend the wedding.

The case of Mr. Q. demonstrates that although relatively healthy patients do well in many forms of treatment, they also often do well without any treatment at all. Not everyone faced with an unfamiliar setting

or developmental task (such as marriage, a promotion, leaving home for
college) nor everyone experiencing a loss (such as the loss of a loved one,
a limb, health, a job) should or could receive psychotherapy. Although
we strongly endorse the effectiveness of crisis intervention in preventing
regression and symptom formation, we believe that before any treatment is recommended there should be at least some evidence that: 1) the
patient already has pathological symptoms or mourning patterns; 2) the
patient has responded pathologically in the past to similar stresses; 3)
the patient is avoiding the crisis, the mourning process, or the developmental task; and 4) nontechnical help from the patient's family,
friends, church, physician, school advisor or whoever is either unavailable or has not worked.

Healthy patients with minor chronic problems

Some potential patients are individuals who are determined to be perfect in every way and regard treatment as a means of eliminating what
may be relatively minor complaints. In these situations, treatment en-
tails the risk of encouraging self-absorption and emotional hypochondriasis. Consider the following vignette.

THE CASE OF THE UNSHAKABLE FANTASIES

Mr. L., a 38-year-old successful television journalist, first sought psychiatric treatment before his marriage at the age of 25. At that time
he was worried that two of his sexual fantasies might interfere with his
role as husband and provider. In one fantasy, his wife is posing seduc-
tively and then having sex with the photographer; in the other fantasy,
Mr. L. is being stepped on by a high-heeled whore. Mr. L. was particularly concerned because both fantasies occurred while having sex and in
fact made the act more exciting and pleasurable. Thirteen years later,
after an exploratory psychotherapy, a group therapy, a behavioral therapy and, most recently, sexual therapy, Mr. L.'s fantasies were the same
as ever. He was now asking the consultant if a more traditional psychoanalysis might be of help.

The consultant learned that at work, at play, both alone and with
others, Mr. L. had no troubling problems and was widely regarded as
an accomplished and loving man. He had learned already that one fantasy represented a longing for another man (his father) by using the
woman as a conduit, and that the other fantasy was used as a punishment for his success and sexual pleasure. This understanding had made
the fantasies less enigmatic, but no less frequent or exciting. Mr. L. was

still concerned that the presence of these fantasies might indicate some severe latent problem that would require close attention and extensive work.

After an extended evaluation, the consultant concluded that Mr. L.'s fantasies were not a serious sign of psychopathology requiring treatment. Mr. L.'s more pressing problem was that he expected to be "perfectly normal" with no warts or blemishes. The consultant informed Mr. L. of this opinion and recommended no treatment. Four years later, the consultant accidently met Mr. L. who thanked him for his advice. The fantasies had not changed; the need to remove them had. Mr. L. felt his life was the same as ever . . . "filled with problems, but no ghosts."

Does such a patient who seeks treatment for seemingly minor problems actually need treatment to diminish his expectation for perfection? Perhaps at times, but the consultant must be cautious about colluding with such a patient and failing to recognize the limitations of treatment, just as the patient has had trouble recognizing and accepting limitations in himself. In general, except perhaps for training purposes, therapy is not warranted for patients who have some minor problems but who are generally emotionally healthy. Of course, the consultant must always be wary of any patient who presents with seemingly trivial problems and a history of adequate or even superior adjustment. In some instances, an extended evaluation reveals more serious problems beneath the facade of health and the apparently minor problem turns out to be an indication of underlying psychopathology that does indeed require treatment.

Research regarding spontaneous improvement

Once a patient is already in treatment, spontaneous improvement is, for obvious reasons, methodologically impossible to measure. Studies have therefore used control groups receiving no treatment in order to measure spontaneous improvement. Reports from such studies indicate that the degree of spontaneous improvement varies markedly depending upon the psychiatric diagnosis. Only 9% of borderline and schizophrenic patients appear to improve spontaneously, whereas up to 54% of patients with other diagnoses improve (Endicott and Endicott, 1963). Bergin and Lambert (1978) summarized 17 well-controlled studies and found a median rate of 43% for spontaneous remissions. The interpretation of these data is complicated because initial evaluations, waiting lists, and other research procedures may themselves constitute a kind of treatment (Malan, Heath, Bacal, and Balfour, 1975). The 43% rate of spontaneous remissions may also be overstated because in most instances the outcome measures tap only the improvement of the presenting symptoms and ignore other kinds of change. For example, a study assessing improvements in anxious patients may find that the control group had no more anxiety after two years than the treatment group — but it remains possible that patients who were treated with psychotherapy may have made substantial changes in their lives or characters that were not measured with the instruments used in the investigation. The high rate of spontaneous improvement reported in a study that depends exclusively on symptom relief outcome measures may therefore be misleading.

4) The Recommendation of No Treatment as a Specific Therapeutic Intervention

Having described clinical situations in which patients are liable to respond negatively to treatment, not respond at all, or to improve just as well without treatment, we now address those situations in which the recommendation of no treatment may in itself be used as a specific therapeutic technique.

Oppositional patients refusing treatment

Haley (1973a) and others have applied systems and communication theory to develop paradoxical injunction as a strategic psychotherapeutic maneuver for dealing with oppositional patients. An oppositional patient who needs treatment but is refusing it can be placed in a useful double bind when the consultant "agrees" with the patient that treatment is likely to be useless or too expensive or difficult or not necessary after all. Oppositional patients often respond to this maneuver by angrily switching fields and trying to convince the consultant that he has made a horrible mistake and that treatment must be provided. This technique, admittedly manipulative, can be helpful for inducting certain patients into therapy who would otherwise take pride in fighting their way out of it, but now take pride in fighting their way into it.

Patients seeking therapeutic regression

Some patients can function on an adequate level on their own but want treatment to justify regression and an escape from the responsibilities in the real world. Refusing to provide treatment can serve as a specific treatment technique that helps to reverse their demoralization, supports the healthier aspects of their functioning, and improves their sense of mastery and competence. Patients who are told that they don't need treatment often gain an increased sense of autonomy and confidence in themselves.

Patients requiring a temporary delay in treatment

Participation in a never-ending chain of therapies does not allow a patient to experience any of the separations fully or to integrate the impact of any one treatment before having begun another. For this reason, patients should not embark on a new therapy just after ending a previous one unless they require maintenance support or unless one therapy has been specifically intended to serve as an induction into another. In addition, there are times when a particular therapy or therapist of choice is unavailable at the moment. In such a case, a recommendation of no treatment at this time may be therapeutic, especially if the patient would enter a treatment prematurely only to fail and therafter be prejudiced against all other kinds of treatment in the future.

Exceptions to Recommendation of No Treatment for Borderline Patients

As mentioned earlier in the chapter, we would like to note four exceptions when therapy might be advisable for a borderline patient, despite a history of repeated failures:

1) Borderline patients who have an isolated, focused problem amenable to brief, circumscribed treatment

The following case illustrates this exception.

THE CASE OF THE FLYING PHYSICIAN

By the time Dr. E. was in his mid fifties, he had established himself as a brilliant and much sought after forensic pathologist. He would pilot his private jet from one famous trial to another and provide incisive testimony that often decided the outcome of the case. While achieving great professional success, Dr. E. had discarded four wives and nine children whom he contemptuously viewed as a burden and the cause of his precarious financial situation. The public was not aware of his vengeful outbursts with associates, his alcohol and drug abuse, and his recurrent brief psychotic episodes that lasted typically for several days and involved delusions of persecution and grandiosity (such as being excluded by the FBI from examining the remains of famous assassinated figures). On a few occasions, a former wife or an older son had tried to have Dr. E. psychiatrically hospitalized, but he would quickly reorganize and present a persuasive legal argument preventing commitment. On only one occasion, when Dr. E. was in his late thirties, did his self-prescribed abuse of medication and near fatal overdose necessitate a more prolonged hospitalization. After withdrawal from all drugs over a three-month period, his diagnosis was still not clear and the attending physicians continued to be unsure of the extent to which his various difficulties could best be accounted for by drug abuse, bipolar affective illness, narcissistic character disorder, or borderline personality disorder.

Except for this one psychiatric involvement, Dr. E.'s relationships with psychiatrists had always been adversarial until by chance he met a kindly psychiatrist at a dinner party. A few months later, when one of Dr. E.'s professional colleagues insisted upon psychiatric consultation because of Dr. E.'s wild piloting and increased suspiciousness, Dr. E. agreed to see his fellow guest at the dinner party. This psychiatrist, unlike his predecessors, wisely did not try to reconstruct Dr. E.'s character, convince Dr. E. that his ego-syntonic personality traits were pathological, or introduce a medication regimen with no hope of compliance. Instead, the psychiatrist focused on the specific stress precipitating the most recent decompensation (a bout of impotence during a one-night sexual encounter), offered empathy and advice, and assured Dr. E. that further psychiatric involvement at this time would not be particularly necessary or profitable. An invitation for future consultations was extended. For the next seven years, Dr. E.'s character problems persisted, but the severity and frequency of his decompensations have decreased. A few times each year, he "drops in" to see his psychiatrist for two or three visits around a circumscribed problem.

>*2) Borderline patients whose lives are so immediately endangered or intolerable that the risks of treatment no matter how great are worth taking*

The case of Mr. F. illustrates this exception.

THE CASE OF THE EMBITTERED SOCIALIST

When Mr. F. graduated from high school, he was voted most likely in his class to succeed. Thirty years later, he was a self-confessed failure, living alone in a windowless basement apartment where he wrote obscure diatribes against the capitalist system.

Mr. F.'s first psychiatric hospitalization occurred when he was a freshman in college and "freaked out on acid." His classmates and the admitting psychiatrist believed that an additional explanation for this brief psychotic episode was Mr. F.'s reaction to being rejected and humiliated by his homosexual lover. Mr. F. refused follow-up treatment and was again hospitalized three years later when he became briefly delusional and convinced that the CIA was attempting to destroy his senior thesis on the American Communist Party. This second psychotic episode was one of many reasons Mr. F. was not graduated from college. Again, Mr. F. refused follow-up psychiatric treatment. Instead, he joined a militant activist group and was soon arrested for planning to dynamite the mayor's home. His third documented psychotic episode occurred while he was in jail awaiting trial and involved similar delusions about government agencies preventing his revolutionary ideas from being heard. The journal he kept while in his cell was a combination of platitudes and gibberish. Because he was unable to participate in his own defense, Mr. F. was psychiatrically hospitalized.

The diagnosis of schizophrenia was considered, but he quickly reorganized completely, without medication, and the diagnosis of a borderline personality disorder seemed more likely. For a variety of reasons, the legal charges were dropped, Mr. F. was discharged from the hospital and again refused follow-up care.

Mr. F. worked for the next several years as the chief gardener on a socialist commune. His enthusiasm for nutrition at times became fanatical, but he was generally accepted as an agreeable eccentric. When the commune dissolved, he was forced to reenter the despised capitalist society that had so repeatedly rejected him. Mr. F. would become involved with one or another radical group while supporting himself with welfare or working as a busboy. Some stress, altercation, or rejection would occur with a co-worker or "comrade" and he would react by becoming bizarre, litigious, suspicious, homicidal, or suicidal. Within a few days, after hospitalization had removed him from the precipitating stress, Mr. F. would reorganize without medication and leave the hospital without accepting further care. The psychiatric staff at several different institutions grew accustomed to his appearing in the Emergency Room in either a violent state or stuporous after an overdosage. Under such circumstances, treatment was obviously mandatory even though all those familiar with Mr. F. realized that within a few days he would most likely again be leaving the hospital, not only ungrateful for having been pulled back from the edge of the cliff, but also angry and contemptuous towards all those who had sold out and worked for the establishment.

3) Borderline patients who for the first time have the opportunity and resources to obtain expert treatment

The case of Mr. S. illustrates this exception.

THE CASE OF THE DISTURBED ARMY BRAT

Mr. S., the son of a career Army officer, was shuffled from one base to another during his first 14 years. His poor school performance, absence of friends, temper tantrums, and compulsive neatness were attributed to the many family moves. The seriousness of his problems could no longer be ignored when, in reaction to a minor slight by a female high school teacher, Mr. S. superficially cut his wrist, nose, and genitals in a bizarre suicidal gesture. He was seen that night by the military physician on call, who recommended psychiatric treatment in the nearby town since there were no trained psychiatrists on base. Mr. S.'s father minimized his son's problems and seemed more concerned about the implications of his son's behavior upon his own career. He refused to complete the necessary paperwork for psychiatric treatment. The mother's reluctance was more complicated. The patient had known for years that his mother, a strikingly beautiful woman, hated her husband and engaged in a series of extramarital affairs. His mother was concerned that psychiatric treatment might make her son less willing to conceal her behavior. For the five years after Mr. S.'s initial psychiatric presentation, he was provided only brief and perfunctory care: school counseling; aborted psychiatric consultation with untrained military personnel; or brief and unsystematic trials of lithium, antidepressants, or neuroleptics. At the age of 21, because of medical complications following a near-fatal suicide attempt, Mr. S. was transferred from a military hospital to a university facility. There, for the first time, he was seen in psychiatric consultation by a well-trained clinician. By this time, Mr. S.'s parents were divorced and his mother was living abroad with her wealthy new husband. She agreed to a prolonged inpatient hospitalization for her son who was placed in a research project examining the benefits of exploratory treatment for borderline patients. Mr. S. was treated for a total of four years, one of which was in the hospital, one in a halfway house facility, and the rest as an outpatient. He did extremely well and although still prone to outbursts and exaggerated sensitivity to criticism, he has been able to marry and establish a reasonably successful career.

4) Borderline patients who have become less impulsive and destructive with advancing age

In our discussion of the pros and cons of treatment for borderline patients, we have used clinical examples to illustrate how the severity of this condition can vary widely from individual to individual and how, within any given individual, the level of functioning can also vary widely from year to year. The case below points out another complicating feature of the borderline condition which also must be considered when designing a treatment plan, namely, that the symptoms of this disorder may change over time. The impulse-ridden, rebellious borderline adolescent may become more accepting and responsive to psychiatric treatment in later years.

THE CASE OF THE LATE-BLOOMING HEIRESS

Ms. J. was raised as a "poor little rich girl," living in elegant style on various estates, shopping for designers' clothes, and entertaining for the fanciest people. This fairytale world collapsed when her mother's severe alcoholism took its toll and resulted in a rather sudden death from the complications of cirrhosis. At age 11 and without a friend in the world, Ms. J. was shipped to a distant aunt who had been assigned her legal guardian, but the many boarding schools she attended and her aunt's employees were in fact forced to assume the parenting role to the extent it was assumed at all. Not surprisingly, Ms. J. did poorly in school and socially, and relied on her wealth and seductiveness to make temporary friends who took advantage of both her money and her developing promiscuity.

By the time Ms. J. was in her late teens she had attended no school for longer than one year, required four abortions, and, just as her mother had also done, fled to Europe to spend money, travel, and drink. The many attempts at psychiatric intervention were brief and in vain. Ms. J. would characteristically defy and devalue her female therapists or attempt to seduce (at times successfully) the male therapists whom she adored and then defeated. Finally, at age 42, after a life "in the jet stream" and countless psychiatric consultations for what she vaguely described as boredom, depression, or loneliness, Ms. J. stopped for a moment and took stock of her life while in the hospital for a benign breast biopsy. The consultation-liaison psychiatrist referred her to an elderly male therapist and she began an intensive exploratory psychotherapy. Despite much pain and, at one point, a brief hospitalization for a profound suicidal depression, Ms. J. remained in this treatment, viewing it as "a last chance for someone who has simmered down but is not yet burned out." After eight years of therapy, her therapist died. By that time Ms. J. had married a divorced elderly man and was spending her days caring for him and taking delight in his young grandchildren as if they were her own. She had clearly benefited from psychiatric treatment, but chose not to resume therapy, since she was satisfied with the way she was feeling and the way her life was going.

METHODOLOGICAL AND ETHICAL CONSIDERATIONS

In the absence of adequate research data to substantiate our suggested indications for no treatment, we have filled this chapter with many illustrative case reports. Although most clinicians would agree that at times no treatment is probably the preferred alternative and could provide their own anecdotal reports to document this belief, there are some who might nevertheless criticize our general approach to this issue. These critics might marshall two pieces of data: 1) The prediction of treatment outcome is admittedly likely to be inaccurate (Luborsky, Mintz, Auberbach, Christoph, Bachrach, Todd, Johnson, Cohen, and O'Brien, 1980) and becomes clearer during a trial treatment; and 2) the consensus of many studies is that treated groups of patients tend on average to fare better than untreated groups (Luborsky, Singer, and Luborsky, 1975; Smith et al., 1980). Perhaps a trial of treatment should be offered to virtually everyone willing to try it. We are not content with this conclusion. Until clearer guidelines emerge from research, the consultant should avoid playing the odds blindly by offering every patient therapy. "No treatment" should be recommended when clinical experience and judgment call out for it and particularly when the patient has failed to respond or has gotten worse with all other previous attempts at treatment.

We realize that the decision to recommend no treatment, especially when the patient's situation appears desperate and chaotic, requires considerable courage and the conviction that this constitutes the best possible course of action, given the particular circumstances. Whenever it is feasible, an additional consultant should also evaluate the patient's condition and thereby share in the responsibility for making a difficult choice and for presenting this decision to the patient. A second opinion reduces the possibility that the recommendation of no treatment has arisen from the first consultant's countertransference feelings. A collaborative effort also conveys more clearly to the patient that the recommendation has been a careful one that has been made with the patient's welfare in mind and is not simply a brush-off.

For the purpose of discussion, we have somewhat artificially presented "no treatment" as though it were an all or none verdict. In actual practice, this is, of course, very rarely the case. In fact, some would argue that the process of evaluating the patient just once and then suggesting no treatment can in itself constitute a treatment with a considerable therapeutic impact. We have therefore deliberately not provided any precise definition of "no treatment" and are well aware that in clinical practice the consultant may be wise to suggest a small amount rather than no treatment at all. This titrated dose may take the form of a follow-up visit, a phone call in a month or so, an extended consultation, a brief therapy, or an arrangement to reevaluate the patient for treatment at some future time.

Rather than the recommendation of no treatment, the consultant may also recommend a different treatment than has been tried in the past: that is, a different setting, format, technique, intensity, duration, or therapist. We have purposely delayed discussing this possibility until now because the consultant too often considers this option first and foremost. The recommendation of some change in the kind of therapy is, in our experience, usually based on the presumption that the wrong kind of treatment was given to the patient. This is often a fair guess, but the consultant should not ignore the possibility that therapy of any kind will be ineffective. Too often, the result is that patients are routinely offered a long series of treatments regardless of impressive evidence that repeated trials have been harmful or have ended in a stalemate.

On the other hand, we do not intend to discount that several variables other than characteristics of the patient may have determined failure in previous treatments. The therapist may have lacked experience or technical skill or may not have been empathically attuned to the patient. The patient may have indeed been in the wrong form of therapy; for example, an anxious and uninsightful phobic patient may have found the uncovering approach in an exploratory therapy too overwhelming, but may go on to be quite suitable for either a behavioral therapy or for the use of psychotropic drugs addressed to specific target symptoms. In addition, the time may not have been right for treatment; patients change over the years in their motivation, circumstances, and ability to use treatment. But before assuming that the previous failure was due to an unskilled therapist, a wrong kind of therapy, or an unsuitable time in the patient's life, the consultant must always keep in mind that patients commonly distort their previous therapy experiences and retrospectively report them in the least favorable light. Along with carefully questioning the patient, the consultant should contact the previous therapists to determine the nature of the previous results as seen from a different and hopefully more objective point of view.

Finally, there are indeed occasions when the clinician is correct to forge ahead in spite of a dire treatment history. Even in the most unlikely circumstances, psychiatric treatment may be indicated because its possible benefits, although remote, outweigh the risks and cost, and nothing better is available.

SUMMARY

Consultants should become less reluctant to recommend no treatment once the potential benefits of such a recommendation are recognized. No treatment may:

1) protect the patient from iatrogenic harm, especially by interrupting a sequence of destructive treatments;
2) protect the patient and clinician from wasting time, effort, and money;
3) delay therapy until a more propitious time;
4) protect and consolidate gains from previous treatments;
5) provide the patient an opportunity to discover that he can do without treatment; and
6) avoid a semblance of treatment when no effective treatment exists.

Because the decision to embark on a psychiatric treatment is so important, the consultant has a responsibility to identify and protect those patients likely to be harmed by treatment. Our first obligation is to follow the injunction *primum non nocere*; our second obligation is the identification of patients we neither help nor hurt; and our third and perhaps most difficult obligation is to allow those patients already on their way to spontaneous improvement to get well without us.

CHAPTER 8

Research and Treatment Planning

This chapter explores the relationship between psychotherapy research and clinical practice and defines our method of reviewing the scientific literature to derive selection criteria for the various treatments. As examples, we present a critical analysis of the designs and conclusions of several of the better known and more influential outcome studies in order to demonstrate the translation of research findings into clinical rules of thumb. We do not attempt to provide any systematic tabulation of research results. This task has already been performed quite well by a number of research reviews whose findings have been used and discussed along the way throughout the book. Our purpose here is much more focused: to discuss the methods and problems of psychotherapy outcome research and to show how one can apply the answers gained from it to the questions raised by differential therapeutics. A recent, quite excellent, and detailed review of many of these same issues has been published by the American Psychiatric Association's Commission on Psychotherapies (1982).

The research on psychotherapy outcome has inevitably been complicated, difficult to control, and ambiguous in its results. Despite inherent obstacles to a scientific understanding of how and when therapy works, there is also cause for reasonable optimism that before long psychotherapy research will become an increasingly fruitful and influential guide to clinical decision-making. Researchers now perform studies with vastly improved methodology and measuring instruments, and can draw upon the seemingly inexhaustible capacity of computers to analyze massive amounts of data. There is also a perceptible change and improvement in the atmosphere surrounding the research-clinical interface. Researchers are becoming more clinically astute and able to address their studies to the questions that interest and puzzle clinicians.

At the same time, clinicians are becoming increasingly rigorous in their training and outlook and better able to complement the art of therapy with an appreciation for what might eventually become its science.

We will begin by describing some of the inherent problems that make it difficult to perform outcome research and limit its application to the clinical situation. This is followed by an outline of the variety of research strategies that have been used in studying psychotherapy outcome. We will discuss the advantages and disadvantages of each method and illustrate these with a critical review of a leading study from each category (where available). Finally, we will describe the parameters that would define the psychotherapy outcome study most ideally suited to answer differential therapeutic questions.

INHERENT LIMITATIONS OF PSYCHOTHERAPY RESEARCH

Although the sophistication of psychotherapy outcome research has advanced dramatically during the past 20 years, the existing literature has many limitations and there are a number of inherent obstacles that make this an especially difficult area for scientific investigation. The following, by no means exhaustive list outlines some of the various problems that must be confronted in the effort to create a research foundation for differential therapeutics.

1) It is often difficult to apply the results of research directly to clinical practice. Studies usually report statistically significant differences in group means. For two reasons this is often not readily translatable into clinical significance for the individual patient: (a) results may achieve statistical significance without having any great clinical meaning or importance; and (b) although a variable may serve as a predictor of outcome for the group as a whole, there is no ready way to know how one variable interacts with others in the individual patient and how powerful a predictor it is in particular circumstances. It always requires clinical judgment to interpret in what ways statistically significant results shed light on the idiosyncracies and complexity of each particular case.

2) Different therapies vary, sometimes dramatically, in their goals and expected outcome but also in ways that are often too subtle to be measured reliably, at least by existing instruments. It has been much easier to devise and validate measures of overt symptoms than to define and measure reliably more subtle changes in self-perception, personality style, or interpersonal relatedness. A depressed patient who has improved in dynamically oriented, individual psychotherapy may be in-

distinguishable in his symptom change score on the Hamilton Depression Scale from another patient who has improved in cognitive therapy, or in one or another form of group or family therapy, but each approach may have conveyed to the patient a very different sense of himself and of the optimal methods to be used in solving problems. The inability of most studies to differentiate the effects of treatments that would seem intuitively to be radically different may reflect, at least in part, on the weakness of currently available instruments to tap important, but difficult to measure, differences in outcome.

3) Related to, but also to some extent independent of, this last point is the fact that different psychotherapies differ in their qualitative value implications in ways that are very difficult or impossible to measure quantitatively and comparatively. For example, what is more valuable – the patient's behavioral change or his subjective relief? And who will decide this – the patient himself, his family, the therapist, the legal system? Ultimately, research cannot provide answers to such value questions. Research is limited to providing data on what is actually achieved by the various therapies and cannot evaluate the differential desirability of these achievements. This explains why it is so difficult to do meaningful cost/benefit analyses of psychotherapy. How do we place a dollar value on an averted suicide? How many dollars for a patient's feelings of satisfaction or pleasure that have replaced previously experienced self-contempt or anhedonia? How much is an orgasm worth to a person who previously could not have one?

4) Psychotherapies, no matter how carefully they are defined, can never be fashioned in forms that are as reproducible as pills. Since psychotherapy contains complex and interacting relationships of many variables, the same procedure can never be delivered twice in exactly the same way even by the same person. The actual interchange between patient and therapist depends, in its most crucial details, upon the timing and nuance of the relationship and context of which the individuals form a part. Psychotherapy is thus inherently to some degree an idiosyncratic activity that poses serious challenges to scientific rigor and generalizability.

5) Similarly, the number and complexity of possibly important patient dimensions are so great that it is difficult, if not impossible, to ensure that the patients who have received different, competing treatments were homogeneous before treatment in all of the ways that might count in predicting subsequent course.

6) To do adequate psychotherapy outcome research requires the patience of a saint, the wealth of Croesus, and a good amount of modesty. This is time-consuming and expensive work and is not likely to lead to

any Nobel prizes or general scientific kudos. This may help to explain why, in spite of the relatively vast resources devoted to the practice of psychotherapy, so very little money, effort, and brainpower have been set aside for its research, development, and evaluation. Moreover, most researchers choose for study those therapies that are the easiest to investigate, i.e., those that are brief, precise, and symptom-oriented, although these may not closely reflect typical community practice and cannot readily be generalized to it.

7) Participant and observer biases can never be fully eliminated in psychotherapy research. The single or double blind study is impossible to do in a situation which usually requires that patient and therapist have at least some idea of what they are about and why.

8) Control groups are often hard to come by in psychotherapy research. Would any sensible patient knowingly accept randomization to either psychoanalysis or brief therapy? Probably not. The commitment is too serious and expensive for a patient to accept decisions made by a roll of the dice. Furthermore, crossover designs which use the patient as his own control have little place in psychotherapy outcome research because the effects of therapy are presumed to persist even after the therapy itself has ended. One can switch from drug A to drug B after an appropriate washout period and hope that drug A is no longer an active agent confounding the trial of B. On the other hand, if psychotherapy A has any ability enduringly to change the patient, then there is no meaningful way to have a washout period to get rid of its effects and return the patient to his pretreatment state.

9) It is difficult (probably impossible) to develop a believable psychotherapy placebo. Putting a patient on a waiting list with minimal contact may have either positive or negative connotations and effects on outcome, depending on how tactfully this is done. A waiting list group does not constitute either a trial of no treatment or a placebo for psychotherapy. An alternative strategy has been to enjoin the therapist from making the specific interventions that are being tested and allowing him instead to engage in nonspecific ways with the patient. This does not constitute a very effective placebo unless the therapist believes that these nonspecific contacts are in some way meaningful; otherwise, he is likely to convey his negative expectations to the patient. On the other hand, if the therapist believes in the therapeutic power of his "nonspecific" interventions, it is no longer clear that they are indeed nonspecific. What is tested under these circumstances is not a placebo but rather a branch of interpersonal therapy. The placebo problem in psychotherapy boils down to this: It is easy enough to create a biologically inert tablet form of placebo for drug studies but it is probably impossi-

ble to create an interpersonally "inert" form of human interaction as a placebo for psychotherapy studies.

10) Measurement of specific therapeutic effects has been less fruitful than expected, in part because of the surprisingly strong and general therapeutic effects of what have been loosely called "nonspecific" aspects of psychotherapy. The background noise of nonspecific effect is sufficiently loud to drown out the impact of specific techniques, at least given the very low amplification of current outcome measures. Clearly, two trends will emerge in the very near future. Nonspecific techniques will be more clearly defined and made specific (since they work so well). At the same time more finely honed instruments will be devised so that we do not lose data on specific therapeutic impacts.

Despite all of these difficulties, psychotherapy outcome research marches on. We will now describe the variety of available strategies.

TYPES OF RESEARCH

There are three general types of research designs used in studies of therapeutic outcome: 1) the naturalistic-correlational; 2) the manipulative-experimental; and 3) a combined factorial design that incorporates both organismic and manipulated independent variables.

Naturalistic-Correlational Studies

This type of investigation stays closest to the actual unmodified clinical situation. In a typical naturalistic-correlational design, a number of patient variables are measured at the outset of treatment (e.g., demographics, diagnosis, symptom patterns and severity, personality characteristics, response to psychological tests or others). These are then correlated with a variety of outcomes (e.g., whether the patient remains in or drops out of therapy, does well or poorly, etc.). If, for example, a study shows that a given type of patient consistently drops out of a particular therapy, this provides some indication to steer such patients away from that therapy. Studies correlating patient characteristics with success or failure in a given treatment have an even more obvious significance for differential therapeutic decisions. In most naturalistic-correlational studies, the patients generally all receive the same treatment and no comparison group or random assignment is used. Treatment variables (e.g., technique, therapist experience) can also be correlated with outcome.

Naturalistic-correlational studies are a first and necessary step in systematically looking at the complexity of clinical phenomena and in generating hypotheses for further (and usually experimental) testing. The clear advantage of the naturalistic approach resides in its closeness to the live, unmanipulated, and natural clinical reality. The research intervention is less likely to influence the therapy it is meant to study. Many factors can be measured and correlated simultaneously to give full justice to the richness and intricacy of psychotherapy interactions. Clinicians often find naturalistic studies more relevant to their practice than the sometimes overly simplified, but better validated, results that emerge from elaborately controlled designs.

These very advantages simultaneously constitute the limitations and disadvantages of naturalistic investigations. Correlational designs are impressionistic and inherently subject to great observer bias in interpretation. Since there is no provision of a control treatment, one can never really be sure that the treatment results are any better or worse than what would have occurred spontaneously without treatment or by using another type of intervention. In other words, naturalistic-correlational studies help to indicate which patients will do well in a particular therapy but not whether they would have done better or worse in some other kind of treatment or in no treatment at all. This obviously limits their value for the differential therapeutic comparison of different treatments. Furthermore, since the variables in naturalistic-correlational studies are uncontrolled, there is no way of determining the extent of causality. When two variables (A and B) are significantly correlated with one another, A may cause B, B may cause A, A and B may be caused by a third and unidentified variable C, or the correlation may result from chance. A naturalistic-correlational design provides no method for deciding the question in a given case except by intuition, and intuition can easily be deceived by bias.

Illustration: A naturalistic-correlational study (Malan)

In the mid-1950s, a group of psychotherapists in London gathered around the esteemed and innovative psychoanalyst, Michael Balint, to form a workshop that would perform and study brief dynamic psychotherapies. One of the charter members, David Malan, later became head of the workshop and over the years has presented its findings in three beautifully written and widely quoted books. Malan and his Tavistock group have chosen a completely naturalistic research strategy which stays close to their (always sensitive and often brilliant) clinical work, but avoids any experimental manipulations or control groups. Malan's work demonstrates the most sophisticated use of the naturalistic-correlational approach in studying the relationship between psychotherapy process and outcome. His studies clearly illustrate the simultaneous great advantages and serious limitations of naturalistic-correlational methods.

Malan's strategy was to study the clinical situation on its own terms. His research interventions were designed to be unobtrusive and to upset only minimally the delivery of focal therapy by workshop members. His close scrutiny and limited interference with actual clinical practice allowed him to generate and test hypotheses of immediate clinical interest and importance: 1) that a brief psychodynamic treatment can facilitate enduring character change; 2) that this treatment is effective even for patients with longstanding problems; and 3) that one particular type of technical intervention, the linking of the transference to early childhood experience, is most highly correlated with successful outcome. His findings can be immediately translated into guidelines for treatment selection and technique. This is often not the case with larger *n* experimental studies that generate group averages at the expense of a high magnification on each individual patient, and in the process of controlling variables, may bend the clinical situation to an unrecognizable shape.

Malan's group collaborated for over 20 years in two separate investigations of focal therapy (Malan, 1963; 1976) and accumulated a sample of over 60 patients, each of whom was treated in a sophisticated, brief psychodynamic treatment with an experienced and highly motivated clinician. Outcome was evaluated at termination and after prolonged follow-up periods (up to ten years in a number of cases). Process ratings were based on therapists' notes that were dictated after therapy sessions. The data were subjected to statistical procedures that were thorough, to the point of being excessively ingenious in salvaging significant correlations.

Our major focus here is Malan's evaluation of outcome. Malan believes that psychotherapy research has been handicapped by the failure to devise outcome criteria that do justice to the complexity of human personality. He attempts to demonstrate that psychodynamic change can be formulated in operational language, scored with acceptable reliability by judges who are experienced clinicians, and then analyzed statistically to "validate" (his word) psychodynamic psychotherapy. Based on the results of psychiatric and psychological evaluation, Malan defines for each patient a "psychodynamic hypothesis" framed in simple, widely accepted, relatively noninferential, and nonmetapsychological terms. The formulation constitutes a kind of individualized goal attainment scaling and includes statements about:

1) the patient's vulnerability to specific kinds of stress;
2) the criteria to be used in judging recovery (which include the patient's ability to cope with these stresses in a new way without developing symptoms; and,
3) cautions against possible false solutions (or ways the patient may appear symptomatically recovered but only at the expense of avoiding the specific stresses rather than overcoming them).

Criteria for improvement are based on the evaluation of overt behaviors or feelings that can be readily observed on follow-up on the assumption that these accurately reflect resolution of intrapsychic conflicts that are not directly measurable in any other way. To get a good outcome score (with assumed resolution of intrapsychic conflict) the patient must demonstrate that he has replaced inappropriate behaviors and reactions to specific stresses with appropriate ones. Malan's raters used a 0- to 4-point scale of psychodynamic improvement as follows:

0 – a false solution, i.e., symptoms improved at the price of avoidance and emotional disengagement;
1 – symptom improvement without detectable changes in psychodynamic functioning;
2 – resolution of conflicts but not those that interfere with heterosexual relationships;
3 and 4 – varying degrees of conflict resolution in heterosexual relationships.

Scores below 2 are considered nonsatisfactory. Malan's outcome scales are meant to be scored intuitively and globally, based on knowledge of each patient, and do not have clear-cut and standardized anchor points for specific situations. He believes these studies have demonstrated that psychoanalytically trained raters can become relatively reliable in scoring clinically meaningful variables and that the results of psychodynamic research performed in this fashion can be applied usefully to clinical practice.

Malan's first study, which consisted of 21 patients treated in more or less brief psychotherapy, turned up the following results: 1) Motivation for insight was correlated with improvement; 2) severity of pathology (within the rather narrow limits of the selection criteria for patients in the study) and duration of complaints were not related to outcome; and 3) thorough interpretation of the transference was related to favorable outcome, especially the interpretation of the link between transference reactions and early parental interactions.

The patients were selected for the investigation by both exclusion and inclusion criteria. Exclusion criteria included: serious suicide attempts, drug addiction, convinced homosexuality, long-term hospitalization, more than one course of ECT, chronic alcoholism, incapacitating chronic obsessional or phobic symptoms, and gross destructive or self-destructive acting-out. Patients were included in the study who showed the following on evaluation and projective testing: response to interpretations; that some conceivable and feasible psychodynamic focus for therapeutic intervention could be formulated; and that dangers of attempting brief therapy did not seem inevitable.

The summary results of data gathered later in a replication study of 39 patients were as follows. Within the limits of patient pathology accepted for treatment, its nature and duration did not correlate significantly with outcome. This confirms the findings of the first study and allows the authors to conclude that at least some severe and chronic psychiatric conditions respond to brief focal dynamic therapy. It must be noted, however, that the fairly stringent inclusion criteria reduce the generalizability of this statement. Most severely disordered patients who might have failed in focal therapy were screened out beforehand and did not receive it. The patient's initial motivation, measured during the consultation phase and from the data of the projective tests, correlates with outcome at the 10% level of confidence. While this is somewhat outside the usual confidence level accepted for research significance, the finding does deserve some consideration because it is a partial confirmation of a significant correlation in the first study. As Malan points out, however, his measure of motivation is of little practical value in the selection of specific patients in the clinical situation, because using such criteria would eliminate too many successful cases and accept too many unsuccessful ones. In more technical language, the motivation criterion is insufficiently specific and sensitive to guide prediction.

Although there were no consistent correlations of focality with outcome, certain very interesting and practically important groupings reflect the relationships among focality, motivation, and outcome. The brief favorable cases were those that showed high ratings of both motivation and focality. This was in contrast with long, successful cases, which were high on motivation but low on focality, and long unsuccessful ones, which were low on both. This seems intuitively right. As was true in the first study, there was a significant positive correlation between the percentage of transference/parent interpretations and positive outcome. An important additional finding was that although transference/parent interpretations were significantly correlated with greater improvement, there was a cohort of improvers for whom this type of interpretation was relatively absent. Moreover, the percentage of such interpretations in comparison to all interpretations made in the treatment was never very high for any of the patients treated. It seems clear that what Malan defined as personality change occurs not only with, but also at least occasionally without, the specific technique of transference/parent linking interpretation. If these linking interpretations are specifically useful, they must be very potent, because they were made infrequently even in those treatments in which they significantly correlated with changes.

Both the advantages and disadvantages of Malan's naturalistic-correlational study are readily apparent. Let us outline the advantages first before we take him (and the strategy) over the scientific coals. The use of a flexible, naturalistic-correlational design has allowed Malan boldly to provide answers to some of the most fundamental questions in psychotherapy research. His results are of enormous clinical interest and (if believed) would have an immediate and obvious impact on clinical practice. Moreover, they seem to make good clinical, intuitive sense, and to confirm what we have always believed. Using the naturalistic-correlational approach, Malan has produced research findings which allow him to make statements on a number of issues that might have taken many generations to study had he instead opted for a more precise and well-controlled experimental design. His microscopic study of the process and of the outcome of each of the individual cases captures and supports interesting clinical insights that might have been lost in the shuffle of experimental studies (which in the past have sometimes been mindlessly concerned only with group averages). Malan is the paradigm of the clinician turned researcher, and he never forgets to reflect his findings back upon clinical practice.

But all of this has been purchased at a considerable price in rigor. Since there is no control group in this research strategy, the far-reaching conclusions of his elaborate study and replication are simply not proven. Malan has uncovered a number of interesting correlations but really has no basis upon which to assert causality. His research findings do not prove that the outcome of focal therapy is superior to, or even different from, spontaneous remission or the outcome of another treatment. Only a controlled study would do this. In his more optimistic moments, Malan proudly declares that he is providing a validation of psychodynamic theory and practice. He asserts that transference/parent linking interpretations, the essence of all uncovering dynamic treatments, are indeed especially and specifically successful in promoting enduring character change in focal therapy. Unfortunately, the findings, however suggestive and appealing, cannot bear the weight of his claim and can be interpreted equally plausibly in a totally contrary way. Malan assumes that the transference/parent interpretations produce a good treatment process and outcome. It is entirely possible that a good treatment process (patient and therapist getting on well together and doing their best to please one another) produces transference/parent interpretations if the therapist believes that these are important and the patient learns to respond to this with positive reinforcement to the therapist. The naturalistic-correlational design prevents us from determining the direction of causality.

Malan's findings are also shaken by some methodological weaknesses that might have encouraged bias. Perhaps the greatest problem is the source of his data. The information about the treatment process comes from notes written (apparently somewhat erratically) by the therapist after the session. We are forced to depend on the therapist's memory and to see the session through his eyes rather than having an independent rating, as might have been possible through the use of video- or audiotapes. In some of the ratings, the judges were not blind to the patients and certainly they were not blind to the hypotheses. Malan is also perhaps a bit too quick on his statistical feet. Here and there, he somewhat whimsically and on minor pretext chooses to include and exclude individual cases that are inconveniently subtracting from the strength of his correlations. Considering the relatively small sample size, one worries that he is selectively filtering data to confirm his preexisting beliefs.

Nonetheless, certain conclusions for differential therapeutics do emerge fairly clearly from Malan's findings. What Malan calls "static" criteria for inclusion (those that reside within the patient and do not arise out of his interaction with the psychiatric evaluator) are of partial, but definitely limited, value. One should not expect focal treatment to work well for the very severely impaired, the suicidal, the impulse-ridden, or the addicted. Ideally, the patient wants to change himself, not just to complain or receive solace, and psychological insight is sought as a means of such change. Malan especially emphasizes the value of inclusion of "dynamic" patient-therapist interaction criteria. Can the patient and therapist together focus on a problem? Can the therapist formulate a dynamic focus? Does the patient respond to interpretation? Do both the focus and the motivation to explore it increase as treatment progresses? The three best predictors — motivation for change, ability to find a dynamic focus, and response to interpretation — remain hard to operationalize and require fine clinical judgment. Nonetheless, they are clearly helpful reminders for any clinician evaluating a patient for focal therapy.

Where does this leave us? Malan is a brilliant clinician who knows just the right questions to ask but sometimes takes shortcuts in answering them. His naturalistic-correlational design, in bold strokes, permitted intuitively "right" clinical conclusions, but his findings did not eliminate alternative explanations and, thus, are not proven. Pending experimental confirmation, how much weight should we give them now? We think, a good deal. With all its flaws and limitations, Malan's correlational method is a great advance over unsystematic and anecdotal clinical lore. Perhaps he has not "validated" psychodynamic therapy (quite a tall order), but he has taken a systematic and enlightening look at it. The selection criteria based on his findings are the best we presently have. It is also noteworthy that other investigators (somewhat independently but working within the same frame of theory and expectations) have also come to Malan's conclusions.

One last word on an additionally important advantage of naturalistic-correlational studies: They are relatively (although not absolutely) inexpensive to perform, and one can choose to study clinical activities that would have been performed anyway. Naturalistic-correlational studies require replication, preferably experimental, but there is no more effective way systematically to generate hypotheses for further testing.

Manipulative-Experimental Designs

The basic strategy of experimental designs is to manipulate one (or more) of the independent variables while hopefully controlling and holding constant all of the others, in order to isolate and measure the specific effect of the manipulation on outcome. The presence of a control group corrects the major problem inherent in the naturalistic-correlational design: A manipulative-experimental design allows one to estimate the extent of the causal input of the independent variable (the particular treatment offered) on the dependent variable (the patient outcome). A manipulative-experimental design always requires some form of controlled comparison. The patient may be compared with himself, with a no treatment control group, with a placebo control group, with a control group receiving a different and competing active treatment, or with a control group receiving a combination of treatments. Often, several of these possibilities may be included within one design. If one is most interested in comparing treatment A with treatment B, it may still be desirable to include a placebo group to provide a baseline comparison of their effectiveness. It may also be useful to use a control group that combines treatments A and B (say behavior therapy and imipramine) to determine if they have synergistic effects when used together and whether each treatment is differentially effective for different target symptoms.

The great advantage of the manipulative-experimental design is this ability to identify functional relationships between therapist behaviors and patient outcome. There are limitations and difficulties, however. A well-controlled experimental study that attempts to get close to the clinical reality must often choose between asking a very simple question or mounting a very ambitious effort. Suppose a study attempts to compare the effects of two types of psychotherapy, with and without the accompanying use of medication, and against medication and placebo. This requires many treatment cells and a very large patient sample.

Manipulative-experimental studies are also not safe from contaminants of various sorts. It is difficult (perhaps impossible) to measure, much less control, everything in a field as complicated as psychotherapy. Unless findings have been thoroughly replicated, it is entirely possible that the results of even well-designed studies are influenced by unknown and uncontrollable, but powerful, independent variables that have not been measured in the study design. For example, in a behavioral investigation of the treatment of phobias, one may assume that the independent variable (systematic desensitization) caused the improvement in the phobia. However, it may be that uncontrolled and unspecified interaction qualities and characteristics of the therapist were actually most responsible for the improvement in the patient.

This problem may receive clarification from a recent refinement in experimental outcome design – the so-called dismantling and construction strategies. If the overall treatment package is composed of multiple, well-defined, freestanding modular parts, one can tease out the specific effects of each component, and their interaction, by systematically studying the effects on outcome of their dismantling or construction.

In the clinical situation, it is not always possible to conduct a true experimental study in which one controls the assignment of subjects to two or more psychotherapeutic interventions. Random assignment may be impossible because of the wishes of patients and families for a particular type of treatment, or the particular orientation of a specific clinic, or the specifications of funding from third-party payers, or ethical reasons, and so on. In spite of the failure to achieve full control, it may be desirable to go ahead and compare the outcome of patients in the different treatments. This has been called the quasi-experimental design (Campbell and Stanley, 1963). In the typical case, two groups of subjects are assigned not by randomization but according to the exigencies of the clinical world and are then studied with all the care of an experimental design. This can yield valuable information in spite of the fact that differences in outcome may reflect differences in the two groups consequent to biased assignment to treatment.

Combined Factorial Designs

Kiesler (1971) has argued persuasively for studies that combine methods derived from both the naturalistic-correlational and manipulative-experimental approaches. The investigator measures the naturally occurring patient independent variables and then determines how well they predict the impact on outcome of the manipulated independent treatment variables. Such a factorial design investigates, individually and in interaction, at least one therapist comparison (e.g., behavioral versus psychodynamic techniques) and at least one patient comparison (e.g., high versus low anxiety) as these relate to outcome. This method has greatly increased the yield and clinical significance of research results. It not only permits a statement about direct causal relationships between independent and dependent variables, but also enables the researcher to measure the impact of the interaction between patient and treatment variables. The results contribute to an understanding of the best match between patient and treatment techniques.

One can easily imagine expanding from a simple 2×2 design to 2×3, 3×3, and ever onward in the hope of better capturing the complexity of the clinical situation. There are, however, inherent limitations and problems with this. The most simple 2×2 factorial study has already required that each cell be divided in half – a feat that is possible only to the extent that the overall sample size is large enough to survive this division with adequate remaining numbers of subjects in each of the newly formed cells. As one increases the number of variables to be investigated, the number of cells increases multiplicatively and the number of subjects needed to fill them may become awesome, or at least very expensive and time-consuming. Although this is clearly the best and most comprehensive approach, it must be reserved for hypotheses and therapies that have proven some likely special merit in less expensive naturalistic designs.

Illustration: A combined factorial study (Sloane)

Sloane and his colleagues (Sloane, Staples, Cristol, Yorkston, and Whipple, 1975) have performed a study that is an extremely valuable paradigm for differential therapeutics and illustrates the richness and flexibility of the combined design. They selected for investigation a crucial question with wide implications: Which factors differentiate the process and outcome of the behavioral as opposed to the psychodynamic therapies and which factors are shared by both? In many respects, this study approximates the ideal design that is outlined in considerable detail in the next section. At each methodological step, there are careful controls and the selection of appropriate measures.

Since the investigators were interested in comparing the effectiveness of behavioral and psychodynamic brief therapy on a diversified patient population, the inclusion criteria were defined broadly to include all non-psychotic outpatients presenting to a university clinic and expressing willingness to participate. This suggests that the findings will be generalizable to the ordinary conditions of clinical practice with patients who have psychoneurosis or personality disorders, but it simultaneously reduces our ability to make statements on the possibly differential effectiveness of the two treatments on particular, more homogeneously defined patient groups. Patients were randomly assigned to treatment conditions according to a method that stratified for severity. Following assignment, the groups were found to be comparable in sex, age, and level of severity. The choice of a diversified patient population assigned under well-controlled conditions ensures that the two competing treatments are starting from the same baseline.

The therapists providing the behavioral and psychodynamic treatments were equally experienced in both overall clinical practice and the particular mode of therapy, but we have no measures of their ability or charisma. Samples of treatment sessions were taped and analyzed in order to ensure that the behavioral and psychodynamic techniques were indeed different and were provided in accord with the two theoretical orientations being tested. Unfortunately, there is little description of the actual techniques used in the treatments and so it remains difficult to evaluate the extent to which they were delivered reliably and without confounding overlap. The dynamic therapy is particularly poorly defined. It is not clear the extent to which it was primarily anxiety-suppressive (supportive) or anxiety-provoking (uncovering or focal), and whether transference interpretations were made (and, if so, whether they were connected to early life experience). This may seem like hairsplitting, especially since a survey of the patients' attitude toward the treatments did not differentiate even the much more obvious differences between behavioral and dynamic techniques. On the other hand, the very reason why patients did not differentiate might be because there was too much overlap between the treatments.

Assessment of patient variables before treatment, after treatment, and at one- and two-year follow-ups was performed by patient questionnaire, therapist, and independent research team. Outcome measures were applied to multiple areas of functioning, including the overall severity of specific target symptoms and the level of work and social adjustment. The results were interesting. There were three experimental groups: one was subjected to 4 months of behavior therapy, another to 4 months of brief psychodynamic therapy, and a third was kept on a waiting list with relatively minimal contact. At four months, the target symptoms of all three groups had improved, but the two treatment groups were significantly better off than the control waiting list group. There was no significant difference in the effectiveness of the two treatments, although a trend slightly favored behavior therapy. There was no significant difference in social or work adjustment in any of the three groups. The results at one-year follow-up were difficult to assess because of intervening, uncontrolled treatment and life experiences. Most interestingly, the waiting list group had caught up both on therapy and on target symptom improvement. The one-year follow-up demonstrated that improvement was maintained or continued in both the behavior and psychotherapy groups.

The study not only compared the overall effectiveness of the two therapies, but also attempted to discover the interaction effects: Which patient variables would predict favorable outcome in each of the different treatments? Positive results would obviously be enormously useful in providing differential therapeutic guidelines to select a behavioral or psychodynamically oriented treatment. The results were disappointingly negative. Sex, severity of neuroticism, and type of target symptoms were not differentially able to predict outcome in each of the treatments. There were only a few leads. High scores on the hysteria and psychopathic deviate scales of the MMPI predicted poor results in dynamic psychotherapy but not in behavior therapy. Based on this Sloane and his colleagues suggest that acting-out, antisocial, behavioral problem patients may do better in behavior therapy. Behavioral treatments also seem to work somewhat faster and might be selected if rapid response is indicated. The study confirms the universal clinical hunch that motivation and expectation powerfully influence results. On follow-up, all four behavior therapy failures had received psychodynamic therapy and three were pleased with the change.

It is an ill wind that blows no good and even largely negative findings can often be very useful. The Sloane study's failure to find much differentiation between the behavioral and dynamic therapies emphasizes what is similar, shared, and "nonspecific" in these two treatments. In addition to the similar outcome results, there was a remarkable similarity in the patients' perception of what was important in their treatment. Regardless of the specific techniques that were practiced (and probably treasured by the therapists), the patients were most mindful of aspects of the therapeutic relationship – the therapist's personality, his helpfulness, and his encouragement in facing bothersome issues. Of course, it remains possible that had the Sloane study had available to it different and more subtle outcome measures and had it exercised more control of the therapies delivered, there might have been more specific and differentiating results, though the weight of the evidence suggests the differences might be small and subtle, at best. Only further studies can resolve this question.

What differential treatment guidelines can be derived from the Sloane study? For nonpsychotic patients motivated for either a behavioral or dynamic approach, and when time for treatment is limited (e.g., four months or less), either treatment could be recommended if the goal is symptom relief. If fast symptom relief is necessary (e.g., the patient is likely to fail his final examinations unless he can settle down and study), behavior therapy should be recommended. There is some, albeit uncompelling, indication that patients who act out their difficulties should be placed in behavioral rather than dynamic therapy.

METHODS OF REVIEWING AND AGGREGATING RESEARCH STUDIES

It has long been apparent that no single outcome study, no matter how well designed, can by itself provide convincing and comprehensive answers about the comparative effects of different psychotherapeutic interventions (see Table 8-1 for representative studies). As one's perspective broadens beyond the individual study to encompass the whole of psychotherapy outcome research, the importance of methods of interpreting data across studies becomes clear. This has been an area of exciting, recent methodological advance.

Initial review efforts were narrative, impressionistic, subject to considerable bias, and not very helpful (Bergin and Lambert, 1978). Reviewers differed in outlook and in their selection of studies for discussion. Many believed that only "good" studies – those with adequate controls and methodology – should receive consideration, but this allowed for considerable subjectivity in selection and the choice of those studies that supported preexisting points of view. Not surprisingly, early reviewers sharply disagreed in their interpretation of the research literature and reviews sometimes resembled advocacy briefs rather than reasoned and fair-minded judgments.

The next advance was the attempt to quantify the process of research review in order to reduce some of the bias that was inevitable in narrative summaries. Luborsky and associates (Luborsky, Singer, and Luborsky, 1975) introduced what they labeled the "box score" method. The

TABLE 8-1
Illustrative Experimental Research Informative to Differential Therapeutics

	Author	Treatments Compared	Outcome
Technique			
Behavior vs. insight	Sloane, Staples, Cristol, Yorkston, & Whipple, 1975	Behavior therapy and psychodynamic psychotherapy	Both groups improved significantly in comparison to a control group.
	Gelder, Marks, Wolff, & Clarke, 1967	Desensitization vs. group vs. individual psychotherapy for agoraphobic patients	Desensitization best at discharge: no differences at the end of 2-year follow-up
Rogerian vs. traditional psychotherapy	Cartwright, 1966	Client-centered vs. psychodynamic psychotherapy	No differences in degree of experiencing and level of self-observation
Format			
Individual vs. group	Barron & Leary, 1955	Group vs. individual	Similarities greater than the differences
	O'Brien, Hamm, Ray, Pierce, Luborsky, & Mintz, 1972	Group vs. individual for schizophrenic patients	Group therapy patients had better adjustment ratings; rehospitalization rates did not differ

Individual vs. marital/family	Mayadas & Duehn, 1977	Communication modeling, modeling plus video-feedback and verbal counseling for marital problems	Communication modeling superior to communication modeling plus video which was superior to verbal counseling
	Pittman, Langsley, & DeYoung, 1968	Conjoint family crisis intervention vs. individual long-term	Conjoint therapy superior to individual in patient return to work
	Stanton & Todd, 1976	Structural family therapy vs. standard methadone treatments for heroin addicts	Family therapy superior
Duration			
Time limited vs. time unlimited	Reid & Schyne, 1969	Time-limited therapy (maximum of 8 sessions) compared to long-term treatment	The time-limited patients improved more
Somatic Treatment			
Psychopharmacotherapy vs. psychotherapy	Klerman, Paykel, & Prusoff, 1973; Klerman, Dimascio, & Weissman, 1974	Antidepressants and psychotherapy for depressed outpatients	Antidepressants effective on depressive symptomatology; psychotherapy effective on social functioning

criteria upon which studies would be allowed into consideration were determined beforehand in order to reduce the reviewer's tendencies to follow his own preferences. A tally was taken to determine the number of qualifying studies in which each competing treatment was significantly superior to the other and also the number of tie scores. In this way, Luborsky and associates were able to make a number of interesting comparisons.

The box score method was a major advance in research review but was still cumbersome and potentially misleading in a number of important ways. The single summary scoreboard made it sound as if homogeneous entities had competed with one another, whereas in fact the studies reviewed constituted ill-defined collections of heterogeneous techniques, patients, and sample sizes. Moreover, critics question whether a summary scoring of often poorly designed and equivocal studies had any claim to authority. Although the box score method had established rules for study selection, it still allowed for some degree of subjective judgment in excluding or including studies of borderline quality. Perhaps the greatest limitation of the box score method is the amount of information that is lost in its presentation of a summary score. A comparison must be scored in the tie column even if a very strong but nonsignificant trend prevails in favor of one treatment — a difference that might have been significant in a larger sample. Further, a wonderfully designed, large, and generalizable study is scored with equal weight to one that is poorly designed with a small n. This is democratic, but not compellingly scientific.

Many of these problems have been solved by the latest and by far the most sophisticated advance in research review technology — the meta-analysis method that was recently applied by Smith et al. (1980). This is a simple but elegant innovation that treats the results of each study as raw data for further statistical analysis. The authors compute a statistic called the Effect Size by using the following calculation: for each outcome measure, the change score in the treated group minus the change score in the control group divided by the standard deviation of the control group. The Effect Size is wonderfully flexible and saves an enormous amount of information lost in the box score method. Effect Sizes can also be determined for different kinds of patients, therapists, study designs, outcome measures, and so forth. The major limitation of the review by Smith and colleagues lies not with their method of meta-analysis, but rather with the data that are aggregated. Much of the available outcome research they have analyzed has been weak in design and inadequate in the definition of patient groups, treatments, and measures. Smith et al. believe that their overall review is more robust than the individual studies forming its data base. However, some of their findings (e.g., that psychodynamic treatment is especially well-matched to psychotic patients) are so intuitively wrong as to make us cautious about accepting other conclusions pending the application of meta-analysis to better outcome data. Their analysis is also limited by the difficulties encountered in categorizing the bewildering array of different psychotherapies.

The authors have painstakingly reviewed the many outcome measures obtained in 475 psychotherapy studies and in some 150 studies in which psychotherapy and drugs were compared alone and in combination. Only the literature on family therapy is slighted by relative inattention. After analyzing their statistical brew with great care, the authors reach the following conclusions:

1) Psychotherapy is definitely effective. The average patient in the treated group of all types of therapy is as well off as the patient in the 80th percentile of the control group. The benefits are not altogether permanent (they decreased by half in two years), but the authors point out with considerable accuracy that little else in life is permanent.
2) Insofar as they can measure them, different types of psychotherapy do not produce different types of outcome. The authors conclude that the determination of the right therapy for a specific problem in a particular patient is not possible, even with the large number of studies they have analyzed, and that the answer to this question may be long in coming.
3) Difference in psychotherapy format, orientation, length, and experience level of the therapist makes little difference to outcome.
4) Psychotherapy alone has an efficacy almost equal to drug therapy alone, even in the treatment of very serious disorders.
5) The separate effects of psychotherapy and drug therapy are essentially additive when they are combined.

Clinicians will welcome the statistically buttressed conclusions that psychotherapy is effective and mixes well with psychotropic drugs, but will find little else in this analysis to guide them in practical decision-making. The authors have in effect demonstrated that the available outcome research only makes a very limited contribution to clinical judgment. It will require a much more extensive and sophisticated future research effort to produce data of sufficient quality to inform the specifics of clinical art. In all likelihood, however, the technique of meta-analysis will endure for many decades as the best and simplest way of aggregating data across studies.

THE IDEAL STUDY

We will now describe (somewhat wistfully) the constituents of the ideal psychotherapy outcome study – one which would be optimally designed to answer most comprehensively the questions that constantly arise in clinical practice concerning the choice of one treatment modality in preference to another. We are drawing closer to having this ideal realized. In fact, a very well-conceived, NIMH multicenter collaborative study investigating the treatment of outpatient depression (with cognitive vs. interpersonal vs. drug therapy vs. combinations) is now being conducted and includes within its design many of the parameters listed below. Additional close-to-ideal studies are likely to be mounted in the very near future.

A few cautions are in order, however. Difficult and expensive as it is to perform even one well-designed psychotherapy study, it is unlikely that any single piece of work will stand on its own without widespread replication. Specific psychotherapy effects tend to be relatively weak and require confirmation; they do not have the clearcut face validity of the penicillin effect in streptococcal infections or of digitalis in congestive heart failure. Moreover, there are already at least 100 different forms of defined psychotherapy and scores of diagnostic conditions which may be differentially affected by them. A thoroughly comparative investigation of all possibly meaningful permutations to determine what works best for what specific problem would seriously drain the Gross National Product and would probably be of more academic than practical interest. For the present, public policy will doubtless choose instead to fund a few well-designed studies of better known and easy-to-deliver psychotherapies intended for the treatment of those psychiatric conditions that present major and expensive public health problems. An important first goal of this effort will be to demonstrate that specific psychotherapy techniques have differential effects on different types of patient problem – a commonsense, ubiquitous, clinical intuition that has thus far eluded clear documentation. Our presentation of the ideal study will deal separately with its design, patient and treatment variables, instruments, and analysis of data.

Design Factors

The combined factorial design produces results that are especially valuable in pointing toward treatment selection criteria for a particular type of patient. The study will address psychiatric disorder(s) with a wide public health, as well as scientific, significance. To be worthy of such careful study, the comparison treatments must have some demonstrated or presumptive efficacy. If combined treatments (e.g., psychotherapy plus drugs) are likely to be either additive or synergistically useful in their effects, the experimental design must compare each of the treatments done by itself to a combination of the two treatments. There should also be a placebo group to serve as a baseline with which to compare the effects of the specific intervention (although as previously discussed, it is perhaps impossible to conceive of a true psychotherapy placebo).

The sample size in a combined naturalistic-experimental design must generally be quite large. In a straight experimental design, the statistical analysis requires only a simple comparison of the overall effectiveness of the two treatments. The combined naturalistic-experimental approach goes much further in its data analysis in order to determine the patient-treatment interaction effects, i.e., which patient characteristics produce better or worse response to the treatment intervention. In measuring these interaction effects, one is obviously further subdividing each cell. The cells must begin with a large enough sample size to bear the weight of this statistical analysis. The ideal study must, of course, be replicated and, preferably, this should be done under the same conditions and also under different conditions in order to determine generalizability. There is a promising trend toward collaborative psychotherapy outcome studies performed simultaneously at many centers, using the same protocol and carefully controlled conditions. This provides immediate replication and the opportunity to increase the n by pooling data to permit multivariate analysis.

Of course, a combined naturalistic-experimental study is complicated and expensive to conduct. It is ideal only as a culmination of previous attempts using less elaborate designs. Hypothesis generation is less expensive in naturalistic studies.

Patient Variables

In order to meaningfully compare treatments and to give each approach a fair run for its money, the patients involved in each modality must be comparable on those dimensions likely to predict the natural course of the disorder and its response to treatment. To the extent that this is not the case, differences in outcome may be more a function of preexisting differences among the patient groups, rather than a function of the contribution made by the treatments themselves. The formation of relatively homogeneous patient groups has been greatly improved by the availability of the fairly rigorous and operational criteria supplied in the Research Diagnostic Criteria (Spitzer, Endicott, and Robins, 1978) and the Diagnostic and Statistical Manual III (APA, 1980).

To ensure patient comparability in the various cells, assignment to groups must be done randomly or by matching. If one suspects that specific patient dimensions are likely to influence results greatly, it is wise to match patients or to stratify assignments of these dimensions to ensure that they will be equally represented in all of the study groups. The dimensions most commonly calling for matching or stratification include sex, age, and other demographic variables, diagnosis, presenting symptoms, personality features, severity of illness, previous course, level of functioning, prognosis, and level of stress. The practical difficulty involved in matching or stratifying, especially as the number of variables involved in the matching grows, are enormous and serve as a limit to the ideal study. It is just not possible to match or stratify on every potentially significant variable; one or two is the norm. Moreover, one must often settle for comparability of the group mean scores on various dimensions rather than expect close individual matching of patients on more than one or two variables.

All patient dimensions must be analyzed against success or failure in each of the treatments being studied. The more narrowly homogeneous patients under study (e.g., all have unipolar, nonendogenous depression with ratings between 18 and 24 on the Hamilton Rating Scale for Depression), the more likely it is that one can determine the specific impact of the treatments investigated on that particular disorder and degree of severity; and reciprocally, the less likely it is that one can generalize to make statements about the effects of the treatments on patients who do not have that particular disorder and degree of severity.

Real, rather than analog, patients should be used. Many studies (particularly of behavioral techniques) have been performed on college or graduate students or recruited volunteers. The generalizability of results from such studies to clinical work with real patients is highly questionable. Even the practice of advertising for patients (e.g., depressed college students or agoraphobics) is likely to net a sample of afflicted individuals who may differ in important ways (especially motivation) from the larger sample of individuals with the same diagnosis who present spontaneously for psychiatric treatment. Analog studies are useful for hypothesis generation and testing and may play a role similar to that of laboratory testing in medical research. Ultimately, however, a technique must prove itself in a clinical population selected in such a way as to be representative of that larger population of similar patients not engaged in the research.

Therapist or Treatment Variables

Insofar as is possible, the treatments used must be clearly specified and reproducible. It will never be possible to package psychotherapy with the metric precision of psychotropic medication, but it is nonetheless crucial that the specific and differentiating characteristics of the given treatment be delivered in some consistent way. The techniques must have an operationally defined format or program which can be reliably taught to therapists, and monitored systematically, to ensure that the patients in each study group are indeed receiving the specific kinds of treatment that are intended and that these differ from one another as prescribed. This requires an independent content analysis of the therapy sessions, which might include measures of how much each participant talks, what kinds of things they say, who interrupts whom more often, and so on. Patients can be surveyed to determine whether they perceive the different treatments as indeed different or similar.

Unfortunately, this method, although crucial, also has certain inherent limitations and works well only for brief treatments. It is particularly difficult to "package" psychodynamically-oriented therapies because these depend, in an essential way, on the spontaneity, intuition, and empathy of the therapist, resulting in interventions that for obvious reasons cannot conveniently be specified in advance, made to order, and included in a treatment package. Partly for this reason, the treatment packages now being tested embody forms of psychotherapy that are to some extent "hothouse grown" and thus can be very unrepresentative of, and perhaps not generalizable to, the day-to-day treatment delivered at large by most practitioners in the community. With due respect to all of these caveats, however, it is only by continuing the effort to define treatments carefully that we can determine just what works and how.

Therapists delivering each of the treatments under study must have equivalent overall competence, experience, training, and belief. If one therapy is represented by more skilled practitioners, differences in outcome may relate to differences in overall skill of delivery, rather than anything inherent or specific to the techniques that have been employed. In the past, most studies have resorted to the use of relatively inexperienced trainees as therapists because they are more available, willing to participate, and/or cheaper. It seems clear, however, that studies comparing the results achieved by inexperienced therapists do not really put the treatment techniques to their fairest and most representative test, and favor those techniques that are easiest to learn quickly or apply mechanically.

The competing treatments must be equally valued by the therapists performing them. Clinicians who unenthusiastically administer a treatment in which they have little faith are likely to get poor results regardless of the inherent worth of the technique. Those who are zealots, with a religious devotion to their approach, may effect nonspecific and nongeneralizable "cures" that are not closely related to the particular technique they espouse.

It is important to gather data about and compare treatments that may have been received by the patients outside the provisions of the particular research protocol. Clearly, if one group of patients has had more access to psychotropic drugs than the other, this fact can confound the interpretation of results and make unclear what would have been achieved by each of the psychotherapies individually. Many patients, especially those who have had poorer results, seek and obtain additional treatment during the follow-up period, after ending the treatment part of the protocol. This may account for the failure of treatment differences to stand up on follow-up in most studies. One cannot ethically restrict patients from receiving treatments they desire (and probably need), but efforts must be made to report the extent and kind of additional treatment and to estimate the effects of such confounding.

Finally, each treatment must be delivered with a frequency, intensity, and duration that is compatible with its best and usual clinical practice. In addition, the frequency, intensity, and duration of the comparison treatments must be more or less equivalent or else these differences may become a confounding influence.

Process Measures

A distinction is usually made between treatment process and treatment outcome studies. The latter measure the results of treatment, either at termination or follow-up; the former investigate the progression of the treatment, when and how it works. While one can attempt to contrast process and outcome strategies, the two also have many elements in common, and ultimately both measure the effects of interventions upon patient behavior. One difference between the two approaches has to do with the point in time at which these effects are studied. Although the goal of process research, i.e., to examine the basic mechanisms of the therapeutic intervention, is an extremely useful one, outcome research is ultimately more relevant to the development of a differential therapeutic system.

Nonetheless, ratings designed to measure various aspects of the ongoing process of therapy are desirable and help to ensure that different competing treatments are indeed different. These measures might include a content analysis of the treatment sessions, ratings of the patient's motivation, expectation, attachment to the therapist, and satisfaction, and measures of the therapist's sense of direction, understanding, and satisfaction, and measures of the patient-therapist interaction. Consumer satisfaction with treatment provides data that may be especially pertinent to the issue of compliance. Consumer perception of each treatment is useful in determining the extent to which different treatments are distinguishable.

Outcome Measures

Ratings of outcome should be made by the patient, significant others in the patient's life, the therapist, and independent raters blind to the treatment. There should be specific outcome measures geared to the particular goals and techniques of the treatments being compared. These should be applied to all study patients in order to measure if specific treatments are indeed differentially able to accomplish what they have set out to do. For instance, if one treatment modality under study is family therapy, measures should be taken on all individual family members and should also address the family interaction, not just in the family but in the comparison treatment groups.

There should be global measures of improvement, which usually tap the severity of symptoms. Additionally, Strupp, Hadley, and Gomes-Schwartz (1977) have suggested ratings in three areas of functioning: the subjective experience of the patient (particularly his feelings of self-esteem); his interpersonal behaviors; and an assessment of the patient's intrapsychic functioning. Thus far, such measures have been much more difficult to develop than symptom measures. Generally, multiple outcome criteria are desirable.

At least some of the measures should be relatively nonreactive, i.e., not easily influenced in any direction by the biases of the therapist, patient, or independent rater. Reactive instruments measure variables that are easily influenced by the patient's desire to please or to deny change, or by the therapist's or rater's positive bias toward achieving certain goals or modesty in denying that these have been achieved. Certain types of measure are inherently more unreactive or easy to keep blind, e.g., the dexamethasone suppression test. Others are inherently more reactive and impossible to keep blind, e.g., the therapist's ratings of patient improvement. Biologic outcome measures are now being refined for a number of conditions and may become especially useful for depression and panic disorder.

Outcome measures should be taken often during treatment and at follow-up to give some sense of the course of response. For instance, if behavior therapy works faster than dynamic therapy, this can be determined only if ratings are taken early and regularly. Follow-up should be long enough to provide evidence of the likely endurance of results.

Analysis of Data Variables

Hopefully, the sample size will have been large enough to allow for multivariate statistical analysis to determine which treatment variables interact with which patient variables to produce most benefit or most harm from the treatment being considered, and to compare such interactions across treatments in order to develop the indications, enabling factors, and contraindications for each. Especially in view of current financial pressures from government and third-party payers, it is also essential that cost/benefit and cost-effectiveness assessment be done, comparing various psychotherapies in this regard.

The study must make explicit the manner in which the treatment dropouts have been included, excluded, or prorated in analyzing the data. There is often no single most sensible way of analyzing dropouts, and it may be best to use and report the several different possible statistical methods.

SUMMARY

Practical considerations ensure that available studies are not (and probably never will be) complete or ideal, but fortunately this does not diminish their value and necessity. Incomplete, and even flawed, research is better than none at all, so long as the particular limitations of each study are clear. Differential therapeutics is still a largely intuitive enterprise, but we can expect it to become progressively more scientific in the very near future.

CHAPTER 9

Clinical Evaluation for Treatment Selection

The evaluation of a new patient constitutes the most important task in all of clinical practice and the most difficult. For the consultant, each new evaluation is a renewal of clinical skill and a stimulating opportunity to widen clinical experience. For the patient, the moment may be a potential turning point, a time of both opportunity and danger.

Two strangers meet. Quickly, they must establish rapport — a word that describes, but does not explain, the interpersonal chemistry that allows people to work well with one another and cooperate in the job at hand. Implicit in the consultation alliance is that the patient tell all (or most all) about his or her symptoms, hopes, fears, fantasies, disappointments, weaknesses, and strengths. The consultant's job is to combine empathy with expertise. He must listen well, question thoroughly, formulate clearly, and thereby bring order to a situation that previously seemed inchoate and unmanageable. The consultant then teaches the patient something about his/her condition, about its course, and about the advantages and disadvantages of the possible treatment options. There is a negotiation phase that leads to a selection of a particular treatment and therapist (or possibly to the choice of no treatment). Finally, the patient learns what will be expected of him or her in the treatment selected and what he or she in return can expect from it.

Done well, a consultation can be a joy forever. It serves to reduce demoralization, provides a sense of direction, increases motivation, and becomes the foundation for a successful treatment experience. Done poorly, a consultation can be a disaster and one that is not easily reversed. The insensitive or inexpert consultation can make a bad situation even worse, discourage the patient about his future prospects, and convince him that psychiatric treatment is something to avoid at all costs. Unfortunately, first consultations are often performed under circumstances of considerable pressure to all involved and may not bring out the best in either the patient or consultant. This is a task that requires practice and attention.

In this chapter, we will suggest how to approach a consultation. We are not attempting to reduce this extraordinarily complex and variable process to a simple formula; nor are we attempting to consolidate the rich and vast literature on conducting a clinical review (MacKinnon and Michels, 1971). Instead, to maintain the focus of this book, we will attend only to those aspects of the evaluation that impact specifically upon treatment selection.

DEFINING THE CONSULTATION TASK

It is to be hoped that every contact between a clinician and a patient will be in some way therapeutic (or at least helpful). We have already mentioned in Chapter 4 that there is some literature suggesting that even one session can have a prolonged beneficial impact. Nevertheless, it is our strong conviction that under most circumstances it is wise to sharply differentiate the psychiatric consultation from the beginning of the treatment. Many clinicians blur this differentiation in their own minds and/or in their dealings with the patient and act as if a treatment contract begins with the first patient contact. This practice has many other disadvantages, but the major one that we will emphasize here is that it forestalls any meaningful discussion of treatment selection. If the patient and clinician have embarked on what feels like a treatment experience from the very start of their relationship, they will avoid making conscious and well-thought-out decisions about what kind of treatment is indicated for the problem at hand and who is most qualified to provide it.

We are suggesting that the consultation alliance is a very different arrangement than the treatment alliance. The goals of the two situations differ appreciably and the relationship between consultant and client is unlike that between therapist and patient. The alliance may evolve, and the consultant may certainly become therapist if this seems appropriate, but such a transition should be marked by a mutually-agreed-upon decision and not occur automatically or routinely.

Although good consultants very often are also good therapists and vice versa, the skills that are special to each task do not overlap completely. Some good consultants are indeed dreadful therapists and some good therapists are indeed dreadful consultants, at least under particular circumstances. The consultant's task requires that he have a wide knowledge of and ability to elicit psychopathology; be an astute observer and diagnostician; be knowledgeable about the indications for a wide range of biological, psychological, learning, and systems treatments (and their most suitable settings, formats, and durations); be conversant with the use of psychotropic medications; be able to size up situations quickly, formulate them clearly, negotiate convincingly and make decisions decisively; and, finally, that he know what services and people are available to provide treatment and be intuitive in sensing good patient-therapist personality matches. To do all of this well, a skilled consultant must be especially good at interacting with strangers and be expert as a generalist. On the other hand, the skills of a therapist can be more specific and specialized to a particular form of treatment. Someone can be a highly successful psychoanalyst or behavior therapist or group therapist without having the wide scope that is necessary in the consultant. Some consultants are wonderful generalists but not very skillful in delivering any one of the specialized treatment modalities. We assume that most clinicians hope to be or to become excellent both as generalists and specialists, but it is probably wise for each of us to take stock of our expertise (or lack of it) in each direction and attempt to either expand our skills or limit our practices to what we do best.

Patients themselves often do not distinguish between psychiatric consultation and psychiatric treatment. Many patients simply present themselves, explain their problems, and expect the therapist to select the best treatment and then perform it. The advantages of a separate consultation period preceding any decision about treatment must be explained to the patient usually from the outset, i.e., the very first telephone call requesting an appointment. Some few patients (particularly those who are dependent, fearful of rejection, or in considerable turmoil) may find this arrangement difficult, but most patients respond positively to the notion of a consultation. They are relieved to learn that they will have a good deal of say in any treatment decisions that are made and that this issue will be given considerable thought. Often patients ask whether the consultant will also be able to do whatever treatment is necessary. The consultant should indicate whether it is likely that he would have the necessary time, but should also point out that it is impossible, before doing a careful evaluation, to know whether or not his working with the patient would indeed be a good idea. The choice of therapist will in most instances depend upon the nature of the problem and whether the kind of treatment that is most indicated is within the consultant's special expertise. Moreover, it will depend on the patient's preference and the patient may or may not choose to work with the consultant.

In our experience, it is often best to discuss this question in some detail early in the contact with a patient. The first telephone call can set the tone for what happens next. Establishing this structure for the consultation makes it clear from the start that the patient has the freedom and responsibility to make choices, that any decisions require the gathering of a considerable data base, and that the patient has a great deal to learn about the nature of the presenting problem, its underlying causes, and the treatment options. This kind of consultative alliance reduces patient regression and impatience and serves as foundation for both the consultation and for whatever treatment, if any, is ultimately decided upon.

One of the most common, and usually unnoticed, errors made by consultants is the routine application of interviewing techniques that are derived from their treatment experience to the very different demands of the consultation situation. The inflexible psychoanalyst is likely to conduct the consultation interview too much like an unstructured analytic session – to follow the patient's associations wherever they lead, without asking a sufficient number of structured questions that are necessary for gathering an adequate descriptive and historical data base. The inflexible behaviorist is likely to err in just the opposite direction and provide too much structure and direction too early, focusing down prematurely on one specific problem and missing important accessory data. Similarly, the inflexible experiential therapist as consultant might rely so much on establishing a caring relationship and empathizing with the patient's plight in the here and now that crucial historical data are overlooked and the patient may feel "raped" because the clinician has gotten too close too fast. At the other extreme, the inflexible, biologically-oriented clinician might determine only the phenomenology of the illness and even prescribe medication, without establishing an empathic doctor-patient relationship that would enhance compliance and therapeutic effect.

A consultative alliance is actually based on a judicious use of techniques derived from all therapeutic orientations. It must be highly structured at times and ambiguous at others, focused but also general, psychodynamic but also behavioral, cognitive, biological, and systems-oriented. Though intuition is important, the clinician can only develop consultative skills through experience, attention, training, and continuing review by peers and self.

EXPLORING THE PRESENTING PROBLEM

It is our experience that very frequently a consultant gathers an enormously detailed history and yet never finds out why the patient has come for help *now*. The careful pursuit of the question *why now* is necessary to focus the consultation and provides valuable data from a number of different perspectives. First, it is impossible to set treatment goals without considering in an explicit way just what brought the patient to treatment in the first place. Furthermore, in finding out what has tipped the balance, the consultant and patient are likely to discover the patient's special vulnerabilities to particular environmental stressors. This tells the consultant something about the patient's intrapsychic dynamics and also indicates whether environmental manipulations are likely to be indicated or possible. A clearly specified chief complaint will also lead to the tentative hypotheses that can be tested during the rest of the interview.

Often the patient will at first offer only very vague and general responses to the question *why now*, perhaps suggesting that consultation was sought because "I feel empty" or "I'm having a mid-life crisis" or "I've been having trouble with my wife for years" or "I'm not satisfied with how my life is going." All of these are reasonable statements but they do not explain or attempt to explain why help is sought on this particular day. Sometimes, perhaps for unconscious reasons, the patient will indeed be quite unaware of the sources of immediate anxiety. It is valuable to take a parallel history, which can provide clues about precipitants that had never occurred to the patient.

A very useful corollary question is *why didn't the patient come for help previously?* In many instances, patients wait a remarkably long time, suffering in silence or seeking help elsewhere, before accepting the need for psychiatric consultation. In learning why the patient did not come earlier, the consultant will gain clues about the patient's resistances to and reservations about treatment and possible compliance problems. The ways in which the patient was able previously to avoid treatment will also indicate what sources of support (internal and external) were available that made it unnecessary in the past.

Although patients often feel, justifiably, as though their problems are unique, in an important way they are wrong. An experienced clinician with a broad knowledge of psychopathology will appreciate that symptoms fall into certain clusters, i.e., into various syndromes, disorders, or illnesses with their own particular dynamics, causes, and courses. The consultant must gather enough descriptive data about the present episode in order to make a DSM-III diagnosis. Which symptoms are present and what was their onset, course, duration, impact, and response to previous attempts at resolution? What are the pertinent negatives? The syndromal format of DSM-III is useful in educating the clinician about which symptoms tend to correlate with one another and which differential diagnoses are most important to consider.

It is often useful to supplement the data that have been gathered from the patient with the views of others, most typically the family, the internist, and other psychotherapists who have been involved. The most common mistake here is for the consultant to go it alone and to lose crucial data that for one or another reason are unavailable from the patient. It is also important to learn about the patient's reaction to the current episode. Is he or she demoralized? To what degree? Is there secondary gain? What are his or her expectations for treatment?

Most patients are only too willing to discuss the chief complaint, which is, after all, what is most bothersome at the moment. Patients may be less willing to discuss the present illness, which involves far more than the current distress. It includes not just the onset and duration of symptoms, but also their course and impact and how they have or have not responded to previous treatments or attempts by the patient to resolve the difficulty. Most important, the present illness also includes those problems that the consultant – but perhaps not the patient – recognizes as being related to the presenting complaint.

A thorough knowledge of the DSM-III can be a powerful tool in delineating the present illness. Whatever the presenting problem – "forgetfulness," "fear of flying," "too fat" – the DSM-III can guide the consultant toward asking about problems that may be related – for instance, disorientation, agoraphobia, or bulimia. An understanding of psychopathology and psychodynamics is by far the best guide to knowing what phenomena are commonly linked with presenting problems. The psychiatric consultant will ask questions that to the patient may seem irrelevant.

ELICITING RELEVANT BACKGROUND DATA

Does the current episode conform to recurring patterns in the patient's life? How is it similar to or different from previous episodes? What have been the circumstances of previous episodes, the treatments tried, their effects? Perhaps the best predictor of how a patient will do in a recommended treatment is how well or poorly the patient has done in previous treatments. The consultant must therefore make every effort to determine exactly what happened during previous therapeutic encounters – the name of the therapist, the setting, the format, the techniques, the intensity, the duration, the compliance, the reasons for termination, the experience of this termination, the view of treatment at the time and afterwards, and the exact reasons why the patient has not returned to the previous therapist for additional treatment. Psychiatric treatments are particularly susceptible to transferential distortions on the part of both the patient and the therapist. The patient, in fact, can be told that an attempt should be made to distinguish between how s/he feels about the previous treatment and what s/he thinks actually occurred.

Because the background data may seem completely irrelevant to the troubled patient, the consultant should indicate the rationale for asking about childhood, family history, and items on the mental status examination. This exploration will also help the inexperienced consultant, who may be inclined to compile data simply because it is required on a form and not because it is related to treatment selection. At the end of the chapter, the reader will find the evaluation form used at the Payne Whitney Clinic. We fully recognize that some items may need to be given more emphasis and other items omitted depending on the priorities and time limitations of the particular situation. With some patients, especially those compelled to describe in great detail every aspect of their past, the consultant may choose to state aloud that the evaluation period cannot possibly capture the richness and depth of the patient's experiences and that the assigned therapist will no doubt acquire such information over time. This kind of statement will limit the expectations of the patient (and of the consultant) and may make the necessary interruptions more tolerable.

At this point in the evaluation – after defining the task, establishing a consultative alliance, delineating the present illness and determining the precipitating event, and acquiring background data – the consultant may wish to conclude the first evaluation session and arrange for a second appointment. This is usually necessary because of time constraints, but there are also several additional advantages in doing an evaluation in two or more sittings. Patients and consultants alike benefit from mulling over the wealth of accumulating data and reflecting upon what has and what has not been said. In addition, the patient's responses to the first session can be useful information regarding what the patient expects to accomplish from treatment and what kind of benefits and resistances will occur.

MEDICAL EVALUATION

Systematic studies of psychiatric inpatients (Hall, Gardner, Popkin, LeCann, and Stickney, 1981) or outpatients (Hall, Popkin, Devaul, Faillace, and Stickney, 1978; Muecke and Krueger, 1981) reveal the alarmingly high incidence of unrecognized medical problems. An editorial comment (Hall, Faillace, and Perl, 1979) commonly accompanies these reports, imploring psychiatrists to recognize their responsibilities as physicians. Despite these periodic reports and pleas, the majority of psychiatric patients do not undergo a thorough search for an underlying physical condition that may be compounding or even causing the mental disorder. Several reasons (or rationalizations) for "deferring" a complete medical evaluation follow:

1) The history and mental status examination will in most cases reveal evidence for a possible medical disturbance;
2) in the absence of such supporting evidence, a complete medical evaluation of every new psychiatric patient is not cost-effective;
3) the evaluation process, particularly the physical examination, is intrusive, disrupts neutrality, and crosses the necessary barrier of psychotherapy in which physical contact should be avoided;
4) although medically trained, most psychiatrists no longer have the skills and knowledge (or facility) to conduct a medical evaluation;
5) patients often seek consultation at a time of situational crisis and are therefore neither motivated nor able to undergo a physical examination; and
6) many patients are simply too disorganized at the time of consultation to arrange and follow through with an adequate medical evaluation.

None of these reasons withstand a thoughtful analysis:

1) Some physical problems (e.g., endocrinopathies, cardiovascular disturbances, chronic infection) cannot be detected by even a thorough history and mental status examination.
2) Considering the length and cost of psychiatric treatments and disability, only a small percentage of positive yields would be necessary to justify the expense of a thorough medical evaluation, especially if a medically treatable disorder is disclosed. A treatable dementia is a case in point.
3) Although some kinds of psychotherapy (e.g., psychoanalysis) preclude the direct interventions required for medical evaluation, the consultation process should be distinguished from psychiatric treatment.
4) Even if the consultant lacks the necessary skills, knowledge, and

facilities to conduct the medical evaluation, arrangements can be made for a referral to an internist to perform the necessary examination and laboratory tests.

5) When a situational crisis precludes a thorough medical evaluation, the consultant can at least state explicitly that the consultation process will not be considered complete until a medical evaluation is performed in the near future.

6) Even the most disorganized patient may find the familiar physician-patient relationship provides the necessary structure for role definition and reorganization.

By insuring that a thorough medical evaluation has been performed, the consultant provides a valuable service not only to the patient, but also to the therapist, who will be less worried that an underlying physical problem is producing the symptoms and will have baseline data in the event that somatic therapies are implemented (e.g., lithium, antidepressants). Furthermore, if the therapist is not a physician, the patient's early resistance—"I think all my problems are physical"—will be less worrisome and can be dealt with directly.

A number of laboratory tests have recently received extensive research attention and some clinical use in the differential diagnosis of psychiatric disorders. The dexamethasone suppression test as a marker of depression is perhaps the best studied (Greden, Gardner, King, Grunhaus, Carroll, and Kronfol, 1983; Targum, 1983). Unfortunately, none of the available tests has lived up to their early promise of providing a sensitive and specific independent confirmation of diagnosis and none adds a great deal beyond clinical observation in selecting a treatment. Nonetheless, this is an area of fast-breaking progress and it seems clear that, in the coming decades, laboratory tests will increasingly inform psychiatric diagnostic and treatment decisions, as they have in other medical specialties.

ADDITIONAL SOURCES OF INFORMATION

A decision must be made during each consultation about whether information from additional sources is indicated. These sources include psychological assessment (see Chapter 10), school records, hospital reports, family members, and previous or current therapists. In our experience, there is a general tendency for clinicians not to pursue these sources vigorously. The reasons for this disinclination vary from clinician to clinician and from case to case.

Some clinicians fail to contact doctors, previous therapists, current therapists, relatives, schools, and hospitals because these contacts would "bias" the data, detract from the uncontaminated purity of the consultative process, and deprive the patient of necessary privacy and confidentiality. Although we agree that these sources of additional information should not be used routinely or thoughtlessly, and although we are not naive about the inconvenience and time required to obtain information from outside sources, we strongly urge the consultant to overcome resistances to taking advantage of these additional data in planning a treatment selection. Moreover, each consultant must carefully examine his motives for not contacting others: Does the consultant feel intimidated by (or contemptuous of) the internist and reluctant to deal with the pervasive skepticism about the psychiatric profession in nonpsychiatric medical colleagues? Is the consultant feeling competitive toward past or current therapists and shying away from this rivalry by not discussing the patient with them? Does the consultant simply not want to take the inordinate amount of time to obtain hospital records?

One reason why clinicians fail to take full advantage of additional sources of information is that they fail to make the distinction between a consultation and treatment. For example, the psychoanalytic stance is predicated on the analyst's not touching the patient (as in performing a physical examination) or having the material contaminated and biased by data from outside sources. Similarly, if the goal of treatment for an adolescent is to facilitate individuation, frequent contact between the therapist and the parents may be inadvisable. Nonetheless, the consultant can serve a crucial role by making sure in advance of treatment that no underlying physiological problem is contributing to the psychiatric symptoms or that the family members have been well-informed about why it may be necessary during the course of treatment for them to be "excluded."

By far the best predictor of response to psychiatric treatment is response to previous treatments. Since patients tend to present highly distorted views of what actually happened during the course of a previous therapy, the consultant should make every effort to contact the therapist and get his or her point of view. Therapists themselves may retrospectively distort what occurred, but contrasting impressions can provide crucial information for the consultant in designing a future treatment plan.

THE CONSULTATION PROCESS AS PREDICTOR

Thus far we have discussed the data base that the consultant gathers by listening to and questioning the patient. In this section, we discuss an additional important source of data on which to base predictions, i.e., observations about the patient's behavior in and reaction to the consultation process itself. There is evidence from several different studies (Malan, 1976; Morgan, Luborsky, Crits-Christoph, Curtis, and Solomon, 1982) that static measures tapping patient characteristics independent of their interaction with treatment are much less useful as predictors of ultimate treatment outcome than are the more dynamic measures of therapist-patient interaction gathered shortly after the treatment has begun. This should not occasion any great surprise. It is easier to predict how well an interaction will work after trying it out than to base predictions on hypothetical and static patient selection criteria.

Although we have emphasized the importance of distinguishing between consultation and treatment, we would also strongly recommend that the characteristic techniques likely to be used in any treatment under consideration be tried during the consultation in order to get some idea of how well or poorly they are likely to work. For example, it makes no sense to recommend a psychodynamic treatment if tentative interpretations have not first been tried during the consultation process so that reactions to them can be monitored. Equally, it makes no sense to recommend a family treatment unless this has been preceded by a family evaluation to see how the family members work together with one another. And similarly, a behavioral or cognitive treatment should be preceded by trials of behavioral or cognitive interventions in order to determine the patient's ability to use them. This kind of situational testing has been found to be most predictive of job performance in selecting candidates for vocational placement, and the same principle applies equally well in selecting patients for psychiatric treatments. This is particularly important in evaluating the patient's enabling factors for various treatments and motivation for participation in them.

The use of the consultation process as a predictor of response to various treatment means that the evaluation will often have to occupy two or more sessions and in some instances will have to be extended to brief therapy length. It is especially useful to see how the patient has responded to the first visit. Did he or she think about it? Has it stimulated new thoughts and memories? Has any homework been done? Has the patient gotten better? Or worse (a hint of proneness to negative therapeutic reaction)? By observing the manner in which the patient handles the evaluation interviews, the consultant learns how much structure and direction he is likely to need in treatment, his ability to use psychological insights and explorations, typical resistances, and early transferences, and so on.

In order to get optimum benefit from the consultation process, it is crucial that the consultant continually frame testable hypotheses based on what has been revealed so far in the evaluation. Lazare, Eisenthal, and Frank (1976) have pointed out that the hypothesis will necessarily include questions concerning the biological, psychological, learning, and social systems implications of the patient's disorder and its treatment. The consultant then tests these hypotheses by listening for what happens next and by making the various kinds of interventions most likely to verify or disqualify them. Moreover, as choices narrow concerning the most appropriate setting, format, orientation and duration, specific questions arise – the answers to which will help decide how best to proceed. The consultation should, in most instances, be an active intellectual endeavor for both participants.

FORMULATION

A comprehensive formulation includes a description of the patient's psychopathology and hypotheses about its origin and maintenance. All of the separate orientations in psychiatry provide part of this picture, but none is likely to be fully explanatory by itself. Thus, the formulation will include phenomenologic, biologic, psychodynamic, cognitive-behavioral, and systems components.

Descriptive Diagnosis

DSM-III has adopted a multiaxial system that requires data on five different areas of patient functioning – clinical syndrome, personality disorder, contributions from medical illnesses, level of stress, and highest level of adaptive functioning during the past year. In effect, DSM-III has gone beyond straightforward diagnosis and includes within its five areas the beginning of a formulation statement.

Biological Hypotheses

Does the patient have a condition that is definitely the result of a known biological condition, e.g., brain tumor, Huntington's, Alzheimer's, hypothyroidism? What tests are necessary to rule in or out possible medical disorders that may be an important contribution to the presenting psychopathology? Another group of conditions – e.g., the schizophrenias, serious affective disorders, Tourette's syndrome – are presumed to have a strong biological contribution but one that has thus far eluded clear pathophysiological elucidation. These conditions do often respond to biological interventions and it is an important part of the formulation to discern the extent to which the patient has target symptoms that are appropriate for a somatic intervention. It is quite likely that most of the "neuroses" and personality disorders also have a biological substrate, but only in a few instances is somatic treatment indicated (e.g., panic and compulsive disorder).

Psychodynamic Hypotheses

It is convenient to divide these into the dynamic and genetic. Dynamic formulations pertain to the cross-sectional intrapsychic conflicts that are expressed in the patient's symptoms. Psychogenetic formulations refer to longitudinal hypotheses that relate the current conflictual situation with those that have obtained throughout the patient's life, and particularly to those of early life. It is very interesting that the patient's chief complaint and recent dreams are often quite similar in their content, form, and level of object relations to the patient's early or screen memories. This reveals a continuity in life that is often necessary to account for in planning any treatment.

Cognitive/Behavioral Hypotheses

A topographical analysis is done to delineate all currently impaired modalities (e.g., affective, verbal-cognitive, overt motor, social, sensory). This analysis not only describes problem areas, but also identifies cognitive and behavioral indicators of future progress in treatment. Additional to topographical analysis, a functional analysis determines the contingencies that control current behaviors. What interactive exchanges and other environmental stimuli occasion the patient's symptomatic behaviors — reinforce and maintain them?

Systems Hypotheses

How is the individual patient's problem embedded in marital, family, occupational, and community contexts? Do the patient's problems result from systems stress or express system pathology? Have the attempts of the patient and his network to alleviate the problem now become part of the problem? Can treatment leverage be most usefully applied on the system, rather than on the individual patient?

EDUCATION

After the consultant has himself reached some tentative conclusions about treatment selection, the next step is to educate the patient. The single most powerful means of improving the adjustment of many patients to their psychiatric (and medical) disorders is to educate them about what is happening. Ignorance about the cause, meaning, and course of symptoms breeds confusion and secondary symptoms. In most instances, the consultant's direct explanations are remarkably reassuring and provide the patient with the ability to regain control of what had seemed an untenable situation.

The overall morbidity associated with psychiatric disorders is occasioned only in part by the debilitating direct effects of the disorder. The secondary effects are often as devastating to the patient as are the primary manifestations. The patient usually reacts to his or her psychiatric difficulties with a sense of inadequacy, shame, guilt, confusion, humiliation, and demoralization, all of which have the potential to make a bad situation much, much worse. The consultant must recognize — and may choose to put clearly into words to the patient — that adjusting to a psychiatric illness is in itself an enormous stress, particularly when the psychiatric illness is to some degree interfering with the patient's usual methods of coping with stress.

DSM-III is sometimes a helpful adjunct in this educational process. Many patients feel as if they have been uniquely damned and are suffering from some special, unknown, and untreatable curse. Others feel responsible for making themselves sick. When the consultant explains what is happening in a detailed and matter of fact way, this puts the patient's concerns in a more reasonable perspective. The DSM-III descriptions confirm that such problems are well known. Most patients smile when they recognize themselves in the DSM-III diagnostic criteria and are relieved to learn that others have had similar problems. Patients develop the reasonable hope that if their condition is clearly defined, there will be some way of curing it or at least of learning to live with it.

What has been said so far about psychiatric education is much more easily applied to patients who meet criteria for affective, anxiety, and most personality disorders than for those with schizophrenic or organic disorders. Because of the stigma that remains associated with schizophrenia, added to the fact that some schizophrenic patients are difficult to teach by virtue of their symptoms, teaching must be slow and careful. Including the family in the psychiatric education is often a crucial step in increasing the odds that the patient will participate actively and cooperatively in the treatment.

After the diagnosis has been discussed (as in most cases it will be), the next step in psychiatric education is to present the range of possible alternative treatment options. This requires that the consultant be familiar with the rationale, requirements, and techniques of the various possible treatment choices and be able to provide the patient with an account of the advantages and disadvantages of each option. This includes discussion of the possible settings, formats, orientations, durations, and frequencies of treatment, the use of medication, combinations, and the possibility of no treatment. The presentation of possibilities must be done in language that is readily understandable to the patient and devoid of meaningless jargon. In many instances, it is also useful to suggest that the patient read the relevant literature. Depending upon the patient's education and interest, this may be restricted to the reading of articles and books written specifically for patients and their families or it may also include the review of the professional literature. Most patients greatly appreciate the consultant's efforts to inform them thoroughly. The failure to provide sufficient information is probably the most frequent complaint patients make about their physicians.

Although discussing the illness and available treatments with the patient requires truthfulness, it does not require telling everything. The frank and detailed exposition of a bleak prognosis takes too much away from the patient before anything has been given in return. This can be a destructive and demoralizing process. Moreover, it is very rare for situations to be entirely bleak in a predictable and clearcut fashion. Without being deceptive, the consultant should emphasize what is reasonably hopeful in the patient's prognosis and what are the likely immediate or long-term benefits of treatment. If no currently available treatment seems likely to be very helpful in the short term, the consultant can point to the activity of ongoing research into the causes and treatments of various psychiatric disorders. Even in difficult situations, the patient can take reassurance from the fact that effective treatments are constantly being developed and tested. At the same time, patients should be cautioned against putting all of their eggs in the first treatment basket and should be advised that sequential trials of several different treatments may conceivably be necessary before the most effective one is discovered. The consultant will be most helpful in reversing demoralization to the extent that he is expert and clear in his presentation of the facts. Patients will sense if he is insincere or patronizing. The consultant should ensure that the patient has correctly understood what has been said. Often patients nod knowingly without really following the flow of information.

There are exceptions to every rule and some patients and families are probably best off if they do not receive any extensive psychiatric education. Some people have a great need not to know about their psychiatric (and medical) conditions. This should be respected if not knowing does not interfere with treatment compliance and if the knowledge gained is more likely to be unsettling than reassuring. It is our impression that most consultants err primarily in the other direction, i.e., they provide far too little information to the patient and the family. Only very rarely in our experience does it seem that too much information has been exchanged.

NEGOTIATIONS ABOUT TREATMENT

As documented by the clinical research of Lazare (1979), patients come for evaluation with their own perspective, definition of the problem, goals, and expectations about the kinds of treatments they think are most appropriate. Clinical interviews with several hundred patients in a walk-in clinic resulted in the following typology of patient requests: administrative or legal assistance; advice; clarification about feelings, thoughts, and behaviors; requesting information as to where in the community he can get proper help; confession of guilt about thoughts or deeds; control for impulses; medical help; psychological expertise; insight; contact with reality; social intervention; succor; and ventilation of feelings and affects. Lazare and Eisenthal (1979) argue that eliciting the patient's expectations about the kind of help they feel they need is a very important step in the negotiation with the patient. Finding out about the patient's point of view takes on added urgency when one considers the large number of patients who fail to comply with treatment recommendations (Eisenthal, Emery, Lazare, and Udin, 1978), those dissatisfied with their therapy (Strupp, Fox, and Lessler, 1969), and those who terminate treatment prematurely (Baekeland and Lundwall, 1975; Lorion, 1974). It is certainly possible that one cause of difficulty is a misunderstanding between consultant and patient over the choice of treatment (Frank, Eisenthal, and Lazare, 1977). Lazare, Eisenthal, and Frank (1976) list several areas of possible conflict: conflict over the goals, methods, and conditions of treatment, and over the relationship with the therapist.

The patient is to be regarded as an active participant and, in most instances, a full voting partner in the process of treatment selection. The consultant does not decide unilaterally which treatment is best or which selection criteria the patient has met. He does not hand a prescription to the patient who is then expected meekly to follow it. As has been mentioned several times already, patients are good at not following decisions they do not like. Patients often (almost always) make up their own minds anyway about what they think is best for themselves.

It is therefore highly desirable to find out what is on the patient's mind. How has he or she responded to the possibilities that have been raised? What are his goals, expectations, fears, preferences, and beliefs about treatment? What treatment does he think will work, how long does he expect it to take, how much of a commitment is he prepared to make? What will be the reaction of significant others to possible treatment options? Treatment selection is a shared decision made by the patient and consultant working together (and sometimes including the family).

The patient is regarded as a "customer" of psychiatric services who has the right and responsibility to become an informed consumer. This does not mean that the customer is always right – particularly those customers who suffer from severe psychiatric disturbances that sometimes impair judgment about the possible benefits of treatment. Examples are the depressed patient who wants to avoid treatment altogether because he is convinced that he deserves to die, or the manic patient who believes he does not need treatment because he is already talking to God. But even under what appear to be very unfavorable circumstances, the customer can be educated and almost always remains competent to participate in some fashion in the decisions that are to be made.

In most instances, the consultant will feel that a number of alternative psychiatric treatments are possible – all of which have some chance of success and none of which is clearly and certainly the only sensible choice. The consultant may have certain favorites among the possibilities; however, if he is open-minded, he will generally have to admit that, since our ability to predict the best treatment is not totally reliable, other options deserve consideration. The "customer" is presented with the range of options and informed about the advantages, disadvantages, and costs of each. Insofar as the patient shares responsibility for choosing the treatment selected, he is much more likely to follow through and give it its best chance of being effective. Expectations are very important in influencing outcome.

The process of negotiation is very simple, straightforward, and bilateral in some situations, but much more problematic in others. Negotiation runs smoothly when the consultant and patient agree completely about what to do next. There is also very little problem when the patient is an informed and competent consumer and decides to select a treatment that is reasonable, but not the consultant's first choice. On some occasions, the patient is a fairly incompetent consumer but there is no really effective psychiatric treatment. This is a sad but relatively straightforward situation. We need not pressure people to participate in treatment if we have little reason to think it will be helpful. The toughest negotiations occur when a specific interaction is likely to be very helpful (lithium for a manic patient), but the patient's psychiatric disorder impairs his ability to act as would a prudent person.

Occasionally, the process of negotiation breaks down. Depending on the circumstances, the patient is either forced into treatment involuntarily or is allowed to end the discussion. This is unfortunate and should be a rare event. Extensive negotiations, done sensitively, are often successful, even in situations which at their outset seemed strictly confrontational. The patient should always be given the maximum possible responsibility for treatment selection that is reasonable under the circumstances. Even in those situations which require some coercion, the consultant should preserve some of the patient's freedom of choice (for example, the choice whether to sign into a hospital voluntarily or be committed involuntarily is in its own paradoxical way still a choice). The consultant, even under these extreme conditions, should make only those decisions that are clearly important for the patient, and it should be made clear that this delegation of responsibility is meant to be temporary. Once the patient's judgment returns, he will be given more responsibility.

In those situations in which the consultant disagrees with the patient's preference about treatment selection but the patient is not so incompetent or at risk as to warrant imposing a decision, the question sometimes arises whether to compromise with the patient or to stand firm on the initial recommendation. These situations are too variable to be comprehended in any single discussion; and, of course, there will be times when it makes sense to compromise, others when it is best to stand firm. An alternative that is often very useful is the suggestion that the patient seek additional opinions from one or more independent consultants. If the patient hears the same recommendation from another consultant, he may be more likely to give it credence and follow it.

There are some occasions in which the customer-centered approach is not very helpful and instead can be harmful. Certain patients, particularly dependent and obsessive ones, simply cannot make decisions for themselves, especially if they are in the midst of a regression. Such people may be thrown into a further panic when the consultant offers them what may seem a bewildering variety of choices. It is sometimes the better part of wisdom for the consultant to decisively but unobtrusively take charge and make only one recommendation. However, this should be a conscious decision tailored specifically to the needs of the given patient and should not become part of routine practice with everyone.

ROLE INDUCTION

The different psychiatric treatments make different demands on the patient and present different stressors and opportunities. Almost all treatments are somewhat unusual from the patient's point of view. If they reproduced the usual social conventions and did not have their own idiosyncratic rules, treatments would probably be no more effective than the many nontechnical interventions the patient has already received from family, friends, the bartender, or priest.

Treatments vary in the degree of role induction they require in direct proportion to how much they differ from the patient's average expectable environment and require from him something different than his average expectable behavior. A psychoanalyst expects a patient to lie on a couch and, deprived of the usual social cues, say whatever comes to mind however embarrassing this may be. The patient can expect very little response from the analyst and yet must try and reveal everything – and do this for several years. A patient about to enter psychoanalysis will form a better treatment alliance if he is provided with a thorough and nontechnical explanation of why the analytic setting requires a lack of external cues (in order to permit the emergence of fantasy), why the analyst says so little (to encourage the patient to project distortions), and why it takes so long (to allow the working through and resolution of many deeply ingrained patterns of behavior).

A group therapist also makes what appears to be rather strange demands, although of a different kind. The patient presents with a very specific and personal problem and seemingly, before he knows what has happened, he is in a room with six or seven other people who are talking about their own problems and interrelationships and seem either oblivious to him or openly hostile. The goals, methods, expectations, and advantages of group therapy must be explained in a manner that is understandable and agreeable to the patient if he is to stay around long enough to become part of the group and to participate meaningfully in its process.

Treatment dropout and failure often result from the fact that the patient did not understand what was going on nor how best to respond to it. Providing the patient with a cognitive grasp of the rationale of the specific treatment and a clear sense of the role expectations involved increases the chances of success. Role induction goes hand-in-hand with treatment selection and psychiatric education.

FAMILY/MARITAL INTERVIEW

We have assumed so far that the evaluation interview would be conducted with the patient alone. There are a number of occasions in which a consultant should attempt to interview the family either in the first evaluation interview or in a subsequent one. These conditions would include the following: a symptomatic child or adolescent; recent clear stress to whole family unit; psychiatric hospitalization is being considered for one family member; marital or family problems are presented as such without a clearly symptomatic individual (Clarkin, Frances, and Glick, 1981).

Just as there is an outline for the assessment of an individual patient that is blazoned into the head of every psychology intern and psychiatric resident in training (chief complaint, present illness, past history of illness, etc.), so there is a family assessment outline that one should have in mind before the assessment interview. This is useful in later recording the interview, in giving oneself a checklist of what data should be gathered, and in presenting the case to others. Such an outline, analogous to that on an individual patient but with more focus on interpersonal aspects, would include: family complaint and problem; perception of the problem by all members of the family; history of the problem including history of therapeutic attempts and problem-solving by the family itself; interactional patterns and styles of the family, especially those around the problem behaviors; diagnoses of individual members and evaluation of family interactional pathology and resources; motivation and resources for intervention (Glick and Kessler, 1980).

The overall goal of the family evaluation is to assess the indications and enabling factors for the possibility of family intervention around the problem or problems that bring the family to the consultant. Most usually, the family brings an identified patient (IP), usually a symptomatic or acting-out child or adolescent, or sometimes an obviously symptomatic spouse. At other times, couples present with marital difficulties. Since family intervention is most appropriate when *current* family interaction patterns are causing or maintaining the problem situation, it is those interactions which must be assessed in this family evaluation.

There are a number of overall strategies that are somewhat different in family evaluation than individual evaluation. First, most family therapists will attempt to meet with the large family unit – usually parents and all children – in the first session. Experiences suggest that, unless all members are brought in to very early sessions, it is difficult to get them to come later. The reverse is not so. If one wishes to meet with the large family unit and then in a second evaluation session meet with the parents/parental and spouse subsystem (mother and father and husband and wife), this is often indicated and easily done. Meeting with the large family unit gives one an in-the-room experience of the interactions when the total group is present and, likewise, meeting with the spouse subsystem alone enables information-gathering (e.g., sexual information) that should not be shared in the larger family unit. Thus, even in the evaluation itself the interviews can be arranged in such a way as to enable the therapist to draw appropriate boundaries between subunits of the family in order to provide data and to instigate improved functioning.

Another general strategy in family evaluation is the observation of nonverbal cues. Where each family member sits, in what subgroups, who talks to whom, the nonverbal turning away from certain people – all are extremely valuable information in the assessment phase. The evaluation is usually begun by asking the family – not a particular individual – about the problem that the family is experiencing. The overall intent is to get each person's view of the difficulty but not let the identified patient take all the weight and responsibility for the problem and its solution. While some situations (e.g., an acute schizophrenic breakdown in one particular family member) demarcate an identified patient, the goal of family evaluation is to explore the interaction patterns of the whole family around this particular person. This gives the family evaluation a different flavor and orientation from the typical individual evaluation. Another guiding principle and strategy in the evaluation is to explore the context (Wynne, Gurman, Ravitch, and Boszormenyi-Nagy, 1980) of the problem as presented. This means that the family evaluator will attempt to place the problem in the context of repetitive family interaction patterns. Indeed, some family evaluators would want to have the family problem in some way acted out in the evaluation session itself so that the live interaction patterns are elicited. A dramatic example of this is the evaluation of an anorexic daughter by Minuchin (1974) in which the family has a meal with the evaluator and is directed to get the anorexic daughter to eat.

Another quality of the family evaluation is that the family evaluator is relatively active. For example, with a large family, the consultant may become the leader of the group and may instruct individuals not to cut off other family members when they are speaking in order to allow one person to talk at a time. The family evaluator must focus the discussion and lead various members in talking in turn about crucial issues. Some family evaluators suggest tasks and intervention techniques in the evaluation itself to see how the family will begin to respond to intervention. While a degree of activity is absolutely necessary for family evaluation to occur, the more active the evaluator the more likely that blurring will occur between the evaluation and the actual treatment. As in the individual evaluation, the family evaluation should include negotiation and role induction with the family as a whole. What is each member's view of the problem, what solutions are desired, who desires them, and what goals are seen as appropriate and obtainable? Often this is more important and complex in family than in individual evaluation. The family member who most desires change or has most power to keep the family in or out of treatment may not be the identified patient.

TERMINATION

The termination of a consultation will be somewhat different if the consultant plans to refer the patient rather than become the designated therapist. We will discuss these two situations separately.

No matter how definite the consultant has been in distinguishing the consultation process from treatment, most patients will inevitably form an attachment to the consultant and feel hurt, sad, or angry about being referred elsewhere. Even if feelings are not openly expressed, the consultant should expect their presence and ask about them specifically. The consultant might also instruct the patient that residual feelings toward the consultant often influence the early phase of treatment with another therapist and that the patient should realize that any strong positive or negative feelings toward the new therapist might be a result of unresolved or unexpressed feelings toward the consultant.

If the patient will be entering a treatment that differs markedly from the consultation process – such as a psychoanalytic psychotherapy – the consultant should again warn the patient that the assigned therapist's mode and style will necessarily be quite different from the consultant's. Some of this work will have been done during the role induction phase of the consultation, but can be reinforced at termination.

The consultant should be explicit about what contact, if any, the patient and consultant will have once treatment with another therapist has begun. The consultant can honestly state that an important educational process for the consultant is learning what recommendations have or have not been helpful and that a call or a letter from the patient in a few weeks would be appreciated, but that any more involvement might detract from the recommended therapy and be an inadvisable way of avoiding the difficulties of saying a final goodbye.

The consultant should also make explicit that the designated therapist will probably contact the consultant to acquire some information and opinion, but that the patient will need to repeat large portions of the material that has been discussed. The patient should not leave with the fantasy that the consultant will have continuing discussions with the therapist during the course of treatment, because this is another way of failing to say goodbye.

Some of the feelings about termination will emerge when the fee is openly discussed. At some point during the evaluation process, such as when logistical arrangements are being made for the second appointment, the consultant should have discussed his fee. We recommend an arrangement for a consultation fee that is unlike the standard practice of charging a set amount for each therapeutic session. Using the model of attorneys, accountants and other such professionals, we charge patients seen in consultation for the actual amount of time—with and without the patient—spent in the evaluation process. We find this arrangement conveys to the patient that the consultation will involve more than the time the two of them spend together. In addition, the consultant will be more inclined to make the necessary phone calls and arrangements if he is being reimbursed for these tasks.

Whatever the financial arrangements made beforehand with the patient for the consultation fee, we suggest the patient be personally handed the bill before the last consultation visit is over and, if possible, that this be paid before the patient leaves. This recommendation is made only in part for mercenary reasons (it does improve fee-collecting), but also because paying the consultant will concretely facilitate the termination process and elicit whatever positive or negative feelings have not been expressed. Unlike the therapist, the consultant has no further opportunity (or leverage) to deal with the patient who does not pay the fee for either conscious or unconscious reasons.

If the consultant will become the therapist, the termination process is of course different, but should still be a well-defined phase of the consultation and not blur indistinguishably into the beginning of treatment. The therapist should make explicit that his therapeutic stance may by design be different than the stance taken during the consultation. This statement is particularly necessary if the consultant has been active and interventive during the evaluation phase and now plans a more neutral position for an exploratory therapy.

Although most patients will state that they are pleased that the consultant will become the therapist, countertransference difficulties may prevent the consultant-therapist from exploring the *disappointment* that the patient is not being referred to someone who is wiser, or more caring, more experienced, more handsome, a different sex, a different religion, and so forth. Additionally, patients may have trouble changing from a consultative to a therapeutic alliance which, though related, is not the same; like clinicians, some patients are excellent at assessing psychiatric problems and deciding what should be done, and not so expert at the arduous task of actually dealing with the problems that have been correctly evaluated and assigned to a specific treatment. The termination phase can be helpful in reminding the patient of this important distinction.

Some of the suggestions made in this chapter regarding the clinical evaluation for treatment selection are controversial—or at least different from common practice. To illustrate how these recommendations can be implemented, we will now summarize an actual consultation by following the headings we have described above. The case example cannot be considered ideal, complete, or typical (no case can), but it will present the different phases of the consultation process and how the task and methods differ from treatment per se.

THE CASE OF THE FATALIST

A Mr. G. called for an appointment, immediately explaining, "My doctor said I should call you." When asked if the problem was urgent, Mr. G. replied, "No, he just thinks I'm too fat."

Without pursuing the matter over the phone, the psychiatrist gave a choice of three times he would be available "for consultation" in the next two weeks. After Mr. G. decided on a time, the psychiatrist ended the phone call by saying, "I'll look forward to discussing this problem with you. We can then decide if psychiatric treatment is advisable and if so, what kinds of treatment and with whom."

Defining The Task

When Mr. G. arrived for his scheduled appointment, he was exactly as he described—too fat. In his mid-thirties, he appeared somewhat younger because of his soft skin and round baby face, yet his 300-plus pounds caused him to move and puff like an old man. His marked obesity also gave him a slovenly appearance, with his shirt bulging at the buttons and revealing the rolls of fat underneath.

Because Mr. G. looked so unkempt and lugubrious, the psychiatrist was somewhat surprised when Mr. G. began the interview in a direct, assertive, and articulate manner: He had been seeing his doctor, an endocrinologist, for the past four years because of a benign pituitary tumor. Radiotherapy had cured his headaches and blurry vision, "But I'm still too fat. What can you do for me?"

The psychiatrist took this early opportunity to define the consultation task and answered with the same kind of comment he had made on the phone: Acting as a consultant, he would be pleased to review Mr. G.'s problems with him and together, over the next two or more meetings, they could determine if psychiatric treatment is advisable and if so, what kind of treatment and with whom. To get as full an understanding as possible, he would be inquiring about aspects of Mr. G.'s life which may not seem directly relevant, but which would help place the problem in perspective. The psychiatrist added that, as a first attempt to establish a consultation alliance, the more the consultant knew about Mr. G. — his strengths and weaknesses, his past life and future expectations — the more informed would be any recommendations regarding treatment at this time; the psychiatrist would therefore hope that Mr. G. would volunteer whatever information he thought would be valuable, while understanding that many interruptions would be necessary and that some areas might not be pursued in elaborate detail.

Mr. G. was a bit taken back by the psychiatrist's remarks. He volunteered that he was expecting only to be "scolded and starved to death" but would be willing to talk about himself if that was what was necessary to decide what to do.

Exploring the Presenting Problem

Because Mr. G. was expecting to be "fed questions" and was bewildered by where to begin, the psychiatrist offered some direction during the early phase of the consultation and suggested, "Let's start with your telling me about your present problem. I'd be interested in hearing whatever you think would be important for me to know."

Mr. G. at first focused only on his obesity. He explained that, although he had been chubby as a child and between ten and 20 pounds overweight as a teenager, his immense obesity began in his early twenties and increased during the next few years until he had reached his current weight of over 300 pounds, before he was 30. There had been little fluctuations in his weight during the past few years. His only explanation for this obesity was, "I drink lots of Coca Cola."

Because of the paucity of information supplied spontaneously by Mr. G., the consultant had to ask specific questions to learn that "lots of Coca Cola" meant ten to 15 sodas per day, compounded by nightly raids to his mother's well-stocked refrigerator for salami, Polish sausage, cheese, and pies. He had never lived away from home except for one three-month period during his early twenties when he was on a summer tour for the National Reserve and when, incidentally, he lost about 30 pounds because "the food was so bad."

Although Mr. G. was more than willing to describe his current diet, bite by bite, he was not able to offer any reason for his voracious appetite. To him, it was a complete mystery. The consultant, using the DSM-III as a mental guide, therefore devoted the middle portion of this initial consultation to asking specific questions that might disclose an explanatory, underlying Axis I diagnosis. Mr. G. responded with relief to this provision of structure and cooperated fully, but the yield was only a series of important negatives. There was no confirmatory evidence of primary affective illness, schizophrenia, panic episodes, phobias, substance abuse, or of cognitive impairment on formal mental status examination.

Having failed to uncover any pressing symptoms related to an Axis I diagnosis, the consultant then returned to the chief complaint, for it was still not clear why Mr. G. had sought treatment for a very chronic problem at this particular time. Mr. G.'s response was at first no different than before: He was here because his endocrinologist thought it was a good idea. The consultant, reminded that Mr. G. up to this point in the interview had still not discussed his pituitary tumor and its effects upon his life, noted this conspicuous omission: "You have not yet told me about your medical problems. I imagine that they also have had some influence on you."

Mr. G. at first shrugged off this obvious omission. With seeming indifference, he then described the onset of headaches and impaired vision three years before, the various misdiagnoses by family physicians, the eventual documentation of a "brain tumor," and gradually the "shrinkage" after numerous doctor visits, radiotherapy, and follow-up diagnostic tests.

Mr. G.'s perfunctory description was hard to accept. His nonchalance was the attitude of a child whistling in the dark. Accordingly, the consultant commented on the contrast between Mr. G.'s unemotional presentation and the frightening experiences he had endured. This comment was all that was necessary to get beyond the fragile veneer of Mr. G.'s indifference. Breaking into tears, he acknowledged that for the past three years — ever since he began to go blind because of a growth in his head — he was convinced that he was going to die. As a result of this conviction, he had not bothered to think much of his future; he did not even think he would have one. He lived (and ate) as though each day would be his last. Being obese was the least of his problems.

In order to learn more about "why now?" and "why *not* now?", the consultant concentrated on exactly what had occurred that made Mr. G. telephone for a psychiatric consultation. He discovered that the phone call was made the very day that Mr. G. learned from his endocrinologist that the pituitary tumor was now unquestionably under control. Instead of feeling great relief, Mr. G. felt anxious, left the doctor's office, and wandered the streets asking himself, "Now what?" Feeling desperate and confused, he then called the psychiatrist from a telephone booth in a restaurant, having actually been given the phone number of the consultant by the endocrinologist several months before.

Eliciting Relevant Background Data

After poignantly conveying his fatalistic attitude, Mr. G. appeared emotionally engaged but not overwhelmed. The consultant took advantage of this established rapport to arrange the next appointment. He realized that Mr. G.'s motivation for treatment might wane and he did not want to leave the scheduling until the hurried concluding moments of the session. When told that another appointment would be necessary, Mr. G. agreed – though he looked somewhat dismayed and felt that there was little else left to say. Mr. G. also granted permission for the consultant to contact the endocrinologist; in fact, he said that he was pleased that the psychiatrist was willing to take such an initiative and "call the shots." While making these arrangements, the consultant also stated his hourly fee and explained that this would include the time spent contacting others and formulating a treatment plan. Mr. G. said the fee was similar to that of the endocrinologist and, without indicating specifically his financial resources, believed the estimated expense would not be a problem.

With the fee settled and the next appointment reasonably assured, the psychiatrist used the remaining 20 minutes of the first session to obtain a relevant developmental history. Because Mr. G. was still somewhat passive and reticent in supplying information and was primarily interested only in his problem of obesity, the consultant raised questions about the patient's past in ways that related to the chief complaint: "I can imagine that this problem of being overweight has affected many aspects of your life over the years. Exactly how has your obesity influenced your relationships with your family and friends, your schooling and your work?"

In response to this more open-ended question, Mr. G. explained that he had always been "a loner," preferring since childhood to stay at home with his stamp and coin collections because he did not want to endure the ridicule from his peers for being overweight. With no encouragement from his family and with no ambitions of his own, he had maintained a B average, despite being delinquent in his homework assignments and, on many occasions, staying home from school to watch quiz shows on TV. He did extremely well on his college boards, however, and with "nothing better to do," attended a local city college, while continuing to live with his parents. He did not recall ever imagining what he would do when he "grew up" and by the time of his senior year, he simply stopped attending classes mid-semester to avoid appearing in public and began spending his days babysitting for his younger sibling. Because of his marked obesity, he was "too embarrassed" to look for work or even travel far from the confines of his home—and, of course, dating was out of the question.

His father, an uneducated immigrant mill worker, had long ago stopped reprimanding his son for being "a dreamer" and, now retired, spent his time visiting his other children who were married, successful, and far more accepting and acceptable. Mr. G.'s mother, a lonely Polish-speaking woman, had never exerted any pressure on her son. In contrast to the father's rejection of Mr. G. and devotion to the other children, the mother seemed to enjoy having her son around the house. In fact, after the father would retire for the night, she and Mr. G. would spend hours together in the kitchen (eating), while they discussed the events of the day.

Mr. G.'s one other interest—besides eating, daydreaming, and talking with his mother—was in rare coins, which he had studied in detail and begun trading by mail order during his early adolescence. By his mid-twenties, after dropping out of college, he began to buy and sell these coins more regularly; by chance and not design, his assets had accumulated to an estimated worth of over $200,000. Like his daily excursions to the bakery, Mr. G. had kept his coin dealings a secret so that his family still had no idea of his private estate. Because Mr. G. was too ashamed of his appearance to attend annual coin shows and made all of his transactions by phone or mail, among numismatists he had become a legendary phantom figure who was known only by a post office box number. It was typical of Mr. G.'s lifelong attitude that he preferred to view his coin collecting as nothing more than a "hobby." He had no plans to use his knowledge and expertise as a vocation and means of financial support. He simply planned to live with (and off of) his parents "forever."

As the first session drew to a close, the consultant briefly summarized what he had learned so far: Hampered by his obesity and his reluctance to leave home, to risk establishing peer relationships, and to plan for the future, Mr. G. had drifted along day by day and meal by meal. The pituitary tumor had compounded his chronic lifestyle and reinforced Mr. G.'s fatalistic attitude toward the future. The recent report by the endocrinologist, in many ways quite reassuring, had actually forced Mr. G. to look at himself and his life in a way for which he was emotionally unprepared. The consultant, without offering false reassurance, closed the first session by stating that this current crisis, though understandably upsetting, held the potential for unrealized opportunity. In addition, he suggested that as a "homework assignment" Mr. G. think about what the two of them had discussed, consider what other information would be relevant and, more specifically, note what events – emotional or situational – immediately preceded his binge-eating episodes. On this seemingly hopeful note, the first session ended.

Medical Evaluation

Having obtained permission, the consultant phoned the endocrinologist, who confirmed much of what Mr. G. had reported: A benign pituitary tumor had indeed responded remarkably well to radiotherapy and although a recurrence was possible, the overall prognosis was now quite good. Extensive laboratory tests over the years had never disclosed any physiological cause for the obesity which had antedated the symptoms of the pituitary tumor by several years.

After giving a full medical report, the endocrinologist then volunteered that he considered Mr. G. "a big baby." He missed at least half of his scheduled appointments, refused to go to his outpatient treatments or blood tests unless accompanied by his mother, and never took responsibility for paying his bills. He always needed to be prodded, no matter what the issue.

In closing, the endocrinologist said that he was pleased, though actually quite surprised, that Mr. G. had finally made an appointment for consultation and added, almost as an aside, "I guess he got fed up with the other guy." The consultant then learned that Mr. G. had actually been in "counseling" with a social worker at a mental health center near his home. The endocrinologist did not know the type or frequency of treatment for he had never actually spoken with Mr. G.'s counselor but he did know that the treatment had been going on "for years."

Additional Sources of Information

Mr. G. arrived a half-hour late for his second appointment, explaining only that the subway took longer than he had planned. If possible, his appearance was even more slovenly and the assertiveness that had characterized the opening phase of the first session was absent, as well. When asked about his thoughts regarding the first visit, he said that he left feeling "empty" and again with the fear that the psychiatrist would want to "starve him to death." Mr. G. could recall no specific comment made by the consultant that indicated that this was his intention: "It was just the feeling I got." The consultant then learned that Mr. G. had dealt with this feeling by gorging himself the moment he left the office at a coffee shop on the ground floor of the psychiatrist's office building and had spent the meal, as well as the rest of the week, contemplating whether or not he should bother to return for the second appointment.

With the limited time available, the psychiatrist chose as a top priority a further exploration of Mr. G.'s reluctance to return. The patient revealed that he was afraid that treatment could not help and even more frightened about what treatment would require and what would be expected of him – professionally, sexually and personally – if he were ever to lose weight. His reaction to these fears was a typical avoidance and passive resignation: "It's no use. I've just lost too much time over the years."

Mr. G. had completely forgotten about his "homework assignment." He could not even remember what exactly the two of them had discussed during the first meeting. The consultant then informed Mr. G. about his discussion with the endocrinologist and his "surprise" at discovering that Mr. G. had been in a form of psychiatric treatment for some time.

In a manner that appeared more indifferent than defensive, Mr. G. explained that he had not intended to withhold such information, but just did not see how it was important: "The fellow's not really treating me for my weight. He's just a friendly guy and we talk every once in a while about this or that, mostly about coins. He's getting real interested in them." The consultant's attempts to learn more about the treatment – what problems had led to Mr. G.'s seeking help, what actually had transpired during the sessions, how long they lasted, what they cost, what he expected, and how he felt about the therapist and the therapy – were to little avail. The consultant did learn that the therapist was social worker in his mid-thirties who saw Mr. G. on the average of once a month whenever he called for an appointment: "We just talk with each other for an hour or so about this and that."

As the shortened session came to a close, Mr. G. gave permission for the consultant to contact his therapist, but did not see what "the fellow" would possibly have to offer that would be of any help. Although the psychiatrist felt that this second visit was rather brief and perfunctory with little emotional engagement, Mr. G. – for some unclear reason – actually felt less discouraged at the end of the session and spontaneously offered, "I'm not nearly as hungry as I was the last time." On this note, the two of them agreed that the next appointment would be spent beginning to discuss what treatment options would be advisable.

When the social worker was phoned, he spoke quite fondly of Mr. G., although he had not seen him "for several weeks." He said that Mr. G. had originally been referred to the clinic by his mother's physician for treatment of obesity; in fact, the doctor had referred both Mr. G. and his mother for their shared problem, but only Mr. G. had kept his appointment. Because Mr. G. did not seem at all motivated to lose weight and because he seemed like "such a lonely guy," the social worker chose to see Mr. G. whenever the patient wanted, "Just for him to have some contact with someone, you know, sort of a big brother."

The social worker had no idea that Mr. G. was now seeing someone else in consultation and, furthermore, had only a vague and superficial understanding of Mr. G.'s "brain tumor." When asked about his working diagnosis, the social worker said that he expected Mr. G. was schizophrenic – "most of our patients are" – but he offered no supporting evidence other than Mr. G.'s social isolation and "obsession over coins." The consultant was left with the impression that the social worker was a well-meaning but rather inexperienced man who had relied heavily on experiential techniques.

The Consultation Process as Predictor

The consultation process with Mr. G., though limited in time and range, already supplied important data regarding treatment selection. On the positive side, the patient had kept both appointments, albeit tardily, and during the sessions had presented personal material in an articulate manner without insurmountable reserve or suspicion. He was willing not only to have the consultant contact the endocrinologist and social worker, but also to reveal to a stranger very personal facts about himself, such as his secret coin collection, his eating habits, his embarrassment about his weight, and his previously unshared beliefs that he would die of a brain tumor.

On the more negative side, except for his initial assertiveness when describing his chief complaint, Mr. G. had remained excessively passive throughout the consultation, required direct and structured questions, and assumed little responsibility during or between sessions for the decision regarding treatment selection. Having been given a "test dose" of various treatment techniques, Mr. G. had not responded to any of them:

He had not noted antecedent stimuli for his binge eating (behavioral therapy); he had not done his "homework assignment" (cognitive therapy); he had not responded to any suggestion that his obesity might have psychological determinants (exploratory therapy); and he had not felt comforted or reassured by the shared emotional experience during the first session (experiential therapy). Most worrisome, Mr. G. had actually felt much worse – "empty" – after the first visit and appeared to have deteriorated further during the week before his second appointment. This decline raised the possibility of a negative therapeutic reaction to any treatment, a concern compounded by Mr. G.'s distorted notion of the consultant "wanting to starve him to death." The fact that Mr. G. felt worse after exposing so much during the first session and felt better after the superficial second session suggested that he simply was not able to tolerate any intense interpersonal involvement at this time.

The potential for negative countertransference reactions was also an important consideration regarding Mr. G. His appearance and passivity could possibly elicit contempt, helplessness, and frustration in the therapist, who might then develop rescue fantasies as a reaction formation against these feelings.

Formulation

In preparation for Mr. G.'s third appointment, the consultant outlined a tentative formulation as a guide toward treatment selection:

I. *Descriptive diagnosis*
    Axis I.   None
    Axis II. 301.82 Avoidant personality disorder
                 301.60 Dependent personality disorder
    Axis III. Benign pituitary tumor
    Axis IV. Moderate stress – good medical prognosis – 4
    Axis V. Highest level of adaptive functioning past year – poor – 5

II. *Biological hypothesis*
    Genetic and constitutional predisposition toward obesity suggested by chronicity of problem since childhood and by obesity in patient's mother. Possible role of CNS tumor.

III. *Psychodynamic hypothesis*
    The patient's Polish-speaking mother, herself an obese loner excluded from familial and social relationships, has encouraged a

dependent bond with Mr. G. The patient's rejecting father has not been a strong source of identification to intercept this mother-child bond. Growing up and leaving may unconsciously represent to Mr. G. an abandonment of his mother, an identification with the hated father, and a symbolic starvation.

IV. *Cognitive/behavioral hypothesis*
Mr. G. is locked into a vicious cycle of reinforcement: His obesity elicits rejection and embarrassment; he assuages these distressing feelings by overeating with his mother; his obesity thereby increases, while avoidant behavioral patterns are reinforced and maintained.

V. *Systems hypothesis*
The social and familial ostracism of the mother has literally fed Mr. G. The "support and care" provided (understandably) by the social worker and the endocrinologist have also maintained Mr. G.'s passive, dependent style and allowed him not to take responsibility for his life. The resignation of the patient's father and siblings has enabled Mr. G. to remain an isolated loner; they may inadvertently want Mr. G. to stay with his mother so that they can "abandon" her with less guilt.

VI. *Treatment alternatives*
A. Setting
1. residential treatment ("fat farm")
for: – maximum structure, external control
– break current reinforcement cycle, e.g., with mother
– establish new eating habits
– nutritional education
– lost weight before when left home (National Reserve)
– early accelerated weight loss provides further incentive

against: – probably not acceptable to Mr. G. at present
– abrupt "weaning" too stressful
– social/peer demands too great
– perhaps sabotaged by mother/family
– no adequate maintenance upon return
2. hospitalization (partial or full)
for: – necessary structure, external control
– remove from home

against: —doubtful cost-effectiveness
   —infantalizing, regressive
   —not acceptable to Mr. G.
   —not targeted for obesity per se
3. outpatient
   for: —most acceptable to Mr. G.
   —least expensive

   against: —less day-to-day structure, control, monitoring
      poor compliance in past (social worker/endocri-
      nologist)
B. Format
   1. individual
      for: —probably most acceptable to Mr. G.
      —similar to medical model with which Mr. G. is
      familiar
      —best opportunity to uncover well-concealed fan-
      tasy life

      against: —not successful in past (social worker)
         —little leverage with family
         —limits interpersonal involvements
         —most potential for regression, infantilization, en-
         hanced passivity
         —greatest chance of countertransference problems
   2. family
      for: —intercept scapegoating by father/siblings
      —intervene directly with mother-patient overde-
      pendency
      —healthy members improve compliance and pro-
      vide intersession structure/controls

      against: —enhance Mr. G.'s view of self as child, not adult
         —mother implicitly excluded if therapist is not
         Polish-speaking
         —bring Mr. G. closer to family rather than sep-
         arate, individuate
   3. heterogeneous group
      for: —supply both confrontation and support
      —decrease intensity of countertransference
      —directly observe and improve peer interactions

      against: —no intersession controls
         —no immediate focus on obesity
         —too overwhelming, exposing

4. homogeneous group (e.g., Weight Watchers)
  for: – initial acceptance by other members
  – proven efficacy
  – inexpensive
  – structure, control, monitoring
  – no threatening intimacy
  – focused on chief complaint

  against: – avoid personality problems
  – even minimal interpersonal involvement may be too threatening

C. Time
  1. frequency
  once/week – least threatening, little intersession monitoring
  twice/week – more structure, perhaps too intimate
  three/week – more close control, potentially infantilizing
  2. duration of sessions
  20 minutes – simulates medical model, superficial
  45 minutes – more involvement, perhaps intimacy and exposure too threatening
  90 minutes – more gradual exploration, expensive
  3. duration of treatment
    3 months – intense focus combat daydreaming and passivity, but perhaps too much too fast
    6 months – concentrate on set termination to confront procrastination and failure to separate, but then no prolonged follow-up
    open-ended – provide continuing care to assure tasks completed, but encourage endless procrastination without necessary focus on future

D. Techniques
  1. exploratory
  for: – lifelong personality problems requiring gradual uncovering
  – intelligent, articulate

  against: – not psychologically-minded
  – potentially too regressive
  – insufficient structure, support
  2. directive
  for: – closest to Mr. G.'s expectations
  – supplies structure, monitoring
  – intercepts problem of "daydreaming"

against: – encourages need for control/direction from others
– specific antecedent stimuli hard to discern
– resists "homework"

3. experiential

for: – least threatening
– accepted in past (social worker)

against: – not structured
– insufficient in past to implement change

E. Somatic Therapies

1. antidepressants/lithium – no evidence of affective illness, panic attacks
2. major tranquilizers – no current indications
3. minor tranquilizers – possibility if anxiety proves antecedent to binge eating, but potentially habit forming in this dependent man
4. diet pills – doubtful efficacy, potential for abuse
5. surgery (jejuno-ileostomy) – future possibility if other treatments unsuccessful

F. No Treatment as Recommendation of Choice

for: – refractory to treatment in past
– potential high for regression and enhanced passivity
– obesity not often responsive to psychotherapy

against: – no adequate trial to date
– potential strengths of patient worth risks/expense of treatment
– doubtful spontaneous remission

VII. *Relevant Literature*

Booth, B. A. Satiety and appetite are conditioned reactions. *Psychosomatic Medicine,* 1976, *39,* 76.

Bray, G. *The obese patient.* Philadelphia: W. B. Saunders, 1976.

Mahoney, M. J. & Mahoney, K. *Permanent weight control: A total solution to the dieter's dilemma.* New York: W. W. Norton, 1976.

Stunkard, A. J. (Ed.). *Obesity: Basic mechanisms and treatment.* Philadelphia: W. B. Saunders, 1978.

Education

Having outlined the above formulation, the consultant was prepared for Mr. G. when he arrived for his third appointment and sluggishly lowered his massive frame into a chair before asking, "So what do you want to do with me?" After Mr. G. admitted that he himself had given no further thought to the matter and had not yet told anyone that he was seeking help, the consultant was tempted simply to accept Mr. G.'s passivity at face value and to take charge by making specific treatment recommendations. Instead, the consultant realized that if there was any hope of eventual acceptance and compliance, it would be crucial for Mr. G. to become a more active participant in this treatment selection process. Education would be an important component of Mr. G.'s assuming more responsibility for his fate.

The following is a paraphrased version of how the consultant attempted to teach Mr. G. about his problems and their possible solutions. During the actual session, there were many interruptions, clarifications, and elaborations, but the main themes of the consultant's discourse are included in their entirety to convey the effort, time, and tone taken to strengthen the fragile consultative alliance with Mr. G:

> Although there are many features of your problems and of your life that I do not yet fully understand, my impression after our first two meetings is that you have spent the last three years convinced that you were going to die; however, because your pituitary tumor has responded to radiotherapy and you have been given a good prognosis, you are confronted with a personal crisis, that is, you are now suddenly faced not with dying, but with living. You do not want to spend the rest of your life being excessively fat, friendless, and a failure. You would like to get your life on track, but don't know how. You also fear that it is too late to change and that any treatment will be too demanding.
>
> This current crisis in your life is compounded by difficulties you had even before the brain tumor. You've never been very comfortable outside the home and when you started to put on even more weight during your college years, after returning from your summer tour with the National Reserve, you were even more embarrassed about your appearance and more uncomfortable socializing. You have been avoiding social contacts ever since. The only thing that filled the emptiness in your life and made you feel temporarily comforted was a full stomach — but of course overeating just perpetuated the vicious cycle. Because you've never had a fulfilling social or sexual life, you've filled your days with unrealizable dreams and never made specific plans for the future.
>
> When you discovered that you had a brain tumor and became secretly convinced that you would have no future, even your dreams were taken away. Since you have always been the kind of person who tended to put things off for another day, it was understandable that you would react to the stress of having a serious illness with the same coping strategy that you had always used, name-

ly, putting things off even more and living day by day. In your mind, you had even less reason to overcome your fears or to go on a diet or to plan a career or even to leave home. You became more fatalistic.

Fortunately, your endocrinologist has found that you have a good prognosis and that there is no indication that the tumor will be fatal. Although that is good news, you are now faced with a future that you did not expect and that you did not plan for. You are understandably worried how you will manage without a career, without social skills, without friends, and with a serious problem of being overweight. Although your prospects seem to you quite discouraging and even frightening, I do not share your grim view — though I understand that you are tempted to view your fate with passive resignation.

If you agree with my impression, let me first describe your diagnosis and what I would consider possible treatments. (Mr. G. agrees.) We can then discuss these various alternatives together and work out a mutually agreeable plan.

Your psychiatric diagnosis is what we call a personality disorder. This term means that your characteristic way of dealing with life is not sufficiently flexible and adaptive. There are many types of personality disorders, which tend to overlap. You would best be described as an avoidant personality in that you withdraw from opportunities for developing close relationships because you are afraid of being belittled or humiliated. In addition, you have some features of a dependent personality, in that you have allowed others to assume responsibility for the major areas of your life and have lacked the self-confidence to function more independently. I realize that I may be overwhelming you with a lot of information at once so, before you leave today, you might find it interesting to read a description of your personality types. You can then see how many features you share with others who have similar problems.

You may be wondering what all of this has to do with your obesity, which after all is the main reason you are here. Although obesity is not in itself a psychiatric problem, your personality difficulties contribute to your overeating. There are most likely other reasons for your obesity as well. Some of the problem may be hereditary or relate to the way you were fed as a child. There is no indication that anything physically wrong is contributing to your being overweight at this time, but I suspect that some of your obesity is related to your basic physical predisposition. Just as we do not know all the reasons why people develop personality disorders, we do not know all the reasons why people develop obesity. Fortunately, however, as with your pituitary tumor, we can treat these problems, even if we do not know all of their causes.

Let us now consider what are the best ways to treat your two problems – your personality disorder and your obesity. Because the two of them are interrelated, we should try to design a treatment that will help both problems.

Let's first consider *where* your treatment could be. One possibility is a "fat farm," that is, a special facility, usually located in the countryside, where obese people go to lose weight. An advantage of such a place for you would be that the environment would prevent you from hanging around coffee shops or your stuffed refrigerator and overeating. While discipline was being supplied for you by the surroundings, you could learn new eating habits. Furthermore, many people find that once they see that weight loss is possible they become encouraged and continue losing weight after the three-to-six weeks they spend at such a facility.

But there are two disadvantages of such a place for you at this time. First, as you described, the idea of being "starved to death" is frightening to you and you are worried about the demands that would be placed upon you once you became less fat. Until some of these concerns are dealt with, you might not be able to keep your weight down after you return home and might fall into old patterns. The second disadvantage of a "fat farm" is that such a residential treatment setting does not usually deal with specific personality problems. Your tendency to wallow about in a life filled with dreams and your fears of leaving home and living more independently will probably continue, unless they are specifically treated; and if they continue, your weight loss would be hard to maintain.

Because your overeating is very much linked with your day-to-day activities and your personality problems, I would suggest that you be treated at present in an outpatient setting, rather than being hospitalized or going to a residential treatment facility; however, I would suggest that you keep these alternative settings in mind for the future. They may be advisable options somewhere down the road.

Now, let me discuss the format of your treatment, that is, whether you should be in treatment alone, or with your family, or in some kind of group. I would recommend that your treatment involve a combination of all three of these different formats. You could be seen individually by a therapist who would get to know you personally and privately, while mapping out a very specific day-to-day plan of how to improve your situation. I would also suggest that you and your therapist meet with your family because I suspect from what you have said that they inadvertently are "feeding" into your problems and making it more difficult for you to lose weight and leave home.

After you feel some support from your therapist and after sessions with your family have helped you break some bad habits, I would then suggest that you enter a self-help group, that is, a group of people who have problems similar to yours. I realize that you are very reluctant to enter any group at this time and reveal yourself to others, but these groups can be quite helpful in providing specific instructions and encouragement. The members tend to be very supportive without making great personal demands. Finally, somewhere down the road, after you have lost some weight, are not so embarrassed, and have a good working relationship with your therapist, you may consider entering a group therapy. By working with people who have all sorts of problems and who come from different walks of life, you can improve your social skills and learn more about how you come across to others and how they affect you. I want to repeat that at the present time you would probably be too uncomfortable to expose yourself in such a group, but I am mentioning to you what alternatives are available for the future.

Having discussed where the treatment should be and with whom, let me now discuss what kind of psychiatric treatments are available for your kind of problems. One common method is "exploratory." In this kind of treatment, the therapist and patient work together in order to understand the nature of the problem and its derivatives, some of which may be outside of awareness (unconscious) and based on important relationships and feelings in one's past. Although I would hope that you and your therapist would acquire a good perspective on your life as treatment evolves, I doubt that simply understanding your problems will motivate you to change.

Another method of treatment available for your problems is "experiential." In this kind of treatment, you and the therapist would work toward a shared emotional experience, similar to but perhaps somewhat more intense than the one you have developed with your social worker. Although I believe that you should certainly have some emotional involvement with your therapist, I suspect that this emotional involvement will not in itself motivate you to change. You might be inclined to use such a relationship in place of establishing social relationships outside of treatment. Furthermore, I doubt that any therapeutic relationship would be sufficient to fill the emptiness in your stomach and your life.

A third method of treatment is "behavioral." In this kind of treatment, the therapist helps you to alter maladaptive behavior such as overeating, unassertiveness, and avoidance of social interactions. I would suggest this method of treatment for you, especially assertiveness training. None of these treatments are given in a "pure" form. The other techniques will be used from time to time as indicated, but I would recommend that the behavioral mode be the main technique in the earlier phases of treatment.

I have not mentioned the use of medication for your obesity and personality problems because at this time I cannot see how any drugs would be helpful. Diet pills have not been shown to be helpful for your kind of obesity in the long run. Other kinds of psychiatric medication – tranquilizers or antidepressants – may be indicated in the future if specific symptoms of depression or anxiety develop, but do not appear warranted at present. You may want to keep in mind that surgery has been used in some patients who are extremely obese. Sections of the intestine are removed so that less food is absorbed. Such a treatment is, of course, a major step and I would suggest that other more conservative methods be tried first; however, you can file the possibility of surgery in the back of your mind as a last resort.

Finally, let me mention how often I would recommend you meet with the therapist and how long treatment should be. I don't know for sure, but I think meeting once or twice a week for a half-hour to 45 minutes would be the right intensity and frequency for you. If sessions were less frequent or shorter in duration, I think they would be too superficial and not provide the structure and direction you need at present. On the other hand, if sessions were more frequent or longer in duration, I would be concerned that you would become more involved in treatment than in your life – and might even find such an intense involvement so upsetting that you would stop treatment altogether. The frequency and duration of treatment might need to be adjusted, for instance, if and when you began sessions with your family or enrolled in a self-help group, such as Weight Watchers or Overeaters Anonymous. How long should treatment be? I would suggest that you and your therapist agree on specific goals that be met at three months, six months, and one year. If it is understood by both of you that treatment will not continue indefinitely, I think you will be more inclined to plan for the future and not expect the present situation to last forever.

Negotiations About Treatment

The educational process paraphrased above took the first half of the third consultation visit. The second half of the session – the negotiation phase – began when the consultant asked Mr. G. what were his initial thoughts about the summary and recommendations.

As might be expected, Mr. G.'s first response was to feel discouraged and overwhelmed: "It's all so much more involved than I had expected." But then, more as an aside than a direct note of appreciation or hope, he mumbled, "I guess you think it's worth all this effort."

Interestingly, Mr. G.'s first doubts were not about his diagnosis (which he accepted with relief because "at least I'm not the only one"), nor about all that might be required for him to do in therapy. Instead, his doubts concerned the cost of treatment. His questions in this regard did not convey an insurmountable resistance but rather that he was taking the consultant's recommendations seriously and assuming some adult responsibilities. He knew that one of his well-to-do sisters had been paying for his medical insurance and that the policy might cover some psychiatric expenses. He volunteered that selling any of his coins would probably be out of the question — "they're all that I have" — but after the consultant pointed out that his hobby might become a more successful career if he overcame his seclusiveness, Mr. G. tentatively considered making a "small investment, one or two coins," in himself.

The other issue raised during the negotiation phase was the possibility of involving his family. This resistance required further exploration and confirmed Mr. G.'s fear of abandoning his socially isolated mother if treatment ultimately led to his leaving home or even becoming interested in activities outside the house. The consultant reminded Mr. G. that family treatment was being recommended for this very reason, namely, outside help would be necessary to redirect destructive forces within the home and that Mr. G. should not assume this responsibility alone. Interestingly, and characteristic of Mr. G.'s schizoid adaptation, he did not mention or indicate any concern about who the therapist might be.

Role Induction

The final few minutes of the third visit were devoted to preparing Mr. G. for the recommended individual and family treatments. Regarding the recommended behavioral techniques, Mr. G. acknowledged that he had never been very good at "doing homework" but worked well in class if the teacher gave specific directions and prodded him "with a kick in the butt." Mr. G. therefore believed that he could accept the role of a "directed" patient.

Mr. G. had far more reservations about participating in any family treatment. The consultant appreciated the strength of this resistance, yet strongly believed that some kind of family intervention would be necessary if Mr. G. were ever to profit from the recommended psychotherapy. He therefore suggested to Mr. G. that another consultation visit be arranged for the entire family so that they could all together be instructed about the requirements and expectations for this component of Mr. G.'s treatment. The consultant instructed Mr. G. to tell all the members of his family that he would like to meet together with them to discuss "the repercussions of Mr. G.'s medical illness and what kinds of treatment would be necessary for the future." When the request for a family interview was phrased in this quasi-medical manner, Mr. G. was more willing to inform his family and bring them to the next consultation.

Family Interview

The following week at the scheduled hour, the consultant was shocked when he walked out into his waiting room and found Mr. G. sitting with his entire family – his father, mother, his two younger brothers, and his two younger sisters with their husbands. Not only was the consultant taken back by the number of family members who had agreed to come, but also by their appearance. In striking contrast to the slovenliness of Mr. G., the siblings and their spouses were tastefully dressed in expensive clothes and looked like highly successful members of society (which, as it turned out, they were). Even the father, though not in a suit, had a neat and sophisticated manner and did not look like the "immigrant mill worker" the patient had portrayed. However, along with Mr. G., the mother looked like an outsider, for she too was obese, disheveled and, slumped in a chair in a corner of the waiting room, was further excluded because she did not speak English.

During the family consultation, many of the consultant's speculations were confirmed. Though concerned about Mr. G. and "wanting to do whatever was necessary," the brothers and sisters and father had all subtly encouraged and reinforced Mr. G.'s bondage with his mother, who they viewed as someone unable to adapt to the American way of life. The family dynamics were revealed in the interview itself, for as the consultant explained Mr. G.'s problems, the family members relied on Mr. G. to translate what was said to his mother.

For purposes of this discussion, a detailed description of the family interview is not necessary and might deflect from the main point: Including the family in the evaluation process enabled the consultant to confirm speculations, to obtain new data, to educate family members about the indications and requirements of psychiatric treatment, and to induce these members into the therapeutic process so that compliance with the recommendations would be enhanced.

Termination

Mr. G. arrived 15 minutes late for his fifth and final consultation appointment. In contrast to the explanation he gave for being late for his second appointment, this time he admitted that he was getting "cold feet" about getting started with the recommended treatment plan. He had found that the family consultation visit had taken "a load off my back" in that he no longer felt responsible "for everything and everyone." He was pleased that members of the family would be attending treatment with him, but was somewhat disappointed – though not distraught – that as they had all discussed during the previous session, the consultant would not be able to schedule these family sessions at a time that was mutually feasible and that Mr. G. would therefore need to be in treatment with another psychiatrist.

The consultant mentioned to Mr. G. that he would appreciate a call in a few weeks to learn how the treatment was progressing. On a pleasant and appreciative note, Mr. G. gave his thanks, paid his bill, and said goodbye. Seven weeks passed before Mr. G. gave the consultant a call. In the meantime, the consultant had heard from the therapist that Mr. G. had begun treatment. The patient stated that, accompanied by his youngest sister, he had entered a weight-watching program and that as a result of family sessions, his mother was no longer stocking the refrigerator. Otherwise, in his view, little had changed but he was willing to stay with it a little while longer. His main reservations about treatment were not the behavioral modifications coordinated with the therapist – these so far had been very undemanding – but instead that he would be forced to sell a valuable coin if his wealthy brother-in-law did not agree to help pay for treatment. The issue of who would pay for what was the current topic during the family sessions.

Further details about Mr. G.'s treatment are not known; however, a year later the endocrinologist called regarding another patient and mentioned that Mr. G., though still overweight, had lost 75 pounds, had moved outside the home and was now living in the back room of his newly established coin and stamp shop. His pituitary tumor had not recurred.

INITIAL EVALUATION SUMMARY

I. *Presenting Situation:* (Use pt.'s words plus why you think pt. is coming now.)

II. *History of Present Illness:*

III. *Past Psychiatric Illness and Treatment and Response:* (Date previous treatments, hospitalization, suicide attempts.)

IV. *Family of Origin:* (Describe members, sibling order, religious and ethnic background, occupations, how family functions, family myths and traditions; psychiatric illness in family members.)

V. *Psychosocial History:* (Include first memories, relevant vignettes from latency, adolescence, adulthood, middle and advancing age. Include but do not repeat data about education, work, sexual life, friendships, recreation, drug use.)

VI. *Current Life:*
   A. *Present Family:* Members of present household: describe current interaction; recent changes such as births, deaths, separations, finances.

   B. How does patient spend a typical week?

   C. What was patient's most recent dream?

VII. A. What specific symptoms and/or life patterns does patient say he or she consciously wants to change (if any).

   B. Patient's perception of what is causing his problem.

   C. Patient's preference for treatment modality (individual, group, etc.) and approach (advice, insight, medication, no treatment, etc.)

   D. Rate patient's motivation for involvement in treatment with us.

   1   2   3   4
   Low   High

VIII. *Mental Status:* (Include direct quotes.)
   1. Appearance, attitude, behavior functioning, speech.

   2. Affect (which ones predominate: their appropriateness, lability, range?)

   3. Thought process and content.

   4. Suicidal or homicidal ideation and behavior.

5. Evaluation of sensorium and intelligence.

6. Interviewer's emotional reaction to patient and patient's emotional reaction to interviewer.

7. Would you like to work with patient: SCORE: 1   2   3   4   5
                     No   Yes

IX. *DSM III Diagnosis:* (Complete all axes at end of first visit.)
   1. Axis 1. _____
           2. _____
           3. _____
           4. 1   2   3   4   5   6   7   0   Stress: _____
           5. 1   2   3   4   5   6   0

2. List in order of importance major areas of behavioral impairment as you see them.

    Short-Term   Long-Term (Characterological)
a.
b.
c.
d.

On the follow-up a year after treatment is complete, what changes in behavior would signify improvement? Grade as to degree of likelihood.

                  Most likely   1.
                                2.
                                3.
                                4.

3. a. What are your hypotheses about the current intrapsychic conflicts which underlie the short- and long-term behavioral impairments (psychodynamic formulation)?

   b. How are current problems a recapitulation of life patterns and how do they relate to the patient's experience of his early life (psychogenetic formulation)?

   c. Level of Integration: _____ Psychotic; _____ Borderline; _____ Neurotic; _____ Healthy.

4.   Social system diagnosis (How are the patient's presenting problem a symptom of family, work and community interactions).

X. *Type of Treatment You (in Consultation with the Patient) Feel is Most Suitable:* (Rank if more than one.)

____ Evaluation Only – no further treatment

____ Crisis Intervention

____ Brief Therapy (mainly insight)

____ Brief Therapy (mainly problem-solving)

____ Individual (for character change)

____ Individual (mainly supportive)

____ Group Therapy (mainly insight)

____ Group Therapy (mainly support-ive)

____ Medication

____ Family

____ Marital

____ Sex Therapy

____ Behavior Therapy

____ Environmental Change

____ Further explora-tion by acute follow-up or addi-tional interview or letter

Based on what indications (also explain rankings):

XI. *Actual Disposition and Action Taken and Why:* (Indicate if patient has been given an appointment or awaits decision of Treatment Committee; if patient referred out, to whom and why.)

XII. *What Research Question Occurred to You with this Patient?*

XIII. Global Assessment Scale Score (GAS) _____
       (Complete at end of first visit)

		M.D.	
_____	_____	_____	_____
Evaluator	Date	Supervisor	Date

CHAPTER 10

Psychological Testing for Treatment Selection

In the previous chapter, we have discussed the time-honored and efficient technique of clinical interviewing as it is used to assess a patient and/or family in order to facilitate the choice from among different treatment interventions. Psychological tests and instruments are also useful in gathering pertinent information for such decisions. In contrast to the unstructured clinical interview, psychological tests are more standardized and reliable — that is, any two testers will administer and score the test in more or less the same way. There is a large variety of psychological tests and instruments (e.g., educational tests which measure achievement, occupational tests which measure career interests and aptitude), but we will be discussing only those instruments used in the clinical situation to measure behaviors relevant to the diagnosis of and treatment selection for mental disorders and emotional problems.

INDICATIONS FOR PSYCHOLOGICAL TESTING

The age and developmental stage of the patient are an important consideration. Children and adolescents (and even some young adults) are in crucial developmental phases and often psychological measurement of their emotional and intellectual development is very helpful. Since children and adolescents have perforce only a truncated past on which to base judgments, testing is most helpful with these age groups. Another indication for psychological testing arises when the consultant is uncertain about the presence or absence of such variables as depression, suicide intent, or thought disorder. In contrast to the unstructured interview situation which generates clinical impressions, test materials yield scores that enable one to compare the patient with others. Such comparison is often helpful in solving otherwise puzzling diagnostic and treatment issues and in assessing change. Patient enabling factors (e.g., motivation for psychotherapy and capacity for insight) can be tapped by specific instruments designed for this purpose. Tests can also be used to focus more clearly and specifically on issues that will be addressed within the context of the general treatment plan (e.g., to provide a particular focus for a brief dynamic therapy or a brief behavioral intervention).

Psychological assessment often serves as a valuable aid in role-inducing the patient into a therapeutic mode of thinking. By sitting down, taking time, and attending to the specific target behaviors being assessed, the patient is encouraged to become an observer of his or her own behavior.

Clinical interviews and psychological testing often concentrate on the weaknesses, problems, and symptoms of the patient. Psychological tests of intelligence, capacity for cooperation, etc. measure assets that significantly affect the choice of certain treatments. Moreover, psychological testing is very useful in allowing the consultant or therapist to compare symptoms or dynamic issues before, during, or after a treatment intervention in order to assess treatment progress and the need for further intervention.

In most instances, the patients in need of careful differential treatment planning (including psychological testing) are neither the most healthy ones, who might spontaneously remit or respond well to most interventions, nor the most ill patients, who respond poorly to many interventions or have obvious treatment needs; rather, they are the patients in the mid-range of symptomatology and adjustment. Indeed, Woody, Luborsky, McLellan, O'Brien, Beck, Blaine, Herman, and Hole (1983) found that drug and alcohol patients with high adjustment tended to profit from treatment regardless of which of six treatment programs they were assigned, and those with the lowest adjustment failed to respond no matter which program they were in. In those 60% of the patients in the mid-range, there was some evidence for meaningful patient-treatment matches. The payoff for careful differential therapeutics, in general, may be in this 60% range.

The gap that exists in many people's minds between the clinical interview and psychological testing is unfortunate. It could be argued that every good clinical workup should include both a clinical interview and some systematic assessment procedures that involve quantification of aspects of the patient's life, whether these be symptoms, problem constellations, psychodynamic conflicts, and/or the environment. The current tendency to regard clinical interviews and testing as very different and separate can be traced to a number of roots. Turf issues in mental health have ways of dividing up the patient and losing sight of integrated evaluation and treatment. The division of labor assigning the psychiatrist for the medication prescription, the psychologist for testing, and the social worker for the family is an exaggerated (but not all that uncommon) manifestation of this fragmentation of efforts.

Therapists and assessors from all disciplines should take advantage of instruments that are simple to give and allow for some quantification. This is especially true for self-report instruments that require some patient, but little professional, time. The use of test instruments should not be an exotic and rare event requiring in all instances a time-consuming referral process. Some tests should probably be included as part of the evaluation for almost every patient. Once important problem areas have been identified in the clinical interview, these can then be followed up with selective instruments. Quantification of the goals of treatment with scaled estimates of areas needing improvement should be done routinely, at least in all brief treatments regardless of their specific techniques and orientation. This would involve either measuring target complaints or goal attainment scaling (Kiresuk and Sherman, 1968).

DEFINITION AND NATURE OF PSYCHOLOGICAL TESTS

A psychological test is a standardized method of sampling behaviors (defined broadly to include feelings, thoughts, symptoms, and intellectual functioning) in a reliable and valid way. The immediate goals of testing are to extrapolate from representative samples of behavior to predict future behaviors or current behaviors other than those being directly sampled by the tests, or to measure change over time.

Tests are given and scored in a standardized manner to ensure reliability, the establishment of norms, and the meaningfulness of comparisons and generalizations. There are various forms of reliability. The test-retest reliability is the correlation between the scores on the same test by the same subject at two different points in time. For most tests, it is desirable to have high test-retest reliability over a short period of time. When a longer period of time, such as six months or more, is under question, one might expect different scores based on changing states, subjective experience, and accumulation of life experience. An alternate form of reliability measures the correlation between scores obtained by the same person on different forms or versions of the same test. And, finally, a third form of reliability is the split-half reliability obtained from correlating an individual's performance on one-half of the test with that on the other half.

The ultimate goal of any assessment instrument is its validity: Does it really tap what it is intended to measure? Validity is determined by the relationship between the score on the test and other external criteria of what the test is designed to measure. For example, a valid test of intelligence might have a positive relationship with school performance as criterion; a valid test of depression might have a high correlation with a clinician's assessment of depression or with response to treatments. There are three major categories of validity: content, criterion-related, and construct validity.

Content validity refers to whether the test content covers an adequate sample of the behavior under question (e.g., the Wechsler Adult Intelligence Scale-Revised, an intelligence test, covers various content areas of intellectual functioning, such as vocabulary, arithmetic skills, and abstracting abilities). A test of depression can be examined to see if the items adequately sample the various types and manifestations of depression (cognitive, vegetative, behavioral, etc.).

Criterion-related validity involves the relationship between the test score and other outside criteria. Such validation can be concurrent validity (correlation with outside criteria in the present) or predictive validity (correlation to future behaviors). A valid test of depression would correlate with the clinician's assessment of depression (concurrent) and might predict future episodes of depression or treatment response (predictive).

Construct validity refers to the ability of the test to measure a particular theoretical construct or trait, such as intelligence or depression. Any aspect of the construct or trait (such as its relationship to developmental changes, its relationship to other behaviors, and its response to experimental intervention) can potentially contribute to the development of construct validity. A theoretical construct such as identity integration (vs. identity diffusion) is illustrative. If one had a test of such a construct, one would expect scores of identity integration in normal subjects to increase with age through the adolescent and early adult periods. The score on identity integration should correlate positively with related constructs (convergent validity), such as that of ego strength, but should not correlate with the behavior of others (discriminant validity), such as anxiety.

By what they described as a multitrait-multimethod matrix, Campbell and Fiske (1959) proposed an experimental model for investigating convergent and discriminant validation. This model calls for the assessment of two or more traits (e.g., anxiety and depression) by two or more methods (e.g., self-report and clinical interview rating). A measure of validity (validity coefficient) would be the correlation of the score for the same trait across two or more methods. Satisfactory validity would be shown if the validity coefficient is higher than the correlation between different traits measured by different methods. It should also be higher than the correlation between different traits across the same method. Finally, the response of the theoretical construct to experimental intervention provides further data in construct validation. For example, one would expect a score on identity integration to improve following psychotherapy intended to facilitate such integration. One would expect depression scores to decrease in those patients treated with antidepressant medication or therapy geared to lessen the depression.

The specific instruments to be discussed in this chapter vary considerably in their technical attributes (reliability, validity). For detailed, specific information on these and other tests, the reader should consult the excellent, available test reviews (such as Anastasi, 1982, or Buros, 1970; 1972; 1978). In Buros, for instance, virtually all of the test instruments that a clinician or researcher would ever consider using are reviewed extensively by one or several experts. These critical reviews are outstanding in their careful analysis of each instrument's theoretical background, construction, use, and reliability and validity.

GOALS OF ASSESSMENT

As noted in the previous chapter, assessment for treatment planning (using the clinical interview and/or psychological testing) must address the following goals:

1) a phenomenological description of the symptoms and behavioral problems;
2) a functional analysis of the problem areas;
3) a monitoring procedure and determination of baseline behaviors;
4) identification of personal and environmental assets;
5) specifications of treatment goals; and
6) establishment of a patient-therapist contract.

Assessment instruments are most helpful in supplementing the work of the interview in achieving each of these goals. While an interview can help describe symptoms and problem areas, instruments such as rating scales and semi-structured interviews are most useful in *quantifying* such areas. Both the interview and test material provide data from which the consultant constructs functional hypotheses of what antecedent events or behaviors and/or hypothetical internal constructs (e.g., conflicts) lead to the pathology. Measurement of baseline behaviors and monitoring can best be done with self-report, using either interview or rating scales, to be compared with subsequent serial self-reports. Tests such as the Wechsler Adult Intelligence Scale-Revised (WAIS-R) and the California Psychological Inventory (CPI) can be used to measure assets. Screening tests, such as the Minnesota Multiphasic Personality Inventory (MMPI), can be helpful in insuring that pathology which should be targeted for intervention was not missed in the clinical interview. In addition, areas of possible intervention, e.g., where there are specific conflicts, can be further explored in projective testing. Explicit treatment goals can be identified and measured using goal attainment scaling (Kiresuk and Sherman, 1968).

TARGETS FOR ASSESSMENT

The targets for differential treatment assessment using instruments are the same as the targets for assessment in the clinical interview. These include any and all of the indications, enabling factors, and contraindications for each of the various treatments that have been summarized throughout this volume.

- patient symptom/problem profile (Axis 1 diagnosis)
- longstanding personality characteristics and interpersonal behavior of the patient that may or may not be the focus of treatment but, in either case, will be a major factor in treatment planning (Axis II)
- the social, intellectual, and behavioral assets of the patient (Axis V)
- enabling factors such as psychological mindedness and motivation for change
- the environment of the patient (especially family, school and work), and special stressors (Axis IV)

It seems obvious, but needs stating, that two individuals with the same DSM-III diagnosis may respond quite differentially to treatment because of the presence or absence of certain assets (e.g., given the same DSM-III diagnosis, one patient may have high IQ and social-relating skills, another may have low IQ and poor social-relating skills). The patient's prior adjustment – particularly in social activities and in work – is a crucial determinant of the type, duration, and setting of the prospective treatment intervention, as well as a strong predictor for prognosis. The living environment of the patient influences what subject matter will arise in psychodynamic treatment (Kernberg et al., 1972). The growing literature on the home environment of the schizophrenic patient indicates that this may strongly influence the course of the disease and may be an important target of intervention.

In 1966, Cole and Magnessen suggested that diagnostic testing procedures be used in "dispositional assessment" to assist the assignment of patients to the most appropriate treatments. Ironically, although this publication was titled, "Where the Action Is," there has been little action since then in the explicit use of psychological tests for treatment planning. Reviews of psychological tests in clinical settings (Kendall and Norton-Ford, 1982; Korchin and Schuldberg, 1981) typically survey the use of clinical testing for diagnosis, assessment of response to therapeutic intervention, research, and training. But one searches in vain for clearly developed models that would guide the use of testing in differential treatment planning.

One interesting exception is the model proposed by Beutler (1979) for differential treatment assignment. Beginning with a review of the prior literature, Beutler hypothesizes three patient dimensions useful in making assignments to appropriate treatments. The first dimension is the dichotomy between those psychiatric conditions whose development is characterized by a specific history and those that involve complex and very general reactions to the environment. As examples of noncomplex symptoms, Beutler lists circumscribed fears and phobias, eating and smoking dysfunctions. Examples of complex symptoms include neurotic conditions, schizophrenias, character disorders, and multisymptomatic phobias. We should comment here that in treatment planning one must certainly attend to this dimension, but with certain variations. For example, although the diagnosis may indeed be a very complex one with mixed and/or unknown etiologies and with a long history of illness (such as is the case with schizophrenia), the treatment planning may involve attention to rather specific, circumscribed problems. However, it is correct to assume that treatment planning must consider where the symptoms fall on the simplicity-complexity dimension.

The second hypothesized dimension is one that describes the patient's characteristic way of coping with intrapsychic conflict. These defensive styles are described as either a disposition toward externalizing defenses (e.g., projection) or a disposition to internal defenses (e.g., intellectualization).

A third hypothetical dimension is one that describes the way the patient copes with demands from the external environment. The concept of reactance, borrowed from social psychology, is used here. A patient high in reactance has a predisposition to resist external influence; in contrast, an individual low in reactance is relatively open to external influence.

It is hypothesized that circumscribed symptoms will respond best to non-insight, behaviorally-based treatments, and complex symptoms will respond best to cognitive modification and insight therapies. Patients with externalized defenses will respond best to behaviorally-based treatments, while those with internalized defenses will respond best to insight treatments. Finally, patients high in reactance will respond best to insight treatments, while those low in this dimension will respond best to non-insight treatments.

Beutler has put these differential treatment hypotheses to several very preliminary tests, using psychotherapy research studies which met minimal criteria for adequate control and design. The psychotherapies used in these investigations were sorted into five categories: cognitive modification, cognitive insight treatments, behavior therapies, behavior modification, and affective insight. In the studies reviewed, there was some support of hypotheses regarding the level of patient reactance. Insight therapy appeared to be superior to behavior therapy among highly reactive patients, whereas less reactive patients were more responsive to behavioral therapies. Other hypotheses either received inconsistent support or were not studied in this post-hoc analysis. In a prospective study of hypotheses about defensive style (externalizing vs. internalizing), Beutler and Mitchell (1981) compared brief psychoanalytic treatment with brief experiential treatment in outpatients treated by psychology interns. Internalizing, depressive patients obtained more benefit from both treatments than did impulsive, externalizing patients. Experiential therapy was better across patient types, and the treatment main effect may have been primarily the result of experiential therapy having greater effectiveness among impulsive, externalizing patients.

While the model certainly needs a great deal of further testing, it does suggest that instruments which measure such targets as defensive style (external vs. internal), reactance (patient's responsiveness to outside influences), and the nature of symptoms should be utilized to assess patients for differential therapeutic planning. In our subsequent review of the most commonly used test instruments, we will attend especially to those that are potentially useful in this regard.

TESTING REFERRAL QUESTIONS

The orientation of the referring consultant, the nature of the treatment setting, and the timing of the referral will influence the type of questions asked of psychological testing by the referring consultant. Behavior therapists working in a phobia clinic, for example, want assessment to measure the severity of fears and to list each and every environmental situation in which the fears arise. A psychoanalyst in an analytic clinic is likely to ask quite different questions of psychological testing and to request impressions about the nature of internal conflicts, defensive patterns, ego strengths necessary for long-term regressive treatment, transference paradigms, and so on.

Psychological testing can be used in conjunction with the clinical interview to assign a patient to the best treatment setting and to provide data on how best to plan further treatment after assignment to that setting. The qualities of the patients preselected to a particular setting influence the sorts of testing questions raised by consultants. In a survey of 168 assessment referral questions made over a six-month sample period in an acute, inpatient division with five units in a private teaching hospital (Sweeney and Clarkin, 1983), it was found that Axis I questions predominated (57%), followed by questions of Axis II disorders (23%), followed by questions concerning treatment planning (including requests about specific recommendations for medication and psychotherapy) and, finally, a few questions about suicide potential and intellectual functioning.

Among the Axis I disorders under question, the major concern was in the assessment of depression, schizophrenia, and psychosis. In contrast, referral questions for testing in day hospital settings often emphasize the assessment of specific cognitive and vocational assets that will enable an adequately diagnosed patient to function and to further treatment planning. In outpatient settings, questions are more often directly related to the patient's internal experience, interpersonal behavior, and fantasy, in order to plan and focus individual exploratory psychotherapy. In family clinics, in child and adolescent clinics, and in some hospital settings, there is a growing recognition of the impact of the environment, especially the family environment, upon the patient and the patient's disturbed behavior; instruments are available to measure and assess this environment. Questions about neuropsychological functioning, including the nature, degree, and location of impairment, are often the major focus of concern with children and adolescents in child clinics, with elderly patients in psychiatric inpatient settings, and in neurology clinics.

METHODS OF ASSESSMENT

Psychological assessment instruments vary in their information source, the way they are constructed (and therefore in their method of obtaining and utilizing information), and in the content of data that are collected.

The source of information may be the report of the patient (self-report), the report of significant others (such as parents, relatives, roommates), and/or the direct behavior of the patient as observed and rated by trained observers. Rating scales, such as the Hamilton Rating Scale for Depression (Hamilton, 1960), usually follow a semi-structured interview format to gather information that is scaled, using anchor points. Objective tests are those instruments that utilize completely structured and standardized formats to obtain data from the subject, which can then be compared to those of normative groups. Examples of typically used objective tests in clinical situations are the MMPI (Hathaway and McKinley, 1942a), the WAIS-R, and the 16-PF (Cattell and Stice, 1950). A final category of instruments, the projective tests, are constructed in such a way as to provide more ambiguous stimuli than is the case with the objective or semi-structured tests. This ambiguity of the projective test stimuli is both an asset and a liability. These tests succeed in eliciting quite diverse, idiosyncratic, and personal behaviors, but this makes it difficult to generate an objective and reliable scoring system and method of interpretation.

The increasing appreciation of course factors as important discriminators of psychiatric diagnoses calls attention to the time perspectives of the various assessment instruments. The Schedule for Affective Disorders and Schizophrenia (SADS) (Endicott and Spitzer, 1978), a semi-structured interview explicitly constructed to yield Research Diagnostic Criteria diagnoses, is the prototypic instrument geared to assessing symptoms reliably and with explicit duration criteria. Other instruments make specific and consistent reference to time, usually limiting the time frame to the recent past. For example, rating scales such as the Hamilton specify the recent past (past week). The MMPI is internally variable in its time frame. Some items ("I have a good appetite") refer to the present. Some items refer to the past and present ("I have never vomited or coughed up blood"). Some items contrast the present with the past ("My judgment is better than it ever was"). Some items, even of a symptomatic content, seem to refer to enduring conditions ("Most of the time I feel blue").

Other tests that sample and measure current behavior, such as the WAIS-R and the Rorschach, provide a cross-sectional reading of the behaviors in question. It is difficult to predict future behaviors with any assurance, or assume past behaviors, from cross-sectional assessments alone. This has an important, often neglected, practical implication: One cannot *diagnose* schizophrenia, which in its DSM-III definition requires symptoms of six months' duration, simply from the behaviors manifested on such cross-sectional tests as the Rorschach and WAIS-R, which do not measure their duration. The tester can indicate that the particular cross-sectional behavior is consistent with schizophrenia or schizophreniform disorders, but can go no further. Moreover, virtually all available psychological tests were developed before DSM-III, and it is not at all clear how applicable are previous efforts using therapist diagnosis.

SPECIFIC ASSESSMENT TOOLS

Table 10-1 lists the major assessment tools used to assist in treatment planning. This is not the place to give a thorough review of the assessment instruments and, fortunately, this has been done very well elsewhere (Anastasi, 1982; Buros, 1978; Golden, 1979; Goldman, L'Engle Stein, and Guerry, 1984; Rapaport, Gill, and Schafer, 1968). However, in order to provide a sense of how the tools are used, we will review some of the available instruments according to methodology and type: self-report instruments; independent ratings using rating scales or semi-structured interviews; objective and projective tests.

Self-report Instruments

Self-report instruments extend the clinical interview by systematically asking the patient about the symptoms, problems, or interpersonal relations as he/she experiences them. These instruments have the advantages of economy and direct standardized measurement of the patient's perception of his/her difficulties and assets. At the same time, of course, the validity of the information obtained by self-report rests on the patient's accurate self-perception and willingness to report with candor. In this regard, the correlation of self-report instruments with independent criteria is not always high. For example, the correlation between self-report measures of depression and clinical ratings ranges from .33 to .56 (Rehm, 1976). This does not mean that self-report is invalid or useless, but that it should not, as a rule, be used alone, especially with very ill patients who are most likely to have less accurate self-perception. Moreover, in some situations the self-report may provide data more valid than those gathered in other ways. The various methods of data collection may supplement one another by providing different types of information.

There are a number of self-report instruments that ask the patient to indicate and rate severity of symptoms. These include the SCL-90 (Derogatis, 1975) for dimensions such as depression, anxiety, psychoticism, hostility, and interpersonal sensitivity; the Beck Depression Inventory (Beck, Ward, Mendelson, Mock, and Erbaugh, 1961) for depression; State-Trait Measure of Anxiety (Spielberger, Gorsuch, and Luchene, 1970) for immediate and enduring tendencies to experience anxiety; and the Fear Survey Schedule (Wolpe and Lang, 1964) for specific feared situations. Horowitz (1979) has pointed out that 76% of applicants for outpatient treatment reported problems that were interpersonal in nature, suggesting that outcome in therapy should often be measured in changes in interpersonal behavior, in addition to changes in symptoms. Self-report instruments that assess interpersonal behavior include the Interpersonal Checklist (Leary, 1957), the Interpersonal Behavior Inventory (IBI) (Lorr and McNair, 1965), the Structural Analysis of Social Behavior Questionnaires (Benjamin, 1974), and the KDS-15 (Kupfer and Detre, 1974) for marital functioning/dysfunction.

Clinical illustration

Benjamin (1977) provides the following clinical illustration involving the use of the Structural Analysis of Interpersonal Behavior Questionnaires to plan and measure progress and outcome of the treatment of a five-year-old male child. This child was abusive and defiant toward his parents, with behavior including kicking, swearing, and threatening to kill his mother. Questionnaire data from the parents, who rated each other, their own parents, and their son in terms of interpersonal behavior, revealed the following system problems. The son's behavior toward the mother was predominantly that of attack, with his own position being that of hostile autonomy. The son was, according to the mother's self-report on the questionnaires, treating the mother as the mother had been treated by her own father. The mother felt supportive toward and supported by her husband and her mother, but felt despair in the face of demanding and critical behavior from her father and her son. The husband remained in a childlike position in relationship to both his wife, who did most of the parenting, and his family of origin.

The test data were used to develop a family therapy treatment plan in which the focus was on assisting the mother to replace her own hostile and controlling behavior toward the son by an encouragement of his autonomous actions. Such a shift in the mother's behavior would hopefully result in a change in the son's behavior from that of hostile opposition to friendly emancipation. The plan met with initial success. The mother engaged in positive activities with the son, as suggested by the therapist, and the father began to be a more active co-parent. However, following this success, a year into the therapy the mother

TABLE 10-1
Assessment Targets and Instruments

	Self-Report	Independent Rater	Objective	Projective
Symptoms and Symptom Constellations (Axis I)				
Depression	Beck Depression Inventory (Beck et al., 1961); SCL-90 (Derogatis, 1975)	Hamilton Rating Scale for Depression (Hamilton, 1960); SADS (Endicott & Spitzer, 1978)	MMPI, D-scale (Hathaway & McKinley, 1942a)	
Suicidal Behavior		Suicide Intent Scale (Beck, Schuyler, & Herman, 1974); SADS		Rorschach (Exner, 1974)
Anxiety	SCL-90; STAI (Spielberger, Gorsuch, & Luchene, 1970)			
Thought Disorder		SADS	MMPI	Rorschach
Personality Variables				
Personality Disorders		DIB (Gunderson, Kolb, & Austin, 1981)	MMCI (Millon, 1977)	
Quality of Interpersonal Relations	IBI (Lorr & McNair, 1965)			
	KDS-15 (Kupfer & Detre, 1974)			

Ego Strength	Washington University Sentence Completion Test (Loevinger, Wessler & Redmore, 1970)			Es Scale, MMPI	
Patterning of Defenses	Defense Mechanisms Inventory (Gleser & Ihilevich, 1969)			MMPI; WAIS-R (Wechsler, 1981)	
Intrapsychic Conflicts					TAT (Henry, 1956) Rorschach
Transference Paradigms					TAT Rorschach
Assets/Prior Adjustment Intelligence			WAIS-R		
Social Functioning	SAS-SR (Weissman, Prusoff, Thompson, Harding, & Myers, 1978)	GAS (Endicott, Spitzer, Fleiss, & Cohen, 1976)			
Work Functioning	SAS-SR	GAS			
Environment	Olson Family Environment Scale	Camberwell Family Interview (Brown & Rutter, 1966)			
	DSP (Derogatis, 1982)				
Therapy Goals/ Monitoring	Goal Attainment Scaling (Kiresuk & Sherman, 1968)				

showed signs of depression, with complaints of lack of enjoyment, excessive use of alcohol, nonperformance of household chores, and much lower self-esteem. This was seen by the therapist as resistance, and treated with a focus on a fuller relationship between husband and wife, one which would allow assertiveness from the husband, and reception of warmth and assistance on the part of the wife. The wife's depression began to lift, followed by more independence. In the meantime, the son was responding well to a behavior therapy program, with a reduction in verbal abuse and increasing self-care behavior. Retesting showed that the son's autonomy had increased appreciably, matched by the mother's decrease in hostile control.

There is growing awareness that the interaction of the patient with the environment has a profound impact on behavior and psychiatric symptoms. Adversive family environment correlates with rehospitalization of schizophrenics (Brown, Birley, and Wing, 1972). The environment of depressives is hypothesized to be lacking in positive but rich in negative reinforcers, and these can be measured by self-report questionnaires (Lewinsohn and Arconad, 1981). In the area of personality assessment, Mischel (1968) has emphasized the interaction of the individual with the setting, and that testing of the individual apart from the setting leads to data with low validity coefficients.

Life events as presumptive, stress-inducing stimuli arising from the environment have been shown to play a role in health deterioration (Rahe, 1968), sudden cardiac death (Rahe and Lind, 1971), complications with birth and pregnancy (Gorsuch and Key, 1974), depression (Ilfeld, 1977; Paykel, Myers, Dienett, Klerman, Lindenthal, and Pepper, 1969; Warheit, 1979), and psychiatric disorder in general (Dekker and Webb, 1974; Myers, Lindenthal, and Pepper, 1971; Uhlenhuth and Paykel, 1973).

Stress is now acknowledged in the diagnostic system by a rating in Axis IV. In assessing stress and coping, one can measure the stress stimuli, the response to the stress, or the interaction of the organism and stress. Stimulus-oriented measures of stress would include Recent Life Changes Questionnaire (RLCQ) (Rahe, 1974), the Social Readjustment Rating Scale (SRRS) (Holmes, 1979), and the Life Experiences Survey (LES) (Sarason, Johnson, and Siegel, 1979). To capture the subjective reaction to the life events, Horowitz and colleagues have developed another life events scale (Horowitz, Wilner, and Alvarez, 1979). Response to stress or response-oriented measures would include many of the self-report instruments covered elsewhere in this chapter, such as the MMPI, the SCL-90, the BDI and the STAI. The Jenkins Activity Survey (JAS) (Jenkins, Rosenman, and Friedman, 1967) is the proto-type of an interaction measure of stress, as it focuses on the cognitive and perceptual characteristics of the individual that mediate responses to stress. This instrument has shown predictive validity for coronary heart disease (Jenkins, 1971, 1976; Jenkins, Rosenman, and Zyzanski, 1974). Obviously, measures using an interactional approach are needed for general areas of psychiatry. The Derogatis Stress Profile (DSP) (Derogatis, 1982), which measures stimuli arising from job, home, and health, together with characteristic attitudes and coping mechanisms, may be helpful in this area but needs validation work.

Clinical illustration

An 18-year-old female, the first of two children born to a lower-middle-class, white family, was hospitalized with a schizophreniform disorder involving acute delusional symptoms. While the family's religion was Jewish, the patient had "converted" to Catholicism with delusions of be-ing a Catholic nun. The diagnosis of the patient seemed clear – schizo-phreniform disorder, first break, with moderate premorbid function-ing – but assessment of the home environment was needed to plan dis-charge and future treatment. While the patient had achieved some autonomy from the family following high school by moving to an apart-ment and beginning college, three months prior to hospitalization she had moved back, and fights with father and mother over house rules had ensued. A modified version of the Kreisman, Simmens, and Joy (1979) self-report measure of family hostility and over-involvement with the patient was administered, along with a modified version of the Holmes-Rahe Life Events Schedule. Data from these instruments, plus additional probing by interview suggested that the move back home by the patient was experienced as a major stress on the family, especially the mother, who felt that the patient's behavior was intruding on her personal life. The score on the Kreisman, Simmens and Joy instrument was high, indicating that the family had considerable expressed hostility toward the patient. This was made the focus for psychoeducational family intervention during the hospitalization. The diagnosis of schizo-phreniform disorder was explained to the parents and daughter, re-sulting in subsequent relief on the part of the parents and some hope that proper treatment would be helpful. The awareness that her daughter was ill and not "bad" enabled the mother to lower her hostil-ity. Subsequent clarification about which of the daughter's behaviors were strivings for autonomy versus other behaviors that were manifes-tations of the illness (e.g., the delusions) also helped decrease the hostility of the family toward the patient and enabled them to provide support and reassurance.

The suicidal potential of the patient has obvious treatment planning implications, whether it be for outpatient management from a behavioral (Linehan, 1981) or psychodynamic point of view (Kernberg, 1975), for potential family intervention, or for hospitalization (Kirstein, Weissman, and Prusoff, 1975) or readiness for discharge from hospitalization. Review of recent literature indicates that suicidal threats, suicide planning and/or preparation, suicidal ideation, and recent parasuicidal behavior are direct indicators of current risk (Linehan, 1981). These factors should be assessed in detail in a clinical interview. Self-report instruments, which focus specific and detailed attention on important aspects and allow one to obtain a score to compare with others, may be of additional help. Such scales would include the Suicide Intent Scale (SIS) and the Scale for Suicide Ideation, both developed by Beck and his associates (Beck, Schuyler, and Herman, 1974; Beck, Kovacs, and Weissman, 1979). Especially troublesome and difficult for adequate treatment and intervention is assessment of suicide potential with the patient who denies suspected depression and suicidal ideation. In such instances, projective tests such as the Rorschach are sometimes used in hope that the patient's responses will indicate such ideation without his/her conscious intent or awareness.

Independent Ratings

Ratings of patient symptomatology and behavior, derived from either an interview (semi-structured or unstructured) or observations of behavior, can play an important role in assessment and treatment planning. Some of the most used instruments include the Global Assessment Scale (GAS) (Endicott, Spitzer, Fleiss, and Cohen, 1976), the Brief Psychiatric Rating Scale (BPRS) (Overall and Gorham, 1962), the Hamilton Rating Scale for Depression (Hamilton, 1960), and the Katz Adjustment Scale (KAS) (Katz and Lyerly, 1963; Katz, Lowery, and Cole, 1967).

Hamilton Rating Scale for Depression

The Hamilton Psychiatric Rating Scale for Depression is designed for rating the severity and kind of depression in patients already known to be depressed. The 17 variables are each rated on a 4-point anchored scale. The content places emphasis on behavioral and somatic symptoms of depression, at the expense of cognitive and affective dimensions of depression, making the scale more appropriate for assessment of severely and biologically depressed patients. The instrument is a detailed guide used to quantify depression reliably based on data gathered in an interview of about one-half hour's duration.

While the clinical interviewer has the advantage of probing where and when he wants, emphasizing specific areas that seem most important, the semi-structured interview by its format ensures the comprehensive coverage of all relevant areas so that the important questions (that could be missed inadvertantly in even a brilliant clinical interview) are asked in a standard way to yield a rating which can generate a score or a categorization.

Schedule for Affective Disorders and Schizophrenia

The Schedule for Affective Disorders and Schizophrenia (SADS) (Endicott and Spitzer, 1978) is another good example of an independent rating test. The SADS is a semi-structured interview guide that enables the clinician to quantify symptoms and patient functioning during the past week, during the worst period of the most recent episode of illness, and/or during the patient's entire past life. The content of the interview covers symptoms related to affective and thinking disturbances and is most useful in planning treatment intervention when the differential between affective and schizophrenic symptoms is crucial. The data obtained from the semi-structured interview enables the clinician to arrive at a Research Diagnostic Criteria (RDC) categorization. While it is too lengthy and detailed for routine clinical assessment, the SADS is an especially useful interview guide and measure when treatment planning around depression is crucial.

Clinical illustration

A 35-year-old policeman was referred for psychological testing following a leave of absence from work three months earlier due to a depression, which was treated with chemotherapy. The testing was needed to assess resolution of previous pathology, ability to reassume dangerous police responsibilities, and assessment of need for further intervention. The psychologist administered the Hamilton for two time periods, once concerning the depressive episode at its worst three months earlier and again to measure the patient's current condition. Scores indicated that he had suffered a moderate to severe depression with endogenomorphic symptoms three months ago, with remission and no depressive symptomatology currently. In addition, validity scales on the MMPI were currently within normal limits, as was Scale 2 (Depression). A SADS interview done at intake confirmed the diagnosis of depression and ruled out schizophrenia. Other tests (Rorschach, MMPI, WAIS) were used to assess current personality functioning and makeup during this asymptomatic period.

Objective Tests

Butcher (1972) has described three essential differences between the objective tests and the projective tests. Objective tests seek a trait description of the patient, that is, a description of the patient's characteristic behavior or style. The stimuli in objective tests are relatively clear and well-defined and ask for circumscribed answers (e.g., true or false). And, finally, objective tests utilize norms so that the individual patient's scores can be compared to normative samples. In contrast, projective tests are done in such a way as to yield information on personality dynamics; the stimuli are vague so as to elicit idiosyncratic responses from the patient; and much of the test response is interpreted without reference to norms. Two objective tests that traditionally have played an important clinical role in treatment planning are the WAIS-R and the MMPI.

WAIS-R

Intellectual functioning is a crucial asset and one that reflects capacities needed for daily functioning in society, as well as capacities needed for different forms of therapeutic intervention. For these reasons, assessment of intellectual functioning traditionally has been considered an important part of the assessment of a patient for treatment planning. Moreover, intelligence is the single most predictive measure of future mental health and adjustment (Kohlberg, LaCrosse, and Ricks, 1972). It is not assumed that a patient's functioning on an intelligence test, such as the WAIS-R, is a measure of native intellectual capacity. Rather, functioning on the tests is seen as a *sample* of how the patient is *currently* performing in selected areas of intellectual performance (e.g., memory, vocabulary). The test in essence taps the ability of the subject to learn from past experience and to reproduce the effects of such learning in the present context.

The relationship of intelligence and the ability to profit from the various types of therapy is a complicated one. Candidates for psychoanalysis are usually of higher levels of intelligence (Hamburg, Bibring, Fisher,

Stanton, Wallerstein, and Haggard, 1967; Siegel, 1962) while behavior therapists have shown little concern with patients' level of intelligence. In a review by Luborsky, Chandler, Auerbach, Cohen, and Bachrach (1971) ten of 13 studies showed a positive correlation (.24 to .46) between intelligence and outcome in psychotherapy. Since psychotherapy is a learning process, there are probably different levels of intelligence (in strong interaction with other variables) needed for the different types of therapy that call for various types of learning. Specificity about minimum levels and type of intelligence needed for various therapies are not established at this time.

The WAIS-R is a revised version (Wechsler, 1981) of the Wechsler Adult Intelligence Scale, which was first published in 1955. The forerunner of the WAIS was the Wechsler-Bellevue Intelligence Scale published in 1939. The WAIS and WAIS-R comprise 11 subtests, six of which (Information, Comprehension, Arithmetic, Similarities, Digit Span, and Vocabulary) are grouped into a Verbal Scale, and five of which (Digit Symbol, Picture Completion, Block Design, Picture Arrangement, and Object Assembly) are grouped into a Performance Scale. Raw scores on each of the subtests are transformed into standard scores. Subtest scores are used to generate scaled scores for Verbal, Performance, and Full Scale scores. The normative sample for the WAIS was a carefully chosen sample of 1,700 subjects, matching proportions according to the 1950 United States Census with respect to area of country, urban-rural location, race, occupational level, and education. Likewise, the normative sample for the WAIS-R included over 1,800 subjects, with matching proportions chosen according to the 1970 United States Census providing the bases for stratification according to age, sex, race, geographical region, occupation, education, and urban-rural residence.

The test can be used in treatment planning by matching the estimate of the patient's overall and specific scores on intelligence with hypotheses or clinical experience as to minimal intelligence needed for specific treatments. In addition, differential performance in various subtests can manifest defensive styles or assess liabilities in areas that need intervention.

MMPI

Devised in the 1940s by Hathaway and McKinley (1942a) the MMPI is a self-report personality inventory with items taken from lists of psychiatric symptoms and complaints compiled from textbooks of psychiatry, previous personality inventories, and the authors' own clinical experience. With a sample of 504 such items, they used the method of contrasting criterion groups to arrive at final scale construction. This empirical approach consisted of giving the item pool to criterion groups, such as diagnosed hypochondriacs, and noting the items that discriminated this group of patients from a group of normals. For Scale 1, hypochondriasis was defined as a neurotic concern over bodily health, and 50 patients with hypochondriasis, uncomplicated by psychosis or other psychiatric features, were selected. Their responses to the MMPI items were contrasted with those of "normals," who consisted of 724 friends or relatives seen at the University Hospitals in Minneapolis. Using this method of criterion-keyed scoring, nine clinical scales were constructed: Scale 1 (hypochondriasis) (McKinley and Hathaway, 1940); Scale 2 (depression) (Hathaway and McKinley, 1942b); Scale 7 (psychasthenia) (McKinley and Hathaway, 1942); Scale 3 (hysteria); Scale 4 (psychopathic deviate); and Scale 9 (hypomania) (McKinley and Hathaway, 1944); Scale 5 (masculinity-femininity); Scale 6 (paranoia); Scale 8 (schizophrenia) (Hathaway, 1956). In addition to the clinical scales, validity scales were constructed in order to assess the test-taking attitudes of the patient.

Meehl and Hathaway (1946) focused on the necessity of assessing two test-taking attitudes of defensiveness or minimizing symptoms and problems ("faking good"), and maximizing problems ("faking bad"). Validity scales were constructed. The L scale was constructed of items that are socially desirable qualities but rare in their occurrence in one individual. Endorsement of a number of these items would suggest maximizing assets or "faking good." The F scale was composed of items with a low frequency of endorsement in the normative sample. Thus, an individual answering in the affirmative to a large number of these items would be likely to be maximizing pathology. The K scale was composed of items that reflect change in response when persons are instructed to "fake" psychopathology when answering.

Clinical experience and systematic observation of the correlation of MMPI profile patterns with specific patients (e.g., Marks and Seeman, 1963) have resulted in symptom, diagnostic, and treatment planning statements such as the following: Psychotherapy should be directed initially toward solving immediate problems and avoid introspective self-analysis (high point codes, 2,7,8/7,2,8); these patients are chronically depressed with little motivation to change, and thus improving social skills through assertiveness training and role playing may be beneficial in helping form some meaningful relationships (high point codes, 2,0/0,2); prognosis for significant change is poor, unless the patient can be engaged in long-term therapy (spike 3); angry, hostile patients who deny or rationalize feelings such that prognosis for change is poor (high point

3,6/6,3); supportive measures to bolster defenses in order to weather any current crisis is in order, and any insight therapy should be used cautiously as there is the possibility of underlying psychotic processes (high point 3,8/8,3); these patients often complain of acute, physical symptoms, defend against examining psychological factors, and will likely leave treatment once the physical symptoms abate (3,9/9,3); since these patients alternate between periods of acting out followed by periods of guilt and self-deprecation, intervention is difficult without a long-term therapeutic relationship (high point 4,7/7,4) (Greene, 1980).

While the MMPI began with three validity scales and nine specific symptom or diagnostic scales, many research scales have subsequently been devised to address specific questions, including those centered around treatment planning and differential therapeutics. Historically important and relevant to differential therapeutics is the Barron Ego Strength (Es) Scale (Barron, 1953). The scale was constructed to predict the response of neurotic outpatients to individual psychotherapy. After six months of psychotherapy, 17 patients were judged as improved and 16 others unimproved. Items out of the MMPI were selected that differentiated the two groups, and the resulting 68 items constituted the Es Scale. Barron cross-validated the scale on three additional groups of patients in individual psychotherapy. Much subsequent research (as well as controversy about its usefulness and effectiveness) has gone into the Es Scale. Attempts by other investigators to cross-validate the scale have yielded inconsistent results (Graham, 1977). It seems to work best in predicting response to individual, psychoanalytically-oriented psychotherapy for neurotic patients, and less well for other patient/therapy matches.

Since response to psychotherapy depends not only on the qualities of the patient, but also upon the therapeutic alliance that emerges with the particular therapist (Morgan, Luborsky, Crits-Christoph, Curtis, and Solomon, 1982), it might be fruitful to ask what are the characteristics of the patients who score high on the scale. The information is clearer on this more limited question. High scorers on Es have better general psychological adjustment (Gottesman, 1959; Hawkinson, 1962; Himelstein, 1964; Kleinmuntz, 1960; Quay, 1955; Rosen, 1963; Speigel, 1969; Taft, 1957; Tamkin, 1957; Tamkin and Klett, 1957), and are more aware of internal conflicts (Himelstein, 1964). These are individuals likely to respond to insight-oriented psychotherapy and to form a good therapeutic alliance for this form of treatment.

As suggested by Beutler (1979), specific MMPI scales around defensive patterns, such as the Welsh (1952) internalization ratio, may also be useful in differential therapeutics. As Beutler hypothesizes, patients with defensive patterns favoring internalization might respond best to insight-oriented therapies, while those more externally oriented would be most likely to respond to behavioral interventions. There is related information on this notion from the Sloane study (Sloane, Staples, Cristol, Yorkston, and Whipple, 1975). In that investigation, it was found that patients with MMPI patterns of 4,9 responded better to behavior therapy than to psychodynamic individual psychotherapy. The MMPI is both a self-report questionnaire and an objective test, depending on how it is scored. Content scales, such as those by Wiggins (1966), illustrate the self-report methodology and are based on the manifest content of the items. In contrast, scales derived through actuarial methods conform to the objective test methodology.

The MMPI is the workhorse of the assessment instruments and is the most widely utilized test in hospital and outpatient clinical settings. It has also been used in literally thousands of research studies. Skinner (1979) has compared the MMPI to a 1941 Chevrolet. Its design is old. The recent attention to factorial features, response styles, and the more reliable classification scheme of DSM-III point to serious flaws in the MMPI. However, like old reliable cars that earn our affection over the years, the MMPI is rich in experience and will not quickly yield to sleeker, modern models. More recent instruments do demand attention, however. The Millon Multiaxial Clinical Inventory (MMCI) (Millon, 1977) is an objective, self-report personality inventory that measures 20 clinical syndromes derived from the author's theory of psychopathology (Millon, 1981). While this is an interesting instrument because of its relationship to a systematic and detailed theory of personality psychopathology, as well as its matching to many of the criteria in DSM-III, Axis II, the MMCI has been criticized on structural grounds, as the scales have many overlapping items (Wiggins, 1982). The MMCI has not yet been utilized sufficiently in clinical settings, so its usefulness remains in question.

Projective Tests

Projective techniques, such as the Rorschach and the Thematic Apperception Test (TAT), are by their nature relatively unstructured tasks which call forth from the subject a wide variety of possible responses, thus giving the opportunity for individualized and idiosyncratic material to emerge. Not only are the test stimuli ambiguous and therefore open to a multitude of responses, but also the interpretation or meaning of the response to the tester is relatively unknown to the patient. This is in contrast to the knowledge of the patient concerning the meaning of his response to others when he is asked, for example, on the SCL-90 whether or not he hears voices.

Projective instruments, as indicated on Table 1, are probably most useful in assessment of the presence and degree of current thought disorder, and in the assessment of such personality variables as the quality of interpersonal relationships, ego strengths, patterning of defenses, the presence and nature of intrapsychic conflict, and the presence and quality of transference paradigms.

Rorschach

This projective instrument was developed in 1921 by a Swiss psychiatrist named Hermann Rorschach (Rorschach, 1921). He administered a number of inkblots to different psychiatric groups and observed those responses that differentiated subjects into the various diagnostic categories. Scoring systems were further developed by followers such as Beck (1937) and Klopfer and Kelly (1942). Exner (1974) has recently described a scoring system which hopefully integrates the best aspects of the previous systems. In Exner's system, scores on the location of the response, the determinants of the response (form, movement, color, and shading), form quality, and content categories are explicated in detail. This scoring system is used to generate descriptions of symptom patterns and patient characteristics such as personality and ego strength. Exner indicates that while the Rorschach data may be used in detecting aspects or features of the patient that should be altered through psychotherapy, the data do not identify the treatment format and techniques (Exner, 1978). Nonetheless, the Rorschach may offer some information about the expected changes of patients in different forms of treatment. As an example, Exner suggests that certain formal characteristics of response to the blots (Experience Actual and Experience Potential) predict duration needed in reconstructive treatment. Judging by the results of an outpatient study conducted by Exner (1978), patients with an excessively high or low egocentricity index on the Rorschach had a significantly lower probability of being rated improved after two years in psychotherapy. In addition, Exner suggests that an imbalance of activity to passivity orientation, as judged by Rorschach responses, correlates with difficulty in making ideational shifts, and this can be an obstacle to therapists orienting treatment toward insight. Exner's Rorschach findings are an important beginning in applying the test as a selection instrument for insight-oriented psychotherapy, but need further research.

Probably the most sophisticated use of such projective instruments in a research design was in the Menninger Psychotherapy Research Project (Appelbaum, 1977). In this intensive study of the long-term treatment of 42 patients, the following dimensions or patient variables were rated by two clinical psychologists utilizing test material: anxiety; symptoms; somatization; depression; conscious guilt; unconscious guilt; alloplasticity; core neurotic conflicts; self-concept; patterning of defenses; affect organization; thought organization; anxiety tolerance; insight; externalization; ego strength; intelligence; psychological-mindedness; sublimation; honesty; extent of desire to change; secondary gain; quality of interpersonal relations; and transference paradigms. The responses to the psychological test battery were rated by psychologists on the variables listed above. There were also formulations about treatment recommendations, the nature of the problems to arise in psychotherapy, and prognosis.

Results indicated that the psychologists using the data from the battery of tests were significantly more often in agreement with criterion outcome than was the psychiatrist using history and interview material. Furthermore, those variables which seemed to be crucial in enabling the psychologist and the test material to be a more accurate predictor included the dimensions of ego strengths, transference paradigms, core neurotic conflicts, quality of interpersonal relations, patterning of defenses, self-concept, and psychological-mindedness. The extent to which the psychologists based their predictions upon projective material from the Rorschach and the TAT is unclear, but their writing and presentations certainly emphasize the value of such material.

As noted by several reviewers (Goldfried, Stricker, and Weiner, 1971; Korchin and Schuldberg, 1981), the most substantial findings yielded by the Rorschach are those that utilize specific quantified scales such as the Rorschach Prognostic Rating Scale (RPRS) (Klopfer, Kirkner, Wisham, and Baker, 1951) and Friedman's Developmental Level Scoring (Friedman, 1952).

Correlations of the RPRS with positive therapy outcome have been reported for 21 retardates in play therapy (Johnson, 1953), subjects in behavior therapy and rational-emotive therapy (Newmark, Finkelstein, and Frerking, 1974), and various other psychotherapies (Bloom, 1956; Endicott and Endicott, 1964; Kirkner, Wisham and Giedt, 1953; Klopfer et al., 1951; Luborsky, Mintz, Auerbach, Christoph, Bachrach, Todd, Johnson, Cohen, and O'Brien, 1980; Mindess, 1953; Sheehan, Frederick, Rosevear, and Spiegelman, 1954). However, as one reviewer has pointed out (Garfield, 1978), for every two positive studies one can find a negative study. In addition, there is noticeable overlap of scores in the improved and unimproved groups. The criteria for judging improvement in the studies used in support of RPRS vary considerably. And, possibly of most importance, while the scale predicts outcome in about two-thirds of the cases, this is approximately the base rate of expected improvement in therapy, a prediction that can be made without use of the instrument.

Critics and supporters alike have stated that the Rorschach is more like a semi-structured interview than a psychological test. Aronow and Reznikoff (1976) have pointed to the Rorschach as a meaningful way of interviewing the patient. For instance, Reznikoff assesses patient insight by quizzing about the meaning of responses and applies these data to treatment planning. He views the projective instrument as a microcosm of the treatment interaction. It remains for future research to determine the extent to which such procedures add valuable data to the information gathered in clinical interviews.

Situational Tests

The most direct way to "test" how well one can play baseball or teach a sophmore college class is to watch the subject play in a baseball game or observe him/her teaching a class. This common sense approach is related to situational tests, those that place the subject in a situation which closely approximates the actual criterion situation (Anastasi, 1982). Among the earliest situational tests were those devised to study character development in children (Hartshorne and May, 1928; Hartshorne, May, and Maller, 1929; Hartshorne, May, and Shuttleworth, 1930). For example, in order to investigate cheating behavior, the children were given pencil-and-paper tests of arithmetic. Subsequently, the children were given a copy of their original test paper and asked to correct it. Any changes made by the child were situational evidence of cheating. Situational tests were subsequently used by the Office of Strategic Services during World War II (Murray and MacKinnon, 1946; OSS Assessment Staff, 1948). Candidates for assignment to military intelligence were put through a three-day situational test of living together and responding to stress situations presented by the examiners.

In the area of differential therapeutics, probably the best test of patient response to a particular therapeutic format or technique is a measure of how well things progress in the first few sessions. Indeed, brief therapy can be seen as a situational test of the patient's ability, motivation, and response to therapy (Clarkin and Frances, 1983). There is some evidence to suggest that initial performance in therapy is predictive of later behavior and response. In a study of snake phobia (Bandura, Jeffrey, and Wright, 1974), measures of fear reduction after the first session were predictive of subsequent change, while severity of phobic behavior, attitudes toward snakes, and fear-proneness were not predictive. In another study of the treatment of phobic patients (Mathews, Johnston, Shaw, and Gelder, 1974), measures of anxiety early in treatment were correlated with subsequent outcome, while severity of symptoms, high anxiety and neuroticism, low expectancy and low-rated motivation for treatment were not related to outcome. Early progress on the criterion variable (reduction of fear) predicted later progress on the criterion variable.

Luborsky and colleagues (1980), in the Penn Psychotherapy Project investigating dynamically-oriented individual therapy, studied patient characteristics and relationship with therapist as early predictors of subsequent positive outcome. Pretreatment patient measures on the Health-Sickness Rating Scale (HSRS) and emotional freedom had predictive value but accounted for only about 10% of the outcome variance. In order to investigate the predictive power of the quality of the patient-therapist alliance, the ten most and ten least improved patients of the 73 audiotaped cases in the Penn Psychotherapy Project were selected. Treatment length for these nonpsychotic outpatients was 61 weeks (median) for the improved group and 43 weeks (median) for the less improved group. Process ratings of the fifth therapy session measured two types of positive helping alliance. Type I is an alliance in which the patient experiences the relationship as warm and helping, with the patient a cooperative but passive recipient. Type 2 is an alliance based on the assumption of cooperative work, with the patient as an active, involved participant. While helping alliance Type 2 increased from early to later sessions for the most improved patients, this was not significant. Both Type 1 ($r=.47$) and Type 2 ($r=.46$) correlated significantly with outcome. These correlations of relationship quality are as high as any of the patient pre-therapy predictors. For example, correlation with outcome was .48 with the Rorschach Prognostic Rating Scale, .46 with the emotional freedom composite on the Prognostic Index Interview, $-.49$ on the interests section of the Prognostic Index Interview, and .47 with HSRS. A multiple correlation of .62 betweenHSRS plus treatment alliance and outcome indicates that favorable outcome in brief, dynamically-oriented, individual psychotherapy is most likely for patients with relatively less severe pathology, who also form a positive helping alliance with the therapist.

PSYCHOLOGICAL TESTING AND DIFFERENTIAL THERAPEUTICS: THE PAST AND THE FUTURE

In a recent review of clinical testing, Korchin and Schulberg (1981) argue that the main aim of testing has been to make characterological (rather than psychiatric) diagnoses in order to describe the individual in as full and multifaceted a manner as possible. They point out that the most used tests have been the Wechsler Intelligence Scale for Children, Bender Gestalt, WAIS, MMPI, Rorschach, TAT, Sentence Completion Tests of various sorts, Draw-A-Person, and the Stanford-Binet. There are a number of reasons why there has been a steady decline in the amount of testing done by psychologists—from 44% of their time in 1959, to 28% in 1969, to 10% in 1976—but we will mention only a few here, as they relate to differential therapeutics.

1) The most used tests, listed above, reflect variable technical qualities. The projective tests (Rorschach, TAT, Sentence Completion, Bender, Draw-A-Person) call for quite subjective interpretation by the psychologist; and while such subjective interpretation may be a true art form in the hands of very talented clinicians, it cannot be depended upon in the ordinary clinical operation to provide reliable data for treatment decision-making. It is interesting to note that these most used tests were all constructed by 1943. Much development in drug therapy, different modalities and formats of psychotherapy, therapy research, and differential treatment planning has occurred since then. There has been much instrument development in the interim, but most new instruments apparently have not been picked up in routine clinical practice. Newer instrument development which deserves consideration includes the following: (a) semi-structured interviews; (b) specific observational techniques; (c) self-report instruments in the behavioral tradition; (d) objective personality questionnaires that show technical development in test construction (e.g., Jackson, 1968); and (e) interpersonal behavior assessment (e.g., Wiggins, 1982).

2) As long as the major or sole aim of testing is to describe the person in full, multifaceted detail, psychologists will reduce their cost/benefit ratio (cost will be high due to expensive psychologist time and benefit low if there is reliance on broad-based statements from projective tests) and possibly lose sight of specific areas of assessment, tailored to the individual case, that will allow treatment planning decisions. Testing of the whole person in each and every clinical situation is

analogous to treatment perfectionism in the analytic treatment tradition (Malan, 1963).

3) As long as therapy was focused on long-term psychodynamic intervention, the traditional testing battery with the goal of multilevel assessment of the whole person had much isomorphism with the intervention philosophy, goals, strategies and techniques. However, as treatment strategies become more varied and differentiated, and as clinical and research guidelines for selection criteria are more precise, the old testing battery with its global goals will not suffice.

What is needed? It is easier to see the faults and anachronisms in what is available than to make realistic suggestions for improvement. While the solutions and directions are not clear, we suggest that the future of psychological assessment and testing for clinical decision-making must involve some of the following developments. The goals of testing must become less ambitious, and instead must focus on specific areas of symptomatology and/or personality that predict response to specific treatments. There should be less global emphasis on projective techniques, with their intent of uncovering unconscious and preconscious aspects of the person, and more emphasis on objective instruments with good reliability and narrower predictive validity for decision-making. A wider range of tests should be used discriminatively and selectively, depending on the treatment decision at hand, rather than giving a standard battery of tests to every patient no matter what the referral question. There is a need for model development, hypothesizing what patient variables in interaction with which treatment variables will result in treatment response, in order to guide future treatment assignment. Such model-building may show the way for the needed test development of currently unspecified areas. Testing should not focus solely on the individual and his/her intrapsychic world, as much of the variance of human behavior is related to the environment. Tests and rating scales should therefore be used to assess the patient's intra-family environment, and, at times, school or job environment. In an effort to describe the whole person, only lip service has been given to the goal of using the testing to inform specific clinical decisions. In fact, very rarely does the clinician get feedback on how accurately the tests predict response to treatment. Local data bases should be developed to predict specific phenomena (Wiggins, 1973).

In summary, then, we would predict that assessment devices will become increasingly more specific and sophisticated in measuring patient variables that are helpful in selecting among the treatment alternatives.

CHAPTER 11

Teaching Differential Therapeutics

We will begin our considerations by exploring the reasons why there has been so little attention to the question of differential treatment selection in the psychotherapy literature and in psychiatric training programs. In the process, we will try to demonstrate why we believe that this is a topic of increasing importance and interest, despite the many difficulties and uncertainties it occasions. Finally, we will offer specific suggestions, based on our experience at the Payne Whitney Clinic, on how best to incorporate training in the art and science of differential therapeutics into what is usually an already overburdened curriculum.

THE OBSTACLES AND LIMITATIONS

A critic of training in differential therapeutics might post the following series of difficult questions and objections. Unless we can answer these doubts to our own satisfaction, there will be no particular reason to proceed with the inquiry.

Question 1: Is there a sufficient body of knowledge about differential therapeutics to make training in it worthwhile?

The answer to this question depends very much on one's point of view concerning the available psychotherapy outcome literature. It is certainly true that, to date, there has been a disappointing inability of outcome studies to distinguish which patient variables are best able to predict good or bad response to one or another treatment modality – a step that is necessary to derive empirically based indications for different treatments. Moreover, even on a more basic level of resolution, it has not yet been demonstrated in any substantial way that different treatments have different effects. One could argue that, until there is a greatly expanded data base to inform differential therapeutics, there is not very much to teach on the subject. What we pass on in the way of clinical lore and opinion may be just as wide of the mark as were earlier medical controversies over the respective merits of leeches and bleeding cups. Even further, it could be argued that it is the shared, nonspecific aspects that make psychotherapies effective and the choice of one or another treatment does not mean all that much anyway.

Our reply. First of all, the available psychotherapy outcome research has labored under very severe limitations in design (the emphasis on group means rather than on individual response), in instruments (the emphasis on gross measures of symptom relief), and in the difficulty of defining operationally the different treatments and ensuring that they have been delivered in a reproducible and nonoverlapping fashion. The latest studies have become much more sophisticated methodologically, and it seems probable (or at least possible) that clinically significant differential indications will someday be empirically established. Moreover, although nonspecific effects are certainly powerful, it is still reasonable to hope that, once we have increased the amplifying power of our research tools, we will be able to demonstrate that there are also meaningful specific effects of the different psychotherapies.

No one (and certainly none of the investigators who have been engaged in psychotherapy outcome research) has suggested that patients would best be assigned by lottery to different therapists and to different therapies. Even in the absence of hard scientific criteria, everyone would prefer to rely on clinical judgment in preference to blind chance. It seems clear that we have an obligation to inform that clinical judgment as best we can. Clinicians must be taught the skills necessary to evaluate a patient's goals, expectations, and the enabling factors that will make him/her more or less suitable or unsuitable for one or another type of therapy. An additional benefit to be gained from teaching differential therapeutics is that it will help to stimulate the research necessary to make that teaching more meaningful and will help to frame increasingly useful research questions.

Question 2: Is there a place to teach differential therapeutics? Do our treatment environments offer a sufficiently wide range of alternative modalities so that the choice among them is meaningful? Can we teach differential therapeutics in a setting that does not provide such choices?

Many clinics and outpatient departments offer a relatively narrow range of treatment alternatives either because this is all that is available for practical reasons (limited financial resources or an absence of therapists skilled in the alternative treatments) or because it is part of the staff's belief system that only this narrow range is really necessary or worthwhile or is the mission of the clinic. In a system that refers every patient to individual therapy (or to group or family therapy, etc.), differential therapeutics is unnoticed or is an academic exercise not enriched by the tension of clinical decision-making and feedback about what actually happens.

Our reply. Indeed, it is true that differential therapeutics can be taught optimally only in treatment settings that allow for a reasonable range of choices. This requirement would suggest that rather dramatic changes are necessary in the delivery of service in certain clinics, beyond what might be possible or felt to be desirable by their staffs, if they are to successfully teach differential therapeutics. One alternative for specialized clinics is for them to forge referral agreements with other clinics that provide the missing range of services and to take seriously the necessity of referring those patients who do not meet the selection criteria for the specific treatment that clinic is specialized to deliver.

This recommendation is not pertinent to those clinics that do already have a wide range of services. Moreover, it has been our experience that once a clinic begins to carefully consider differential therapeutics for each of its patients, this tends to lead it to broaden its services. In our clinic, it was only after we became interested in this topic and defined specific patient needs we were not meeting well that we added homogeneous group therapy for a number of targeted problems, specialty clinics for affective, anxiety, and sleep disorders, and expanded our family and behavior therapy. The best way to ensure that a clinic is sensitive to the needs of its patients (rather than following a logic all its own) is to consider carefully the differential treatment options that would be optimal for each patient and then compare these with what is actually being offered.

Question 3: Are there people available to teach differential therapeutics?

Differential therapeutics is the domain of the jack of all trades (who may admittedly be absolute master of none). It could be argued that since the psychiatric literature is so vast already and growing exponentially, its very size and scope surpass the ability of any one person to keep abreast of treatment developments across a wide enough spectrum to be really competent to teach differential therapeutics. Moreover, those who strive for such versatility may sacrifice their ability to be an expert in any one area.

Our reply. Indeed, if a particular program consists only of subspecialists, it is likely that no one will be left to teach differential therapeutics. Unfortunately, in this situation, trainees will also lack a role model for the view that flexibility in therapeutic skills and in treatment assignment is important. Psychiatry, like all medical specialties, must have its broad generalists and its narrow sub-subspecialists, as well as people whose expertise lies between these poles. A training program that consists only of generalists is likely to be superficial and is unlikely to contribute to the growth of new knowledge. On the other hand, a training program that consists only of specialists is likely to be fragmented and may produce graduates who follow dogmatically the precepts of the particular specialist who has served as mentor.

It is probably impossible for any teacher or student to make a serious study of differential therapeutics without being broadened in outlook and gaining a more flexible attitude toward treatment selection and technique. Moreover, once a program becomes interested in teaching this topic, there tends to be an increased dialogue among therapists of the different persuasions. Each group is called upon to become more precise in defining its notions about patient selection and to attempt to define its boundaries and overlaps with other forms of therapy.

Question 4: Are the students ready to learn differential therapeutics?

It seems paradoxical to teach trainees about differential treatment selection before they have had any extensive personal experience in performing any or most of the treatments they will be recommending. It is difficult, perhaps impossible, to learn the selection criteria for various treatments in any meaningful way when one does not yet have any intimate knowledge and feel for that treatment's setting, techniques, or vicissitudes.

Our reply. What are the alternatives? One cannot really wait for someone to become accomplished in a number of modalities before tackling the question of how to choose among them. Furthermore, it is necessary that clinical trainees learn when it is best to refer patients to other therapists for specific treatments they themselves do not provide.

If we encourage trainees to begin their clinical experience by learning intensively one or just a few modalities, without also considering when it is best to refer a patient for something else, we are likely to allow them premature closure about treatment selection. Thus, there may be great value in exposing trainees at the outset of their careers to the undogmatic notion that many treatments are possible and that clinicians should try to determine which is likely to be optimal, even if they do not know how to do it. Learning when and how to refer is a crucial part of clinical training.

Of course, there is great variation among trainees in this regard. Some beginners are more receptive to being taught at this early stage than they will be later in their careers, and instilling the notion of flexibility at an early juncture is crucial. If one were to wait until they are more expert in one or several modalities of treatment, this particular message could be much more difficult or impossible to convey. There are other trainees, however, who begin the program with a quite remarkable assurance that they already know what is right (e.g., the psychoanalyst or behavior therapist in foeto) and may not be particularly open to influence even at this early stage or see the value of any but their preconceived favorite model. Even with such trainees, a training progam risks hardening their premature dogmatism if it is itself dogmatic. There is also the inevitable, but often unfortunate, self-selection process that matches relatively narrow programs with prematurely opinionated trainees who have come to and have been selected by the program precisely because its narrow orientation matches theirs. Certainly the consideration of differential therapeutics is a very small antidote to this problem but is nonetheless a step in the right direction.

Question 5: Do patients present treatment selection dilemmas that are sufficiently complicated or controversial to make the teaching of differential therapeutics worthwhile?

Our reply. This question is the least difficult to answer. Although there may be occasional settings in which the newly evaluated patients are so homogeneous and obvious in their needs as to make treatment selection easy, this is very rarely the case in general clinical practice, at least in outpatient departments. There are so many patient variables that might importantly influence treatment decisions and so many different possible alternative treatments that it is rarely very obvious what is best for any patient. Any given patient sample is likely to be heterogeneous on enough variables to stir up all sorts of interesting debates about what to do next. The only ways in which the patient sample ever limits the teaching of differential therapeutics is if there are just not enough patients (which is very rare) or if the patients all suffer from a severe, incapacitating disorder (e.g.,chronic schizophrenia or chronic dementia), which makes them very much more alike than otherwise. An interest in teaching differential therapeutics is likely to greatly benefit patient care by making it more flexible and individualized.

In summary, we have raised a number of possible objections to the teaching of differential therapeutics. Perhaps there is not really a body of knowledge to teach, or a setting suitable for teaching it, or suitable teachers, or prepared students, or challenging enough patients. Although some of the arguments have great force generally, and some might apply in given times and places, it should occasion no great surprise that we have decided to forge onward. While teaching differential therapeutics poses many problems, we believe that it needs to be done. The question remains – How?

HOW TO TEACH DIFFERENTIAL THERAPEUTICS?

In our experience, there is no one right way of teaching differential therapeutics. An integrated program that combines several different didactic and clinical approaches is probably most useful. We will discuss the following components of a teaching program: the treatment planning conference, the curriculum, the clinical experience, and the supervisors.

The Treatment Planning Conference

For seven years, we have used a weekly Treatment Planning Conference to review and advise on all dispositions made on patients evaluated during that week in our outpatient department. The staff assigned to the service – i.e., psychiatric residents, psychology interns, medical students, social workers, nurses, and activities therapists – present their patients to one of three attendings, each of whom sits in a different corner of a large room that comes to resemble a three-ring circus. The presentation, discussion, and decision of each case must all be achieved within ten highly focused minutes, and then on to the next problem.

The conference serves various purposes. In some instances, the evaluating trainee and his or her supervisor have already made what seems to them to be the obvious decision and the trainee comes to the conference hoping to receive fairly quick confirmation for a fait accompli. We usually, but not always, find ourselves in agreement and, in cases of disagreement, we must decide whether it is worth reopening the issue with the patient. In many instances, however, the evaluating clinician and his or her supervisor are perplexed about what to recommend, and the conference becomes a fascinating opportunity to ponder the uncertainties occasioned by tough treatment decisions. Presiding at this conference is also the single best way of becoming expert in differential therapeutics – the teacher learns as he or she ponders and teaches.

The conference serves as a clinical clearinghouse matching patient need and agency resources. It also provides an in vivo opportunity to teach residents and staff the principles of differential therapeutics and their practical application within the realm of the possible. Moreover, the conference constitutes perhaps the best form of quality control. The clinical leaders of the service ensure that they give input into all major clinical decisions and that policies and procedures are being followed (including record-keeping). The discussion of treatment decisions provides an excellent opportunity to evaluate trainee and staff performance and clinical judgment, as well as to focus on areas for additional training. The conference also serves as a kind of information program evaluation. One spots areas in which the clinic is providing an insufficient range or quantity of service and can attempt remedial action. Several years ago, for instance, we discovered that many more of our patients needed and wanted brief treatment than could be accommodated within our then existing assignment of staff resources to this modality. This awareness encouraged us to learn about, to teach, and to divert resources to brief therapy in order to make it sufficiently available. Finally, the conference is a wonderful facilitator of the smooth recruitment and flow of suitable patients to various research protocols and specialized clinical programs.

The Curriculum

In the optimal situation, the curriculum will include a separate course that focuses exclusively on the question of differential therapeutics. The curriculum will also require instructors teaching courses on psychiatric treatments to emphasize the patient selection criteria for each and how these interact with that treatment's goals, techniques, and setting.

Our course on differential therapeutics consists of five sessions given during the summer of the third year of the psychiatric residency. We also invite psychology and social work trainees, as well as other clinic staff, to attend and participate. Having access to additional sessions beyond the five now available would be highly desirable, but this is not possible within the time constraints of our system. The first session provides an overview of the available research in psychotherapy outcome and its relationship to differential therapeutics. The most pertinent findings from the literature are summarized, with heavy emphasis on those research reviews that have aggregated results across a large number of studies (particularly those of Smith, Glass, and Miller, 1980, and of Luborsky, Singer, and Luborsky, 1975). The methodological limitations of the available research are spelled out in considerable detail. Finally, there is a discussion of the parameters that would define an ideal study for differential therapeutics and the ways in which findings might then be used to guide clinical practice.

During the next three meetings of the course, the group takes a much more specific look at each of the steps that comprise the decision tree that is implicit in all differential therapeutic recommendations. For example, what should be the setting of treatment (e.g., inpatient, partial hospital, outpatient)? the format (individual, group, family)? the orientation (psychodynamic, learning, systems, biological)? the frequency and duration? the match of therapist to patient? For each of the choices on each step of the algorithm, the pertinent systematic research (if there is any), the variety of clinical opinions reported in the literature, and our own clinical experience are combined to arrive at a set of indications, contraindications, and enabling factors. There follows a discussion of how recommendations are made from among the competing alternatives and the ways in which different approaches may best be combined.

The fifth and last meeting of the course is used for a detailed discussion of three different cases. The class is encouraged to share opinions, and often differences, on how to apply the data presented in the previous sessions to the complexity of the clinical situation. It is this part of the course that is in many ways the most interesting and exciting. It is unfortunately cramped into one session and could benefit from a more leisurely pace and from the discussion of a larger number of patients.

The Clinical Experience

Since we regard the skillful evaluation of a new patient as the most crucial of all psychiatric competences, we provide a number of different clinical experiences throughout the training program to ensure that all graduates are thoroughly grounded in this activity. Virtually all mental health professionals, however else they spend their time, are engaged throughout their careers in doing consultations. We believe that training in differential therapeutics is an important perspective for this activity and should occur in every year of the training program. Our Post-

Graduate Year (PGY) I residents have a rotation on an evaluation and walk-in service during which they are carefully supervised in interviewing techniques, diagnostic skills, and in differential treatment selection. During their PGY II year, the same residents evaluate many new inpatients and are supervised in multidisciplinary treatment planning. PGY III residents return to the evaluation service for additional experiences with and supervision in initial consultation—this time with an even greater emphasis on differential treatment choice. Moreover, they begin teaching medical students in these very same activities. We are impressed by the value of simultaneously having the resident making some treatment decisions with the help of a supervisor and in other cases being that supervisor to a more junior clinician. This is done in conjunction with the treatment planning conference and the course in differential therapeutics. Some of the residents return for elective time in the PGY IV year to develop this skill still further and to expand their experience in teaching it.

In order for differential therapeutics to come fully alive, the trainees should have supervised clinical experiences in delivering a number of the treatments that they are and have been recommending for their patients. Trainees should have experience with a rich mix of psychodynamic, behavioral, and systems treatments, provided both individually and in group and family contexts; they should also be familiar with both brief and long-term work. Of course, this makes for a busy life and reduces the trainee's possibility of pursuing specific individual interests to the depth that would be most desirable. We have also emphasized evaluation skills, differential treatment planning, and varied treatment experiences in the clinical training given our psychology and social service students.

The discussion of differential treatment choices between supervisor and trainee will have maximum impact to the extent that it leads to a real decision. This implies that the clinic should be prepared to expand its treatments to provide previously lacking services when a need for them has been identified.

The Teachers

If a clinic is to provide the wide range of services that enlivens differential therapeutics, it needs practitioners to deliver those services and, more importantly, it needs teachers to instruct these practitioners and the new trainees. How does a clinic get these teachers? One major avenue is the careful and energetic recruitment of full-time, part-time, and voluntary faculty. It is highly desirable that departments of psychiatry be pluralistic and versatile in their faculties, rather than do what comes more naturally, i.e., select like-minded and homogeneous fellow travellers in their recruiting. If it is necessary to expand into a new area of treatment delivery and recruitment of individuals skilled in that modality is not possible for reasons of finances or availability, it is often helpful to call in an expert consultant on a time-limited basis. Such a step promotes the training of a cadre of indigenous teachers who can then maintain and expand the program by teaching others. In some cases, a program may develop its own self-taught experts. For example, we have become what we hope is reasonably expert in the brief therapies by reading about them, doing them, and teaching them, then reading about them, doing them, and teaching them some more and so on, until we found ourselves writing about them and finally consulting to others.

Another important issue that arises in regard to the teachers has to do with supervisor-trainee assignments. Some supervisors are excellent teachers, but only within the narrow confines of one type of therapy done one particular way with one group of very highly selected patients. Trainees must also be exposed to some supervisors who embody and serve as role models for skill and flexibility with a variety of models. Moreover, we encourage trainees to seek multiple opinions rather than to assume that any of their supervisors has any special monopoly on the truth. In addition, we convey to trainees that they are ultimately responsible (in conjunction with their service director) for whatever decisions are made and cannot beg off by saying, "My supervisor told me to do this." Differences of opinion between supervisor and trainee should be aired and settled in coordination with the service director, and this is often an interesting learning experience for all involved.

THE OUTPUT

What are the possible gains and risks of a training program that pays considerable attention to the question of differential therapeutics? Perhaps we should face the risks first. Might we produce a cohort of broadly based and flexible idiots who possess a confused hodgepodge of half facts and such great openness to new developments in the field that they are prey to every new fad? Is this result any better than the risk in the other direction of producing narrow adherents to a rigid, dogmatic orthodoxy?

Obviously either extreme is undesirable and different programs run closer to one or the other risk. We believe that the ideal of every training program should be that its graduates are widely knowledgeable, broad as well as deep in their interests, and sufficiently curious to keep learning and growing professionally. Our sense is that a careful attention to differential therapeutics furthers this goal and makes good programs better. We are personally grateful for the learning and insights that have come to us through the study of this area and can recommend it highly to others.

References

Ackerman, N. W. *Treating the troubled family.* New York: Basic Books, 1966.

Aledort, S. L. & Jones, M. The Euclid House: A therapeutic community halfway house for prisoners. *American Journal of Psychiatry,* 1973, *130,* 286–289.

Alexander, F. & French, T. *Psychoanalytic therapy.* New York: Ronald Press, 1946.

Allen, J. The clinical psychologist as a diagnostic consultant. *Bulletin of the Menninger Clinic,* 1981, *45,* 247–258.

American Psychiatric Association. *Manual of psychiatric peer review.* Washington, D.C.: American Psychiatric Association, 1976.

American Psychiatric Association. *Diagnostic and statistical manual of mental disorders* (3rd ed.). Washington, D.C., 1980.

American Psychiatric Association Commission on Psychotherapies. *Psychotherapy research: Methodological and efficacy issues.* Washington, D.C., 1982.

Anastasi, A. *Psychological testing* (5th ed.). New York: Macmillan, 1982.

Appelbaum, S. A. *The anatomy of change.* New York: Plenum Press, 1977.

Appleton, W. S. & Davis, J. M. *Practical clinical psychopharmacology.* Baltimore: Williams & Wilkins, 1980.

Aronow, A. E. & Reznikoff, M. *Rorschach content interpretation.* New York: Grune & Stratton, 1976.

Aronson, H. & Weintraub, W. Patient changes during clinical psychoanalysis as a function of initial status and duration of treatment. *Psychiatry,* 1968, *31,* 369–379.

Ayllon, T. & Azrin, N. H. *The token economy: A motivational system for therapy and rehabilitation.* New York: Appleton-Century-Crofts, 1968.

Baekeland, F. & Lundwall, L. Dropping out of treatment: A critical review. *Psychological Bulletin,* 1975, *82,* 738–783.

Baldessarini, R. J. *Chemotherapy in psychiatry.* Cambridge: Harvard Press, 1977.

Bandura, A. *Social learning theory.* New York: General Learning Press, 1977.

Bandura, A., Jeffrey, R., & Wright, C. L. Efficacy of participant modeling as a function of response induction aids. *Journal of Abnormal Psychology,* 1974, *83,* 56–64.

Bandura, A. & Walters, R. H. *Social learning and personality development.* New York: Holt, Rinehart & Winston, 1963.

Barron, F. An ego-strength scale which predicts response to psychotherapy. *Journal of Consulting Psychology,* 1953, *17,* 327–333.

Barron, F. & Leary, T. F. Changes in psychoneurotic patients with and without psychotherapy. *Journal of Consulting Psychology,* 1955, *19,* 239–245.

Bateson, G., Jackson, D. D., Haley, J., & Weakland, J. H. Toward a theory of schizophrenia. *Behavioral Science,* 1956, *1,* 251–264.

Beck, A. T. *Cognitive therapy and the emotional disorders.* New York: International Universities Press, 1976.

Beck, A. T. & Greenberg, R. L. Brief cognitive therapies. In R. B. Sloane & F. R. Staples (Eds.), *The psychiatric clinics of North America: Symposium on brief psychotherapy.* Philadelphia: Saunders, 1979.

Beck, A. T., Kovacs, M., & Weissman, A. Assessment of suicide intention: The scale for suicide ideation. *Journal of Consulting and Clinical Psychology,* 1979, *47,* 343–352.

Beck, A. T., Schuyler, D., & Herman, I. Development of suicidal intent scales. In A. T. Beck, H. L. P. Resnik, & D. J. Lettieri (Eds.), *The prediction of suicide.* Bowie, MD: Charles Press, 1974.

Beck, A. T., Ward, C. H., Mendelson, M., Mock, J., & Erbaugh, J. An inventory for measuring depression. *Archives of General Psychiatry,* 1961, *4,* 561–571.

Beck, S. J. *Introduction to the Rorschach method.* New York: American Orthopsychiatric Association, 1937.

Bednar, R. L. & Kaul, T. J. Experiential group research: Current perspectives. In S. Garfield & A. Bergin (Eds.), *Handbook of psychotherapy and behavior change* (2nd ed.). New York: John Wiley, 1978.

Bellak, L. & Small, L. *Emergency psychotherapy and brief psychotherapy* (2nd ed.). New York: Grune & Stratton, 1978.

Benjamin, L. S. Structural analysis of social behavior. *Psychological Review,* 1974, *81,* 392–425.

Benjamin, L. S. Structural analysis of a family in therapy. *Journal of Consulting and Clinical Psychology,* 1977, *45,* 391–406.

Berger, M. Multifamily psychosocial group treatment with addicts and their families. *Group Process,* 1973, *5,* 31–45.

Bergin, A. E. & Lambert, M. J. The evaluation of psychotherapeutic outcomes. In S. L. Garfield & A. E. Bergin (Eds.), *Handbook of psychotherapy and behavior change: An empirical analysis.* New York: John Wiley, 1978.

Berkovitz, I. H. (Ed.). *Adolescents grow in groups.* New York: Brunner/Mazel, 1972.

Berne, E. *Transactional analysis in psychotherapy.* New York: Grove Press, 1961.

Beutler, L. E. Toward specific psychological therapies for specific conditions. *Journal of Consulting and Clinical Psychology,* 1979, *47,* 882–897.

Beutler, L. E. *Eclectic psychotherapy: A systematic approach.* New York: Pergamon Press, 1983.

Beutler, L. E. & Mitchell, R. Differential psychotherapy outcome among depressed and impulsive patients as a function of analytic and experiential treatment procedures. *Psychiatry,* 1981, *44,* 297–306.

Bibring, E. Contribution to the symposium on the theory of the therapeutic results of psychoanalysis. *International Journal of Psychoanalysis,* 1937, *18,* 170.

Bilodeau, C. B. & Hackett, T. P. Issues raised in a group setting by patients recovering from myocardial infarction. *American Journal of Psychiatry,* 1971, *128,* 73–78.

Blackwell, B. Drug therapy: Patient compliance. *New England Journal of Medicine,* 1973, *289,* 249–252.

Bloom, B. L. Prognostic significance of the underproductive Rorschach. *Journal of Projective Techniques,* 1956, *20,* 366–371.

Bloom, B. L. Focused single-session therapy: Initial development and evaluation. In S. H. Budman (Ed.), *Forms of brief therapy.* New York: Guilford Press, 1981.

Boas, C. Intensive group psychotherapy with married couples. *International Journal of Group Psychotherapy,* 1962, *12,* 142–153.

Bond, G. & Lieberman, M. A. Selection criteria for group therapy. In J. P. Brady & H. K. H. Brodie (Eds.), *Controversy in psychiatry.* Philadelphia: Saunders, 1978.

Bowen, M. *Family therapy in clinical practice.* New York: Jason Aronson, 1978.

Brody, S. Simultaneous psychotherapy of married couples. In J. Masserman (Ed.), *Current psychiatric therapy.* New York: Grune & Stratton, 1961.

Brown, G. W., Birley, J. L. T., & Wing, J. K. Influence of family life on the course of schizophrenic disorder: A replication. *British Journal of Psychiatry,* 1972, *121,* 241–258.

Brown, R., Frances, A., Kocsis, J., & Mann, J. Psychotic and nonpsychotic depression: Differential treatment and response. *Journal of Nervous and Mental Disease*, 1982, *170*, 635-638.

Brown, G. W. & Rutter, M. The measurement of family activities and relationships: A methodological student. *Human Relations*, 1966, *19*, 241-263.

Burhan, A. S. Short-term hospital treatment: A study. *Hospital and Community Psychiatry*, 1969, *20*, 369-370.

Buros, O. K. (Ed.). *Personality tests and reviews*. Highland Park, NJ: Gryphon Press, 1970.

Buros, O. K. (Ed.). *The seventh mental measurements yearbook*. Highland Park, NJ: Gryphon Press, 1972.

Buros, O. K. (Ed.). *The eighth mental measurements yearbook*. Highland Park, NJ: Gryphon Press, 1978.

Butcher, J. N. (Ed.). *Objective personality assessment*. New York: Academic Press, 1972.

Butcher, J. N. & Koss, M. P. Research on brief and crisis-oriented psychotherapies. In S. Garfield & A. Bergin (Eds.), *Handbook of psychotherapy and behavior change* (2nd ed.). New York: John Wiley, 1978.

Caffey, E. M., Galbrecht, C. R. & Klett, C. J. Brief hospitalization and aftercare in the treatment of schizophrenia. *Archives of General Psychiatry*, 1971, *24*, 81-86.

Campbell, D. T. & Fiske, D. W. Convergent and discriminant validation by the multitrait-multimethod matrix. *Psychological Bulletin*, 1959, *56*, 81-105.

Campbell, D. T. & Stanley, J. C. *Experimental and quasi-experimental designs for research*. Chicago: Rand McNally, 1963.

Caplan, G. *Principles of preventive psychiatry*. New York: Basic Books, 1964.

Carkhuff, R. R. & Truax, C. B. Lay mental health counseling: The effects of lay group counseling. *Journal of Consulting Psychology*, 1965, *29*, 426-431.

Cartwright, R. D. A comparison of the response to psychoanalysis and client-centered psychotherapy. In L. Gottschalk and A. Auerbach (Eds.), *Methods of research in psychotherapy*. New York: Appleton-Century-Crofts, 1966.

Cartwright, R. D. & Vogel, J. L. A comparison of changes in psychoneurotic patients during matched periods of therapy and no therapy. *Journal of Consulting Psychology*, 1960, *24*, 121-127.

Cassell, W. A., Smith, C. M., Grunberg, F., Boan, J. A., & Thomas, R. F. Comparing costs of hospital and community care. *Hospital and Community Psychiatry*, 1972, *23*, 197-200.

Castelnuovo-Tedesco, P. *The twenty minute hour*. Boston: Little, Brown, 1965.

Cattell, R. B. & Stice, G. *The sixteen personality factor questionnaire*. Champaign, IL: Institute for Personality and Ability Testing, 1949-1950. (Manual, 1950.)

Ciminero, A. R., Calhoun, K. S. & Adams, H. E. (Eds.). *Handbook of behavioral assessment*. New York: John Wiley, 1977.

Claghorn, J. L., Johnstone, E. E., Cook, T. H., & Itschner, L. Group therapy and maintenance treatment of schizophrenics. *Archives of General Psychiatry*, 1974, *31*, 361-365.

Clarkin, J. F. & Frances, A. The brief therapies. In B. B. Wolman (Ed.), *The therapist's handbook: Treatment methods of mental disorders*. New York: Van Nostrand Reinhold, 1983.

Clarkin, J. F., Frances, A. J., & Glick, I. D. The decision to treat a family: Selection criteria and enabling factors. In L. Wolberg and M. Aronson (Eds.), *Group and family therapy 1981*. New York: Brunner/Mazel, 1981.

Cole, J. & Magnessen, M. Where the action is. *Journal of Consulting Psychology*, 1966, *30*, 539-543.

Covi, L. A group psychotherapy approach to treatment of neurotic symptoms in male and female patients of homosexual preference. *Psychotherapy and Psychosomatics*, 1972, *20*, 176-180.

Davanloo, H. *Basic principles and techniques in short-term dynamic psychotherapy*. New York: Spectrum Books, 1978.

Dekker, D. J. & Webb, J. T. Relationships of the social readjustment rating scale to psychiatric patient status, anxiety, and social desirability. *Journal of Psychosomatic Research*, 1974, *18*, 125–130.

Derogatis, L. R. *The SCL-90*. Baltimore: Clinical Psychometric Research, 1975.

Derogatis, L. R. Self-report measures of stress. In L. Goldberger & S. Breznitz (Eds.), *Handbook of stress*. New York: The Free Press, 1982.

Dieter, J. B., Hanford, D. B., Hummel, R. T., & Lubach, J. E. Brief inpsychiatric treatment: A pilot study. *Mental Hospitals*, 1965, *16*, 95–98.

Eisenthal, S., Emery, R., Lazare, A., & Udin, H. Adherence and the negotiated approach to patienthood. *Archives of General Psychiatry*, 1978, *36*, 393–398.

Eissler, K. The effect of the structure of the ego on psychoanalytic technique. *Journal of the American Psychoanalytic Association*, 1953, *1*, 104–143.

Ellis, A. *Reason and emotion in psychotherapy*. New York: Lyle Stuart Press, 1962.

Emmelkamp, P. M. G. & Wessels, H. Flooding in imagination vs. flooding in vivo. A comparison with agoraphobics. *Behavior Research and Therapy*, 1975, *13*, 7.

Endicott, J., Cohen, J., Nee, J., Fleiss, J. L., & Herz, M. I. Brief vs. standard hospitalization. *Archives of General Psychiatry*, 1979, *36*, 706–712.

Endicott, N. A. & Endicott, J. "Improvement" in untreated psychiatric patients. *Archives of General Psychiatry*, 1963, *9*, 575–585.

Endicott, N. A. & Endicott, J. Prediction of improvement in treated and untreated patients using the Rorschach prognostic rating scale. *Journal of Consulting Psychology*, 1964, *28*, 342–348.

Endicott, J. & Spitzer, R. L. A diagnostic interview: The schedule of affective disorders and schizophrenia. *Archives of General Psychiatry*, 1978, *35*, 837–844.

Endicott, J., Spitzer, R. L., Fleiss, J. L., & Cohen, J. The Global Assessment Scale: A procedure for measuring overall severity of psychiatric disturbance. *Archives of General Psychiatry*, 1976, *33*, 766–771.

Evangelakis, M. G. De-institutionalization of patients (the triad of trifluoperazine-group-psychotherapy-adjunctive therapy). *Diseases of the Nervous System*, 1961, *22*, 26–32.

Ewing, C. P. *Crisis intervention as psychotherapy*. New York: Oxford University Press, 1978.

Eysenck, H. J. The effects of psychotherapy: An evaluation. *Journal of Consulting Psychology*, 1952, *16*, 319–324.

Eysenck, H. J. *Handbook of abnormal psychology*. London: Pitman, 1960.

Eysenck, H. J. *The effects of psychotherapy*. New York: International Science Press, 1966.

Exner, J. E., Jr. *The Rorschach: A comprehensive system* (vol. 1). New York: John Wiley, 1974.

Exner, J. E., Jr. *The Rorschach: A comprehensive system* (vol. 2). New York: John Wiley, 1978.

Fairweather, G., Simon, R., Gebhard, M. E., Weingarten, E., Holland, J. L., Sanders, R., Stone, G. B., & Reahl, J. E. Relative effectiveness of psychotherapeutic programs: A multicriteria comparison of four programs for three different patient groups. *Psychological Monographs: General and Applied*, 1960, *74*(5, Whole No. 492).

Feinsilver, D. L. & Hall, R. C. W. The new crisis psychiatry: An overview. *Psychiatric Annals*, 1982, *12*, 757–761.

Fenichel, O. *Problems of psychoanalytic technique*. Albany, NY: Psychoanalytic Quarterly, 1941.

Fenichel, O. *The psychoanalytic theory of neurosis*. New York: W. W. Norton, 1945.

Fenton, F., Tessier, L., & Struening, E. A comparative trial of home and hospital care. *Archives of General Psychiatry*, 1979, *36*, 1073–1079.

Ferenczi, S. & Rank, O. *The development of psychoanalysis*. New York: Nervous & Mental Disease Publ. Co., 1925.

Fishman, S. & Lubetkin, B. Personal communication, 1980.

Fox, R. Group psychotherapy with alcoholics. *International Journal of Group Psychotherapy*, 1962, *12*, 56–63.

Framo, J. Integration of marital therapy with sessions with family of origin. In A. Gurman & D. Kniskern (Eds.), *Handbook of family therapy*. New York: Brunner/Mazel, 1981.

Frances, A., Clarkin, J. F., & Weldon, E. Focal therapy in the day hospital. *Hospital and Community Psychiatry,* 1979, *30,* 195-199.

Frank, J. D. *Persuasion and healing.* New York: Schocken Books, 1973.

Frank, J. D. *Psychotherapy and the human predicament: A psychosocial approach.* New York: Schocken Books, 1978.

Frank, A., Eisenthal, S., & Lazare, A. Are there social class differences in patients' treatment conceptions? Myths and facts. *Archives of General Psychiatry,* 1977, *35,* 61-69.

Frank, J. D., Gliedman, L. H., Imber, S. D., Stone, A. R., & Nash, E. H. Patients' expectancies and relearning as factors determining improvement in psychotherapy. *American Journal of Psychiatry,* 1959, *115,* 961-968.

Freedman, A. M., Kaplan, H. I., & Sadock, B. J. *Comprehensive textbook of psychiatry — II.* Baltimore: Williams & Wilkins, 1975.

Freud, S. Analysis of a phobia in a five-year-old boy. *Standard edition.* London: Hogarth Press, 1955. (a)

Freud, S. From the history of an infantile neurosis. *Standard edition.* London: Hogarth Press, 1955. (b)

Freud, S. Studies in hysteria. *Standard edition,* Vol. 2. London: Hogarth Press, 1955. (c)

Freud, S. The ego and the id. *Standard edition.* London: Hogarth Press, 1955. (d)

Friedman, H. Perceptual regression in schizophrenia: An hypothesis suggested by use of the Rorschach Test. *Journal of Genetic Psychology,* 1952, *81,* 63-98.

Fromm-Reichmann, F. *Principles of intensive psychotherapy.* Chicago: University of Chicago Press, 1950.

Garfield, S. L. Research on client variables in psychotherapy. In S. L. Garfield & A. E. Bergin (Eds.), *Handbook of psychotherapy and behavior change* (2nd ed.). New York: John Wiley, 1978.

Gelder, M. G. & Marks, I. M. Severe agoraphobia: A controlled prospective trial of behavior therapy. *British Journal of Psychiatry,* 1966, *112,* 309-319.

Gelder, M. G., Marks, I. M., Wolff, H. H., & Clarke, M. Desensitization and psychotherapy in the treatment of phobic states: A controlled inquiry. *British Journal of Psychiatry,* 1967, *113,* 53-73.

Gendlin, E. T. *Focusing.* New York: Everest House, 1978.

Gillan, P. & Rachman, S. An experimental investigation of desensitization in phobic patients. *British Journal of Psychiatry,* 1974, *124,* 392-401.

Gilligan, J. Review of literature. In M. Greenblatt, M. Solomon, A. Evans, & G. Brooks (Eds.), *Drug and social therapy in chronic schizophrenia.* Springfield, IL: Charles C Thomas, 1965.

Gleser, G. C. & Ihilevich, D. An objective instrument for measuring defense mechanisms. *Journal of Consulting and Clinical Psychology,* 1969, *33,* 51-60.

Glick, I. D. & Hargreaves, W. A. *Psychiatric hospital treatment for the 1980s: A controlled study of short versus long hospitalization.* Lexington, MA: D. C. Heath, 1979.

Glick, I. D., Hargreaves, W. A., Drues, J., & Showstack, J. A. Short versus long hospitalization: A prospective controlled study. IV. One-year follow-up results for schizophrenic patients. *American Journal of Psychiatry,* 1976, *133,* 509-514.

Glick, I. D. & Kessler, D. R. *Marital and family therapy,* 2nd edition. New York: Grune & Stratton, 1980.

Golden, C. J. *Clinical interpretation of objective psychological tests.* New York: Grune & Stratton, 1979.

Goldfried, M. R. Toward the delineation of therapeutic change principles. *American Psychologist,* 1980, *35,* 991-999.

Goldfried, M. R., Stricker, G., & Weiner, I. B. *Rorschach handbook of clinical and research applications.* Englewood Cliffs, NJ: Prentice-Hall, 1971.

Goldman, J., L'Engle Stein, C., & Guerry, S. *Psychological methods of child assessment.* New York: Brunner/Mazel, 1984.

Goldstein, M. J., Rodnick, E. H., Evans, J. R., May, P. R. A., & Steinberg, M. R. Drug and family therapy in the aftercare of acute schizophrenics. *Archives of General Psychiatry,* 1978, *35,* 1169-1177.

Gorsuch, R. L. & Key, M. K. Abnormalities of pregnancy as a function of anxiety and life stress. *Psychosomatic Medicine*, 1974, *36*, 352.

Gottesman, I. I. More construct validation of the ego-strength scale. *Journal of Consulting Psychology*, 1959, *23*, 342–346.

Gould, R. L. Preventive psychiatry and the field theory of reality. *Journal of the American Psychoanalytic Association*, 1970, *18*, 440–460.

Graham, J. R. *The MMPI: A practical guide.* New York: Oxford University Press, 1977.

Graham, S. R. Patient evaluation of the effectiveness of limited psychoanalytically-oriented psychotherapy. *Psychological Reports*, 1958, *4*, 231–234.

Greden, J. F., Gardner, R., King, D., Grunhaus, L., Carroll, B. J., & Kronfol, Z. Dexamethasone suppression tests in antidepressant treatment of melancholia: The process of normalization and test-retest reproducibility. *Archives of General Psychiatry*, 1983, *40*, 394–500.

Greene, B. & Solomon, A. Marital disharmony: Concurrent psychoanalytic therapy of husband and wife by the same psychiatrist. *American Journal of Psychotherapy*, 1963, *17*, 443–456.

Greene, R. L. *The MMPI: An interpretive manual.* New York: Grune & Stratton, 1980.

Greenson, R. R. *The technique and practice of psychoanalysis.* New York: International Universities Press, 1967.

Greenspan, S. I., Silver, B., & Allen, M. G. A psychodynamically oriented group training program for early childhood care givers. *American Journal of Psychiatry*, 1977, *134*, 1104–1108.

Group for the Advancement of Psychiatry. *The crisis in a psychiatric hospitalization.* (Report No. 72.) New York: GAP, 1969.

Group for the Advancement of Psychiatry. *Pharmacotherapy and psychotherapy: Paradoxes, problems and progress.* New York: Brunner/Mazel, 1975.

Grunebaum, H. Soft-hearted review of hard-nosed research on groups. *International Journal of Group Psychotherapy*, 1975, *25*, 185–195.

Gunderson, J. G., Kolb, J. E., & Austin, V. The diagnostic interview for borderline patients. *American Journal of Psychiatry*, 1981, *138*, 896–903.

Gurman, A. S. Integrative marital therapy: Toward the development of an interpersonal approach. In S. H. Budman (Ed.), *Forms of brief therapy.* New York: Guilford Press, 1981.

Gurman, A. S. & Kniskern, D. P. Research on marital and family therapy: Progress, perspective and prospect. In S. Garfield & A. Bergin (Eds.), *Handbook of psychotherapy and behavior change* (2nd ed.). New York: John Wiley, 1978.

Guy, W., Gross, M., Hogarty, G., & Dennis, H. A controlled evaluation of day hospital effectiveness. *Archives of General Psychiatry*, 1969, *20*, 329–338.

Hafner, J. & Marks, I. M. Exposure in vivo of agoraphobics: The contribution of diazepam, group exposure and anxiety evocation. *Psychological Medicine*, 1976, *6*, 71–88.

Haley, J. *Strategies of psychotherapy.* New York: Grune & Stratton, 1963.

Haley, J. Beginning and experienced family therapists. In A. Ferber, M. Mendelsohn, & A. Napier (Eds.), *The book of family therapy.* Boston: Houghton Mifflin, 1973. (a)

Haley, J. *Uncommon therapy: The psychiatric techniques of Milton H. Erickson.* New York: W.W. Norton, 1973. (b)

Haley, J. *Problem-solving therapy.* San Francisco: Jossey-Bass, 1976.

Hall, R. C. W., Faillace, L. A., & Perl, M. Role diffusion and "the death of psychiatry." *Psychiatric Opinion*, 1979, July/August, 21–26.

Hall, R. C. W., Gardner, E. R., Popkin, M. K., LeCann, A. F., & Stickney, S. K. Unrecognized physical illness prompting psychiatric admission: A prospective study. *American Journal of Psychiatry*, 1981, *5*, 629–635.

Hall, R. C. W., Popkin, M. K., Devaul, R. A., Faillace, L. A., & Stickney, S. K. Physical illness presenting as psychiatric disease. *Archives of General Psychiatry*, 1978, *35*, 1315–1320.

Hamburg, D., Bibring, G., Fisher, C., Stanton, A., Wallerstein, R., & Haggard, E. Report of ad hoc committee on central fact-gathering data of the American Psychoanalytic

Association. *Journal of the American Psychoanalytic Association,* 1967, *15,* 841–861.

Hamilton, M. A rating scale for depression. *Journal of Neurology, Neurosurgery & Psychiatry,* 1960, *23,* 56–61.

Hand, I., Lamontagne, Y., & Marks, I. M. Group exposure (flooding) in vivo for agoraphobics. *British Journal of Psychiatry,* 1974, *124,* 588.

Harper, R. *The new psychotherapies.* Englewood Cliffs, NJ: Prentice-Hall, 1975.

Hartshorne, H. & May, M. A. *Studies in deceit.* New York: Macmillan, 1928.

Hartshorne, H., May, M. A., & Maller, J. B. *Studies in service and self-control.* New York: Macmillan, 1929.

Hartshorne, H., May, M. A., & Shuttleworth, F. K. *Studies in the organization of character.* New York: Macmillan, 1930.

Hathaway, S. R. Scales 5 (masculinity–femininity), 6 (paranoia), and 8 (schizophrenia). In G. S. Welsh & W. G. Dahlstrom (Eds.), *Basic readings on the MMPI in psychology and medicine.* Minneapolis: University of Minnesota Press, 1956.

Hathaway, S. R. & McKinley, J. C. *Minnesota Multiphasic Personality Inventory.* Minneapolis: University of Minnesota Press, 1942. (a)

Hathaway, S. R. & McKinley, J. C. A multiphasic personality schedule (Minnesota): III. The measurement of symptomatic depression. *Journal of Psychology,* 1942, *14,* 73–84. (b)

Hawkinson, J. R. A study of the construct validity of Barron's ego strength scale with a state mental hospital population. *Dissertation Abstracts International,* 1962, *22,* 4081.

Heilbrunn, G. Results with psychoanalytic therapy and professional commitment. *American Journal of Psychotherapy,* 1966, *20,* 89–99.

Heine, R. W. A comparison of patients' reports on psychotherapeutic experience with psychoanalytic nondirective and Adlerian therapists. *American Journal of Psychotherapy,* 1953, *7,* 16–25.

Heinicke, C. M. Frequency of psychotherapeutic sessions as a factor affecting outcome: Analysis of clinical ratings and test results. *Journal of Abnormal Psychology,* 1969, *74,* 553–560.

Henry, W. E. *The analysis of fantasy: The Thematic Apperception Technique in the study of personality.* New York: John Wiley, 1956.

Henry, W. E. & Shlien, J. Affective complexity and psychotherapy: Some comparisons of time-limited and unlimited treatment. *Journal of Projective Techniques,* 1958, *22,* 153–162.

Herz, M., Endicott, J., & Spitzer, R. Brief versus standard hospitalization: The families. *American Journal of Psychiatry,* 1976, *133,* 795–801.

Herz, M., Endicott, J., & Spitzer, R. Brief hospitalization: A two-year follow-up. *American Journal of Psychiatry,* 1977, *134,* 502–507.

Herz, M., Endicott, J., Spitzer, R., & Mesnikoff, A. Day versus inpatient hospitalization: A controlled study. *American Journal of Psychiatry,* 1971, *127,* 1371–1382.

Himelstein, P. Further evidence of the ego strength scale as a measure of psychological health. *Journal of Consulting Psychology,* 1964, *28,* 90–91.

Hodgson, R., Rachman, S., & Marks, I. The treatment of chronic obsessive-compulsive neurosis: Follow-up and further findings. *Behaviour Research and Therapy,* 1972, *10,* 181–189.

Hogarty, G. Psychiatric day center: Baltimore City Health Department. *Maryland State Medical Journal,* 1968, *17,* 84.

Hogarty, G. E., Goldberg, S. C. & the Collaborative Study Group. Drug and sociotherapy in the aftercare of schizophrenic patients. *Archives of General Psychiatry,* 1973, *28,* 54–64.

Hollon, S. D. & Beck, A. T. Psychotherapy and drug therapy: Comparison and combinations. In S. L. Garfield & A. E. Bergin, *Handbook of psychotherapy and behavior change,* 2nd edition. New York: John Wiley, 1978.

Holmes, T. H. Development and application of a quantitative measure of life change magnitude. In J. E. Barrett (Ed.), *Stress and mental disorder.* New York: Raven, 1979.

Honigfeld, G., Rosenblum, M. P., Blumenthal, I. J., Lambert, H. L., & Roberts, A. J. Behavioral improvement in older schizophrenic patients: Drug and social therapies. *Journal of the American Geriatric Society*, 1965, *13*, 57-72.

Horowitz, L. M. On the cognitive structure of interpersonal problems treated in psychotherapy. *Journal of Consulting and Clinical Psychology*, 1979, *47*, 5-15.

Horowitz, M., Wilner, N., & Alvarez, W. Impact of event scale: A measure of subjective stress. *Psychosomatic Medicine*, 1979, *41*, 209-218.

Hurvitz, N. Marital problems following psychotherapy with one spouse. *Journal of Consulting Psychology*, 1967, *31*, 38-47.

Ilfeld, F. W., Jr. Current social stressors and symptoms of depression. *American Journal of Psychiatry*, 1977, *134*, 161-166.

Imber, S. D., Frank, J. D., Nash, E. H., Stone, A. R., & Gliedman, L. H. Improvement and amount of therapeutic contact: An alternative to the use of no-treatment controls in psychotherapy. *Journal of Consulting Psychology*, 1957, *21*, 309-315.

Jackson, D. N. *Personality research form manual.* Goshen, NY: Research Psychologists Press, 1968.

Jacobson, N. S. & Margolin, G. *Marital therapy: Strategies based on social learning and behavior exchange principles.* New York: Brunner/Mazel, 1979.

Jenkins, C. D. Psychologic and social precursors of coronary disease. *New England Journal of Medicine*, 1971, *284*, 244-317.

Jenkins, C. D. Recent evidence supporting psychologic and social risk factors for coronary disease (in two parts). *New England Journal of Medicine*, 1976, *294*, 987-994.

Jenkins, C. D., Rosenman, R. H., & Friedman, M. Development of an objective psychological test for the determination of the coronary-prone behavior pattern in employed men. *Journal of Chronic Diseases*, 1967, *20*, 371-379.

Jenkins, C. D., Rosenman, R. H., & Zyzanski, S. J. Prediction of clinical coronary-prone behavior pattern. *New England Journal of Medicine*, 1974, *290*, 1271-1275.

Johnson, E. Z. Klopfer's prognostic scale used with Raven's Progressive Matrices in play therapy prognosis. *Journal of Projective Techniques*, 1953, *17*, 320-326.

Jones, E. *The life and work of Sigmund Freud.* New York: Basic Books, 1953.

Kalinowsky, L. B. *Biological treatments in psychiatry.* New York: Grune & Stratton, 1982.

Kalinowsky, L. B., Hippins, H., & Klein, H. E. *Biological treatments in psychiatry.* New York: Grune & Stratton, 1982.

Kaplan, H. S. *The new sex therapy.* New York: Brunner/Mazel, 1974.

Kaplan, H. *Disorders of sexual desire.* New York: Brunner/Mazel, 1979.

Kaplan, H. S., Fyer, A. J., & Novick, A. The treatment of sexual phobias: The combined use of antipanic medication and sex therapy. *Journal of Sex and Marital Therapy*, 1982, *8*, 3-28.

Karasu, T. B. Psychotherapy: An overview. *American Journal of Psychotherapy*, 1977, *134*, 851-863.

Karasu, T. B. Psychotherapy and pharmacotherapy: Toward an integrative model. *American Journal of Psychiatry*, 1982, *139*, 1102-1113.

Katz, M. M., Lowery, H. A., & Cole, J. O. Behavior patterns of schizophrenia in the community. In M. Lorr (Ed.), *Explorations in typing psychotics.* New York: Pergamon Press, 1967.

Katz, M. M. & Lyerly, S. B. Methods for measuring adjustment and social behavior in the community: I. Rationale, description, discriminative validity and scale development. *Psychological Reports*, 1963, *13*, 503-535 (Monogr. Suppl. 4-V13).

Kaufman, E. Group therapy techniques used by the ex-addict therapist. *Group Process*, 1973, *5*, 3-19.

Kaufman, I., Frank, T., Freind, J., Heims, L. W., & Weiss, R. Success and failure in the treatment of childhood schizophrenia. *American Journal of Psychiatry*, 1962, *118*, 909-913.

Kazdin, A. E. & Wilson, G. T. *Evaluation of behavior therapy: Issues, evidence and research strategies.* Cambridge, MA: Ballinger, 1978.

Kendall, P. C. & Norton-Ford, J. D. *Clinical psychology: Scientific and professional dimensions.* New York: John Wiley, 1982.

Kernberg, O. F. *Borderline conditions and pathological narcissism.* New York: Jason Aronson, 1975.

Kernberg, O. F., Bernstein, C. S., Coyne, R., Appelbaum, D. A., Horwitz, H., & Voth, T. J. Psychotherapy and psychoanalysis: Final report of the Menninger Foundation's psychotherapy research project. *Bulletin of the Menninger Clinic,* 1972, *36,* 1-276.

Kessler, D. R. & Glick, I. D. Brief family therapy. In R. B. Sloane & F. R. Staples (Eds.), *The psychiatric clinics of North America: Symposium on brief psychotherapy* (Vol. 2, No. 1). Philadelphia: Saunders, 1979.

Kiesler, D. J. Experimental designs in psychotherapy research. In A. E. Bergin & S. L. Garfield (Eds.), *Handbook of psychotherapy and behavior change.* New York: John Wiley, 1971.

Kingston, W. & Bentovim, A. Creating a focus for brief marital or family therapy. In S. H. Budman (Ed.), *Forms of brief therapy.* New York: Guilford Press, 1981.

Kiresuk, T. J. & Sherman, R. E. Goal attainment scaling: A general method for evaluating comprehensive community mental health programs. *Community Mental Health Journal,* 1968, *4,* 443-453.

Kirkner, F., Wisham, W., & Giedt, H. A report on the validity of the Rorschach prognosis rating scale. *Journal of Projective Techniques,* 1953, *17,* 465-470.

Kirstein, L., Prusoff, B., Weissman, M. M., & Dressler, D. M. Utilization review of treatment for suicide attempters. *American Journal of Psychiatry,* 1975, *132,* 22-27.

Kirstein, L., Weissman, M. M., & Prusoff, B. Utilization review and suicide attempts: Exploring discrepancies between experts' criteria and clinical practice. *Journal of Nervous and Mental Disease,* 1975, *160,* 49-55.

Klar, H., Frances, A., & Clarkin, J. F. Selection criteria for partial hospitalization. *Hospital and Community Psychiatry,* 1982, *33,* 929-933.

Klein, D. F., Gittelman, R., Quitkin, F., & Rifkin, A. *Diagnosis and drug treatment of psychiatric disorders.* Baltimore: Williams & Wilkins, 1980.

Kleinmuntz, B. An extension of the construct validity of the ego strength scale. *Journal of Consulting Psychology,* 1960, *24,* 463-464.

Klerman, G. L., Dimascio, A., & Weissman, M. Treatment of depression by drugs and psychotherapy. *American Journal of Psychiatry,* 1974, *131,* 186-191.

Klerman, G. L., Paykel, E. S., & Prusoff, B. A. Antidepressant drugs and clinical psychopathology. In J. Cole, A. Freeman, & A. Friedhoff (Eds.), *Psychopathology and psychopharmacology.* Baltimore: Johns Hopkins Press, 1973.

Klerman, G. L. & Weissman, M. M. Interpersonal psychotherapy: Theory and research. In A. J. Rush (Ed.), *Short-term psychotherapies for depression.* New York: Guilford Press, 1982.

Klopfer, B. & Kelley, D. M. *The Rorschach technique.* Yonkers, NY: World Book Co., 1942.

Klopfer, B., Kirkner, F., Wisham, W., & Baker, G. Rorschach prognostic rating scale. *Journal of Projective Techniques,* 1951, *15,* 425-428.

Kohlberg, L., LaCrosse, J., & Ricks, D. The predictability of adult mental health from childhood behavior. In B. Wolman (Ed.), *Manual of child psychopathology.* New York: McGraw-Hill, 1972.

Kohut, H. *The analysis of the self.* New York: International Universities Press, 1971.

Korchin, S. J. & Schuldberg, D. The future of clinical assessment. *American Psychologist,* 1981, *36,* 1147-1158.

Koss, M. P. Length of psychotherapy for clients seen in private practice. *Journal of Consulting and Clinical Psychology,* 1979, *47,* 210-212.

Kreisman, D. E., Simmens, S. J., & Joy, V. D. Rejecting the patient: Preliminary validation of a self-report scale. *Schizophrenia Bulletin,* 1979, *5,* 220-222.

Kupfer, D. J. & Detre, T. P. *The KDS-15 — A marital questionnaire.* University of Pittsburgh, PA: KDS Systems, 1974.

Langs, R. *The technique of psychoanalytic psychotherapy.* Vol. 1. New York: Jason Aronson, 1973, p. 215.

Langsley, D. G., Flomenhaft, K., & Machotka, P. Follow-up evaluation of family crisis therapy. *American Journal of Orthopsychiatry,* 1969, *39,* 753-759.

Langsley, D. G. & Kaplan, D. M. *The treatment of families in crisis.* New York: Grune & Stratton, 1968.

Langsley, D. G., Pittman, F. S., Machotka, P., & Flomenhaft, K. Family crisis therapy: Results and implications. *Family Process,* 1968, *7,* 145–158.

Lazare, A. (Ed.). *Outpatient psychiatry: Diagnosis and treatment.* Baltimore: Williams & Wilkins, 1979.

Lazare, A. & Eisenthal, S. A negotiated approach to the clinical encounter. In A. Lazare (Ed.), *Outpatient psychiatry: Diagnosis and treatment.* Baltimore: Williams & Wilkins, 1979.

Lazare, A., Eisenthal, S., & Frank, A. Disposition decisions in a walk-in clinic: Social and psychiatric variables. *American Journal of Orthopsychiatry,* 1976, *46,* 503–509.

Lazarus, A. A. New methods in psychotherapy: A case study. *South African Medical Journal,* 1958, *32,* 660–664.

Lazarus, A. A. The elimination of children's phobias by deconditioning. *South African Medical Proceedings,* 1959, *5,* 261–265.

Lazarus, A. A. Group therapy of phobic disorders by systematic desensitization. *Journal of Abnormal Social Psychology,* 1961, *63,* 504–510.

Lazarus, A. A. The results of behavior therapy in 126 cases of severe neurosis. *Behavior Research and Therapy,* 1973, *1,* 68–79.

Lazarus, A. A. & Rachman, S. The use of systematic desensitization in psychotherapy. *South African Medical Journal,* 1957, *31,* 934–937.

Leary, T. *Interpersonal diagnosis of personality.* New York: Ronald Press, 1957.

Leichter, G. Group psychotherapy of married couples' groups: Some characteristic treatment dynamics. *International Journal of Group Psychotherapy,* 1962, *12,* 154–163.

Levitz, L. S. & Stunkard, A. J. A therapeutic coalition for obesity: Behavior modification and patient self-help. *American Journal of Psychiatry,* 1974, *131,* 423–427.

Lewinsohn, P. M. & Arconad, M. Behavioral treatment of depression: A social learning approach. In J. F. Clarkin & H. I. Glazer (Eds.), *Depression: Behavioral and directive intervention strategies.* New York: Garland Press, 1981.

Lewinsohn, P. M., Biglan, T., & Zeiss, A. Behavioral treatment of depression. In P. Davidson (Ed.), *Behavioral management of anxiety, depression and pain.* New York: Brunner/Mazel, 1976.

Lidz, R. & Lidz, T. The family environment of schizophrenic patients. *American Journal of Psychiatry,* 1949, *106,* 332–345.

Lindemann, E. Symptomatology and management of acute grief. *American Journal of Psychiatry,* 1944, *101,* 141–148.

Linden, W. Examined outcome studies on phobia treatments. *Archives of General Psychiatry,* 1981, *38,* 769–775.

Linehan, M. M. A social-behavioral assessment of suicide and parasuicide: Implications for clinical assessment and treatment. In J. F. Clarkin & H. I. Glazer (Eds.), *Depression: Behavioral and directive intervention strategies.* New York: Garland Press, 1981.

Linn, M., Caffey, E., Klett, J., Hogarty, C., & Lamb, H. R. Day treatment and psychotropic drugs in the aftercare of schizophrenic patients. *Archives of General Psychiatry,* 1979, *36,* 1055–1056.

Lipsedge, M. S., Hajioff, J., Huggins, P., Napier, L., Pearce, J., Pike, D. J., & Rich, M. The management of severe agoraphobia: A comparison of iproniazid and systematic desensitization. *Psychopharmacologia,* 1973, *32,* 67–80.

Liss, R. & Frances, A. A court-mandated treatment: Dilemmas for hospital psychiatry. *American Journal of Psychiatry,* 1975, *132,* 924–927.

Loevinger, J., Wessler, R., & Redmore, C. *Measuring ego development* (2 vols.). San Francisco: Jossey-Bass, 1970.

Lorion, R. P. Patient and therapist variables in the treatment of low-income patients. *Psychological Bulletin,* 1974, *81,* 344–354.

Lorr, M. & McNair, D. M. Expansion of the interpersonal behavior circle. *Journal of Personality and Social Psychology,* 1965, *2,* 823–830.

Lorr, M., McNair, D., Michaux, W., & Raskin, A. Frequency of treatment and change in psychotherapy. *Journal of Abnormal and Social Psychology,* 1962, *64,* 281-292.

Luborsky, L., Chandler, M., Auerbach, A. H., Cohen, J., & Bachrach, H. M. Factors influencing the outcome of psychotherapy: A review of quantitative research. *Psychological Bulletin,* 1971, *75,* 145-185.

Luborsky, L., Mintz, J., Auerbach, A., Christoph, P., Bachrach, H., Todd, T., Johnson, M., Cohen, M., & O'Brien, C. P. Predicting the outcome of psychotherapy: Findings of the Penn Psychotherapy Project. *Archives of General Psychiatry,* 1980, *137,* 471-481.

Luborsky, L., Singer, B., & Luborsky, L. Comparative studies of psychotherapy. Is it true that "everyone has won and all must have prizes"? *Archives of General Psychiatry,* 1975, *132,* 995-1008.

MacKinnon, R. A. & Michels, R. *The psychiatric interview in clinical practice.* Philadelphia: W. B. Saunders, 1971.

Malan, D. H. *A study of brief psychotherapy.* New York: Plenum, 1963.

Malan, D. H. Science and psychotherapy. *International Journal of Psychiatry,* 1973, *11,* 87-90.

Malan, D. H. *The frontier of brief psychotherapy.* New York: Plenum, 1976.

Malan, D. H., Heath, E. S., Bacal, H. A., & Balfour, F. H. G. Psychodynamic changes in untreated neurotic patients: II. Apparently genuine improvements. *Archives of General Psychiatry,* 1975, *32,* 110-126.

Mann, J. *Time-limited psychotherapy.* Cambridge, MA: Harvard University Press, 1973.

Mann, J. J., Frances, A., & Kaplan, R. D. The relative efficacy of L-deprenyl, a selective monoamine oxidate type B inhibitor in endogenous and nonendogenous depression. *Journal of Clinical Psychopharmacology,* 1982, *2,* 54-57.

Marks, I. Behavioral psychotherapy of adult neurosis. In S. L. Garfield & A. E. Bergin (Eds.), *Handbook of psychotherapy and behavior change* (2nd ed.). New York: John Wiley, 1978.

Marks, P. A. & Seeman, W. *The actuarial description of abnormal personality.* Baltimore: Williams & Wilkins, 1963.

Martin, P. A. & Bird, H. W. An approach to the psychotherapy of marriage partners: The stereoscopic technique. *Psychiatry,* 1963, *161,* 123-127.

Masters, W. & Johnson, V. *Human sexual inadequacy.* Boston: Little, Brown, 1970.

Mathews, A. M., Johnston, D. W., Lancashire, M., Munby, D., Shawn, P. M., & Gelder, M. G. Imaginal flooding and exposure to real phobic situations: Treatment outcome with agoraphobic patients. *British Journal of Psychiatry,* 1976, *129,* 362-371.

Mathews, A. M., Johnston, D. W., Shaw, P. M., & Gelder, M. G. Process variables and the prediction of outcome in behavior therapy. *British Journal of Psychiatry,* 1974, *125,* 256-264.

Mattes, J. A., Rosen, B., & Klein, D. F. Comparison of the clinical effectiveness of "short" vs. "long" stay in a psychiatric hospital: II. Results of a three-year posthospital follow-up. *Journal of Nervous and Mental Disease,* 1977, *165,* 387-394.

Mattes, J. A., Rosen, B., Klein, D. F., & Millan, D. Comparison of the clinical effectiveness of "short" versus "long" stay psychiatric hospitalization. III. Further results of a three-year posthospital follow-up. *Journal of Nervous and Mental Disease,* 1977, *165,* 395-402.

May, P. R. A. *Treatment of schizophrenia.* New York: Science House, 1968.

May, P. R. A. Psychotherapy and ataraxic drugs. In A. E. Bergin and S. L. Garfield (Eds.), *Handbook of psychotherapy and behavior change.* New York: John Wiley, 1971.

May, P. R. A. Research in psychotherapy and psychoanalysis. *International Journal of Psychiatry,* 1973, *11,* 78-86.

May, P. R. A. & Tuma, A. H. The effect of psychotherapy and stelazine on length of hospital stay, release rate and supplemental treatment of schizophrenic patients. *Journal of Nervous and Mental Disease,* 1964, *139,* 362-369.

May, P. R. A. & Tuma, A. H. Treatment of schizophrenia. *British Journal of Psychiatry,* 1965, *3,* 503-510.

May, P. R. A., Tuma, A. H., & Dixon, W. J. Schizophrenia—A follow-up study of results of treatment. I. *Archives of General Psychiatry,* 1976, *33,* 474-478.

Mayadas, N. S. & Duehn, W. D. Stimulus-modeling (SM) videotape for marital counseling: Method and application. *Journal of Marriage and Family Counseling,* 1977, *3,* 35-42.

McCaffree, K. M. The cost of mental health care under changing treatment methods. *American Journal of Public Health,* 1966, *56,* 1013.

McKinley, J. C. & Hathaway, S. R. A multiphasic personality schedule (Minnesota). II. A differential study of hypochondriasis. *Journal of Psychology,* 1940, *10,* 255-268.

McKinley, J. C. & Hathaway, S. R. A multiphasic personality schedule (Minnesota). IV. Psychasthenia. *Journal of Applied Psychology,* 1942, *26,* 614-624.

McKinley, J. C. & Hathaway, S. R. The MMPI: V. Hysteria, hypomania and psychopathic deviate. *Journal of Applied Psychology,* 1944, *28,* 153-174.

McLean, P. Remediation of skills and performance deficits in depression: Clinical steps and research findings. In J. F. Clarkin & H. I. Glazer (Eds.), *Depression, behavioral and directive intervention strategies.* New York: Garland Press, 1981.

McNair, D. M. Comments on the Menninger project. In R. L. Spitzer & D. F. Klein (Eds.), *Evaluation of psychological therapies.* Baltimore: Johns Hopkins University Press, 1976.

Meehl, P. E. *Clinical versus statistical prediction.* Minneapolis: University of Minnesota Press, 1954.

Meehl, P. E. & Hathaway, S. R. The K factor as a suppressor variable in the MMPI. *Journal of Applied Psychology,* 1946, *30,* 525-564.

Meltzoff, J. & Blumenthal, R. L. *The day treatment center: Principles, application and evaluation.* Springfield, IL: Charles C Thomas, 1966.

Millon, T. *Millon multiaxial clinical inventory manual.* Minneapolis: National Computer Systems, 1977.

Millon, T. *Disorders of personality: DSM-III, Axis II.* New York: Wiley-Interscience, 1981.

Mindess, M. Predicting patient's response to psychotherapy: A preliminary study designed to investigate the validity of the Rorschach prognostic rating scale. *Journal of Projective Techniques,* 1953, *17,* 327-334.

Mink, O. G. & Isaksen, H. L. A comparison of the effectiveness of nondirective therapy and clinical counseling in the junior high school. *School Counsel,* 1959, *6,* 12-14.

Minuchin, S. *Families and family therapy.* Cambridge, MA: Harvard University Press, 1974.

Mischel, W. *Personality and assessment.* New York: John Wiley, 1968.

Mittelman, B. The concurrent analysis of married couples. *Psychoanalytic Quarterly,* 1948, *17,* 182-197.

Moreno, J. L. Interpersonal therapy and the psychopathology of interpersonality relations. *Sociometry,* 1937, *1,* 9.

Moreno, J. L. *Psychodrama.* New York: Beacon House, 1946.

Morgan, R., Luborsky, L., Crits-Christoph, P., Curtis, H., & Solomon, J. Predicting the outcomes of psychotherapy by the Penn Helping Alliance Rating method. *Archives of General Psychiatry,* 1982, *39,* 397-402.

Mosher, L. R. & Menn, A. Z. Lowered barrier in the community: The soteria model. In L. I. Stein & M. A. Test (Eds.), *Alternatives to mental health treatment.* New York: Plenum, 1978.

Muecke, L. N. & Krueger, D. W. Physical findings in psychiatric outpatient clinic. *American Journal of Psychiatry,* 1981, *9,* 1241-1242.

Muench, G. A. An investigation of the efficacy of time-limited psychotherapy. *Journal of Counseling Psychology,* 1965, *12,* 294-298.

Munro, J. N. & Bach, T. R. Effect of time-limited counseling on client change. *Journal of Counseling Psychology,* 1975, *22,* 395-398.

Murphy, J. G. & Datel, W. E. A cost-benefit analysis of community versus institutional living. *Hospital and Community Psychiatry,* 1976, *27,* 165.

Murray, H. A. & MacKinnon, D. W. Assessment of OSS personnel. *Journal of Consulting Psychology,* 1946, *10,* 76-80.

Myers, J. K., Lindenthal, J. J., & Pepper, M. P. Life events and psychiatric impairment. *Journal of Nervous and Mental Disease,* 1971, *152,* 149-157.

Newmark, C. S., Finkelstein, M., & Frerking, R. A. Comparison of the predictive validity of two measures of psychotherapy prognosis. *Journal of Personality Assessment,* 1974, *38,* 144–148.

Nobler, H. Group therapy with male homosexuals. *Comparative Group Studies,* 1972, *3,* 161–178.

Oberndorf, C. P. Folie à deux. *International Journal of Psychoanalysis,* 1934, *15,* 14–24.

O'Brien, C. P., Hamm, K. B., Ray, B. A., Pierce, J. F., Luborsky, L., & Mintz, J. Group vs. individual psychotherapy with schizophrenics: A controlled outcome study. *Archives of General Psychiatry,* 1972, *27,* 474–478.

Office of Technology Assessment. *The implications of cost-effectiveness analysis of medical technology. Background paper #3: The efficacy and cost effectiveness of psychotherapy.* Washington, D.C.: U.S. Government Printing Office, 1980.

Orlinsky, D. E. & Howard, K. I. The relation of process to outcome in psychotherapy. In S. L. Garfield & A. E. Bergin (Eds.), *Handbook of psychotherapy and behavior change: An empirical analysis* (2nd ed.). New York: John Wiley, 1978.

OSS Assessment Staff. *Assessment of men: Selection of personnel for the Office of Strategic Services.* New York: Holt, Rinehart & Winston, 1948.

Overall, J. E. & Gorham, D. R. The brief psychiatric rating scale. *Psychological Reports,* 1962, *10,* 799–812.

Parloff, M. B. Psychotherapy and research: An anaclitic depression. Frieda Fromm-Reichmann Memorial Lecture, Washington School of Psychiatry, April 1980.

Parloff, M. B. & Dies, R. R. Group psychotherapy outcome research 1966–1975. *International Journal of Group Psychotherapy,* 1977, *27,* 281–319.

Parloff, M. B., Wolfe, B., Hadley, S., & Waskow, I. *Assessment of psychosocial treatment of mental disorders: Current status and prospects.* Springfield, VA: National Technical Information Services, U.S. Dept. of Commerce, 1978.

Pasamanick, B., Scarpitti, F. R., & Dinitz, S. *Schizophrenics in the community: An experimental study in the prevention of hospitalization.* New York: Appleton-Century-Crofts, 1967.

Pascal, G. R. & Zax, M. Psychotherapeutics: Success or failure? *Journal of Consulting Psychology,* 1956, *20,* 325–331.

Paul, G. L., Tobias, L. L., & Holly, B. L. Maintenance psychotropic drugs in the presence of active treatment programs: A "triple-blind" withdrawal study. *Archives of General Psychiatry,* 1972, *27,* 106–115.

Paykel, E. S., Myers, J. K., Dienett, M. N., Klerman, G. L., Lindenthal, J. J., & Pepper, M. P. Life events and depression: A controlled study. *Archives of General Psychiatry,* 1969, *21,* 753–760.

Pendergrass, R. A. & Hodges, M. Deaf students in group problem-solving situations. *American Annals of the Deaf,* 1976, *121,* 327–330.

Perls, F. S. *Gestalt therapy verbatim.* LaFayette, CA: Real People Press, 1969.

Perls, F. S., Hefferline, R. F., & Goodman, P. *Gestalt therapy.* New York: Julian Press, 1951.

Perry, S., Frances, A., Klar, A., & Clarkin, J. Selection criteria for individual dynamic psychotherapies. *Psychiatric Quarterly,* in press.

Pittman, F., Langsley, D., & DeYoung, C. Work and school phobias: A family approach to treatment. *American Journal of Psychiatry,* 1968, *124,* 1535–1541.

Platt, S., Knights, A., & Hirsch, S. Caution and conservatism in the use of a psychiatric day hospital: Evidence from a project that failed. *Psychiatry Research,* 1980, *3,* 123–132.

Polak, P. R. & Kirby, M. W. A model to replace psychiatric hospitals. *Journal of Nervous and Mental Disease,* 1976, *162,* 13–22.

Powers, E. & Witmer, H. *An experiment in the prevention of delinquency.* New York: Columbia University Press, 1951.

Quay, H. The performance of hospitalized psychiatric patients on the ego-strength scale of the MMPI. *Journal of Clinical Psychology,* 1955, *11,* 403–405.

Rabkin, R. *Strategic psychotherapy.* New York: Basic Books, 1977.

Rahe, R. H. Life change measurement as a predictor of illness. *Proceedings of the Royal Society of Medicine,* 1968, *61,* 1124–1126.

Rahe, R. H. The pathway between subjects' recent life changes and their near future illness reports: Representative results and methodological issues. In B. S. Dohrenwend & B. P. Dohrenwend (Eds.), *Stressful life events: Their nature and effects.* New York: John Wiley, 1974.

Rahe, R. H. & Lind, E. Psychosocial factors and sudden cardiac death: A pilot study. *Journal of Psychosomatic Research,* 1971, *15,* 19.

Rapaport, D., Gill, M., & Schafer, R. *Diagnostic psychological testing.* In R. R. Holt (Rev. ed.). New York: International Universities Press, 1968.

Ravaris, C. L., Robinson, D. S., & Ives, J. O. Phenelzine and amitriptyline in the treatment of depression. *Archives of General Psychiatry,* 1980, *37,* 1075–1080.

Rehm, L. P. Assessment of depression. In M. Hersen & A. S. Bellack (Eds.), *Behavioral assessment: A practical handbook.* New York: Pergamon Press, 1976.

Rehm, L. P. A self-control therapy program for treatment of depression. In J. F. Clarkin & H. I. Glazer (Eds.), *Depression: Behavioral and directive intervention strategies.* New York: Garland Press, 1981.

Reid, W. H. *Treatment of the DSM-III psychiatric disorders.* New York: Brunner/Mazel, 1983.

Reid, W. J. & Schyne, A. W. *Brief and extended casework.* New York: Columbia University Press, 1969.

Riessman, C. K., Rabkin, J. G., & Struening, E. L. Brief versus standard psychiatric hospitalization: A critical review of the literature. *Community Mental Health Review,* 1977, *2,* 1–10.

Rittenhouse, J. D. Endurance of effect: Family-unit treatment compared to identified patient treatment. *Proceedings of the 78th Annual Convention of the American Psychological Association,* 1970, *2,* 535–536.

Rogers, C. R. *Counseling and psychotherapy.* Boston: Houghton Mifflin, 1942.

Rorschach, H. *Psychodiagnostics.* New York: Grune & Stratton, 1949 (originally published, 1921).

Rosen, A. Diagnostic differentiation as a construct validity indication for the MMPI ego strength scale. *Journal of General Psychology,* 1963, *69,* 65–68.

Rosenbaum, M., Friedlander, J., & Kaplan, S. Evaluation of results of psychotherapy. *Psychosomatic Medicine,* 1956, *18,* 113–132.

Rosenstock, I. M. Patient's compliance with health regimens. *Journal of the American Medical Association,* 1975, *234,* 402–403.

Rounsaville, B. J. & Chevron, E. Interpersonal psychotherapy: Clinical applications. In A. J. Rush (Ed.), *Short-term psychotherapies for depression.* New York: Guilford Press, 1982.

Rowan, P. R., Paykell, E. S., & Parker, R. R. Tricyclic antidepressant MAO inhibitors. Are there differential effects? In M. B. H. Youdim & E. S. Paykell (Eds.), *Monoamine oxidation inhibitors: The state of the art.* New York: John Wiley, 1981.

Rush, A. J., Beck, A. T., Kovacs, M., & Hollon, S. Comparative efficacy of cognitive therapy and pharmacotherapy in the treatment of depressed outpatients. *Cognitive Therapy and Research,* 1977, *1,* 17–37.

Rush, A. J., Khatami, M., & Beck, A. T. Cognitive and behavioral therapy in chronic depression. *Behavior Therapy,* 1975, *6,* 398–404.

Sadock, B. J. Group psychotherapy. In A. M. Freedman, H. I. Kaplan, & B. J. Sadock (Eds.), *Comprehensive textbook of psychiatry-II.* Baltimore: Williams & Wilkins, 1975.

Sandler, J., Holder, A., & Dave, C. *The patient and the analyst.* New York: International Universities Press, 1973.

Sarason, I. G., Johnson, I. H., & Siegel, J. M. Assessing the impact of life changes. In I. G. Sarason & G. D. Spielberger (Eds.), *Stress and anxiety* (Vol. 6). New York: John Wiley, 1979.

Satir, V. Conjoint marital therapy. In B. C. Greene (Ed.), *The psychotherapy of marital disharmony.* New York: The Free Press, 1965.

Schwager, E. & Spear, W. New perspective on psychological tests as measures of change. *Bulletin of the Menninger Clinic,* 1981, *45,* 527–541.

Schwartz, G. E. Integrating psychobiology and behavior therapy: A systems perspective.

In G. T. Wilson & C. M. Franks (Eds.), *Contemporary behavior therapy: Conceptual and empirical foundations.* New York: Guilford Press, 1982.

Shader, R. I., Grinspoon, L., Ewalt, J. R., & Zahn, D. A. Drug responses in schizophrenia. In D. V. S. Sankar (Ed.), *Schizophrenia: Current concepts and research.* Hicksville, NY: PJD Publications, 1969.

Shapiro, A. K. Placebo effects in medical and psychological therapies. In S. L. Garfield & A. E. Bergin (Eds.), *Handbook of psychotherapy and behavior change* (2nd ed.). New York: John Wiley, 1978.

Shapiro, A. K. & Morris, L. A. Placebo effects in medical and psychological therapies. In S. L. Garfield & A. E. Bergin (Eds.), *Handbook of psychotherapy and behavior change: An empirical analysis* (2nd ed.). New York: John Wiley, 1978.

Sheehan, D. V., Ballenger, J., & Jacobson, G. Relative efficacy of monoamine oxidase inhibitors and tricyclic antidepressants in the treatment of endogenous anxiety. In D. F. Klein & A. Rifkin (Eds.), *Anxiety: New research and changing concepts.* New York: Raven Press, 1981.

Sheehan, J. G., Frederick, C., Rosevear, W., & Spiegelman, M. A validity study of the Rorschach prognostic rating scale. *Journal of Projective Techniques,* 1954, *18,* 233–239.

Shlien, J. M. Time-limited psychotherapy: An experimental investigation of practical values and theoretical implications. *Journal of Counseling Psychology,* 1957, *4,* 318–322.

Shlien, J. M., Mosak, H. H., & Dreikurs, R. Effects of time limits: A comparison of two psychotherapies. *Journal of Counseling Psychology,* 1962, *9,* 31–34.

Sider, R. C. & Clements, C. Family or individual therapy: The ethics of modality choice. *American Journal of Psychiatry,* 1982, *139,* 1455–1458.

Siegel, N. H. Characteristics of patients in psychoanalysis. *Journal of Nervous and Mental Disease,* 1962, *135,* 155–158.

Sifneos, P. *Short-term psychotherapy and emotional crisis.* Cambridge, MA: Harvard University Press, 1972.

Singh, R. N. Brief interviews: Approaches, techniques and effectiveness. *Social Casework,* 1982, *37,* 599–606.

Skinner, B. F. *The behavior of organisms.* New York: Appleton-Century-Crofts, 1938.

Skinner, H. A. A model of psychopathology based on the MMPI. In C. S. Newmark (Ed.), *MMPI: Clinical and research trends.* New York: Praeger, 1979.

Slavson, S. R. & Schiffer, M. *Group psychotherapies for children.* New York: International Universities Press, 1975.

Sloane, R. B., Staples, F. R., Cristol, A. H., Yorkston, N. J., & Whipple, K. *Short-term analytically-oriented psychotherapy vs. behavioral therapy.* Cambridge, MA: Harvard University Press, 1975.

Smith, M. L., Glass, G. V., & Miller, T. I. *The benefits of psychotherapy.* Baltimore: Johns Hopkins University Press, 1980.

Smith, W. G., Kaplan, J., & Siker, D. Community mental health and the seriously disturbed patient: First admission outcomes. *Archives of General Psychiatry,* 1974, *30,* 693–696.

Sobell, M. B. & Sobell, L. C. *Behavioral treatment of alcohol problems.* New York: Plenum Press, 1978.

Solyon, L., Heseltine, G. F. D., McClure, D. J., Solyon, C., Ledridge, B., & Steinberg, G. Behavior therapy vs. drug therapy in the treatment of phobic neurosis. *Canadian Psychiatric Association Journal,* 1973, *18,* 25–31.

Speigel, D. E. SPI and MMPI predictors of psychopathology. *Journal of Projective Techniques and Personality Assessment,* 1969, *33,* 265–273.

Spielberger, C. D., Gorsuch, R. L., & Luchene, R. E. *Manual for the State-Trait Anxiety Inventory (self-evaluation questionnaire).* Palo Alto, CA: Consultant Psychologists Press, 1970.

Spitzer, R. L., Endicott, J., & Robins, E. *Research Diagnostic Criteria for a selected group of functional disorders.* New York: New York State Psychiatric Institute, 1978.

Stanton, M. D. & Todd, T. C. Structural family therapy with heroin addicts: Some outcome data. Paper presented at the Society for Psychotherapy Research, San Diego, June 1976.

Stein, L. I. & Test, M. A. Alternative to mental hospital treatment: I. Conceptual model, treatment program, and clinical evaluation. *Archives of General Psychiatry*, 1980, *37*, 392–397.

Strupp, H. H., Fox, R. E., & Lessler, K. *Patients view their psychotherapy*. Baltimore: Johns Hopkins Press, 1969.

Strupp, H. H., Hadley, S. W., & Gomes-Schwartz, R. *Psychotherapy for better or worse: An analysis of the problem of negative effects*. New York: Jason Aronson, 1977.

Stuart, R. B. *Marital and pre-counseling inventory*. Chicago: Research Press, 1978.

Stuart, R. B. *Helping couples change: A social learning approach to marital therapy*. New York: Guilford Press, 1980.

Stunkard, A. J. Adherence to medical treatment: Overview and lessons from behavioral weight control. *Journal of Psychosomatic Research*, 1981, *25*, 187–197.

Sugar, M. (Ed.). *The adolescent in group and family therapy*. New York: Brunner/Mazel, 1975.

Swartzburg, M. & Schwartz, A. A five-year study of brief hospitalization. *American Journal of Psychiatry*, 1976, *133*, 922–924.

Sweeney, J. & Clarkin, J. F. Current training and practice in psychological assessment: A survey of teaching hospitals. Unpublished manuscript, 1983.

Taft, R. The validity of the Barron ego strength scale and the Welsh anxiety index. *Journal of Consulting Psychology*, 1957, *21*, 247–249.

Talbott, J. A. The chronic mental patient. Problems, solutions and recommendations for a public policy. *American Psychiatric Association*, 1978. (a)

Talbott, J. A. *The death of the asylum*. New York: Grune & Stratton, 1978. (b)

Talbott, J. A. *The chronically mentally ill. Treatment programs, systems*. New York: Human Sciences Press, 1981.

Tamkin, A. S. An evaluation of the construct validity of Barron's ego strength scale. *Journal of Consulting Psychology*, 1957, *13*, 156–158.

Tamkin, A. S. & Klett, C. J. Barron's ego strength scale: A replication of an evaluation of its construct validity. *Journal of Consulting Psychology*, 1957, *21*, 412.

Targum, S. D. Neuroendocrine challenge studies in clinical psychiatry. *Psychiatric Annals*, 1983, *13*, 385–395.

Teasdale, J. D., Walsh, P. A., Lancashire, M., & Mathews, A. M. Group exposure for agoraphobics: A replication study. *British Journal of Psychiatry*, 1977, *130*, 186–193.

Ticho, E. A. Termination of psychoanalysis: Treatment goals, life goals. *Psychoanalytic Quarterly*, 1972, *41*, 315–333.

Uhlenhuth, E. H., Lipman, R. S., & Covi, L. Combined pharmacotherapy and psychotherapy: Controlled studies. *Journal of Nervous and Mental Disease*, 1969, *148*, 52–64.

Uhlenhuth, E. H. & Paykel, E. S. Symptom intensity and life events. *Archives of General Psychiatry*, 1973, *28*, 473–477.

Usdin, E., Davis, J. M., Glassman, A., Greenblatt, D., Perel, J. M., & Shader, R. (Eds.). *Clinical pharmacology in psychiatry*. New York: Elseries, 1981.

Van Slambrouck, S. Relation of structural parameters to treatment outcome. *Dissertation Abstracts International*, 1973, *33*, 5528.

Wallerstein, R. S. & Smelzer, N. J. Psychoanalysis and sociology: Articulations and applications. *International Journal of Psychoanalysis*, 1969, *50*, 693–710.

Warheit, G. L. Life events, coping stress, and depressive symptomatology. *American Journal of Psychiatry*, 1979, *136*, 502–507.

Warner, S. L. Criteria for involuntary hospitalization of psychiatric patients in a public hospital. *Mental Hygiene*, 1961, *45*, 122–128.

Warner, S. L., Fleming, B., & Bullock, S. The Philadelphia program for home psychiatric evaluations, precare and involuntary hospitalization. *American Journal of Public Health*, 1962, *52*, 29–38.

Washburn, S., Vannicelli, M., Longabaugh, R., & Scheff, B. J. A controlled comparison of psychiatric day treatment and inpatient hospitalization. *Journal of Consulting and Clinical Psychology*, 1976, *44*, 665–675.

Washburn, S. L., Vannicelli, M., & Scheff, B. J. Irrational determinants of the place of psychiatric treatment. *Hospital and Community Psychiatry*, 1976, *27*, 179–182.

Watson, J. P., Mullett, G. E., & Pillay, H. The effects of prolonged exposure to phobic situations upon agoraphobic patients treated in groups. *Behavior Research and Therapy,* 1973, *11,* 531.

Weakland, J., Fisch, R., Watzlawick, P., & Bodin, A. M. Brief therapy: Focused problem resolution. *Family Process,* 1974, *13,* 141–168.

Weber, J. J., Elinson, J., & Moss, L. M. The application of ego strength scales to psychoanalytic clinic records. In G. S. Goldman & D. Shapiro (Eds.), *Developments in psychoanalysis at Columbia University: Proceedings of the 20th Anniversary Conference.* New York: Columbia Psychoanalytic Clinic for Training and Research, 1965.

Wechsler, D. *Wechsler Adult Intelligence Scale—Revised.* New York: The Psychological Corp., 1981.

Weisbrod, B. A. Guide to benefit cost analysis, as seen through a controlled experiment in treating the mentally ill (Discussion paper 559-79). Madison, WI: Institute for Research on Poverty, University of Wisconsin, 1979.

Weiss, K. J. & Dubin, W. R. Partial hospitalization: State of the art. *Hospital and Community Psychiatry,* 1982, *33,* 923–927.

Weiss, R. L. Contracts, cognitions and change: A behavioral approach to marital therapy. *The Counseling Psychologist,* 1975, *5,* 15–26.

Weiss, R. L. & Jacobson, N. S. Behavioral marital therapy as brief therapy. In S. H. Budman (Ed.), *Forms of brief therapy.* New York: Guilford Press, 1981.

Weissman, M. M., Prusoff, B. A., Thompson, W. D., Harding, P. S., & Myers, J. K. Social adjustment by self-report in a community sample and in psychiatric outpatients. *Journal of Nervous and Mental Disease,* 1978, *166,* 317.

Weldon, E., Clarkin, J., Hennessy, J., & Frances, A. Day hospital versus outpatient treatment: A controlled study. *Psychiatric Quarterly,* 1979, *51,* 144–150.

Weldon, E. & Frances, A. The day hospital: Structure and functions. *Psychiatric Quarterly,* 1977, *49,* 338–342.

Welsh, G. S. An anxiety index and an internalization ratio for the MMPI. *Journal of Consulting Psychology,* 1952, *16,* 65–72.

Wender, P. H. Vicious and virtuous circles: The role of deviation amplifying feedback. In H. Barten (Ed.), *The origin and perpetuation of behavior in brief therapies.* New York: Behavioral Publications, 1971.

Whittington, H. G. *Psychiatry in the American community.* New York: International Universities Press, 1966.

Wiggins, J. S. Substantive dimensions of self-report in the MMPI item pool. *Psychological Monographs,* 1966, *80* (22, Whole No. 630).

Wiggins, J. S. *Personality and prediction: Principles of personality assessment.* Reading, MA: Addison-Wesley, 1973.

Wiggins, J. S. Circumplex models of interpersonal behavior in clinical psychology. In P. C. Kendall & J. N. Butcher (Eds.), *Handbook of research methods in clinical psychology.* New York: John Wiley, 1982.

Wilder, J. F., Levin, G., & Zwerling, I. A two-year follow-up evaluation of acute psychotic patients treated in a day hospital. *American Journal of Psychiatry,* 1966, *122,* 1095–1101.

Wilson, G. T. Behavior therapy as a short-term therapeutic approach. In S. H. Budman (Ed.), *Forms of brief therapy.* New York: Guilford Press, 1981.

Winnicott, D. W. *The maturational processes and the facilitating environment.* New York: International Universities Press, 1965.

Wolpe, J. *Psychotherapy by reciprocal inhibition.* Stanford, CA: Stanford University Press, 1958.

Wolpe, J. & Lang, P. A fear survey schedule for use in behavior therapy. *Behavior Research and Therapy,* 1964, *2,* 27–30.

Woody, G. E., Luborsky, L., McLellan, A. T., O'Brien, C. P., Beck, A. T., Blaine, J., Herman, J., & Hole, A. Psychotherapy for opiate addicts: Does it help? *Archives of General Psychiatry,* 1983, *40,* 620–625.

Wynne, L. C., Gurman, A., Ravich, R., & Boszormenyi-Nagy, I. The family and marital therapies. In J. M. Lewis & G. Usdin (Eds.), *Treatment planning in psychiatry.* Washington: American Psychiatric Association, 1982.

Wynne, L., Ryckoff, I. M., Day, J., & Hirsch, S. I. Pseudo-mutuality in the family relations of schizophrenics. *Psychiatry,* 1958, *21,* 205–220.

Yablonsky, L. *The tunnel back: Synanon.* New York: Macmillan, 1965.

Yager, J. Psychiatric eclecticism: A cognitive view. *American Journal of Psychiatry,* 1977, *134,* 736–741.

Yalom, I. D. *The theory and practice of group psychotherapy,* 2nd. edition. New York: Basic Books, 1975.

Yalom, I. D. & Greaves, C. Group therapy with the terminally ill. *American Journal of Psychiatry,* 1977, *134,* 396–400.

Zirkle, G. A. Five-minute psychotherapy. *American Journal of Psychiatry,* 1961, *118,* 544–546.

Zitrin, C. M., Klein, D. F., Lindemann, C., Tobak, P., Rock, M., Kaplan, J. H., & Ganz, V. H. Comparisons of short-term treatment regimens in phobic patients. In R. L. Spitzer and D. F. Klein (Eds.), *Evaluation of psychological therapies.* Baltimore: Johns Hopkins University Press, 1976.

Name Index

Subject Index

389

Medication, psychotropic *(continued)*
  overdosing, 185–186
  psychotherapy combined with, 33–34,
    195, 197, 198, 199, 200–210, 269
  selection of, 180–183
  side effects, 182, 184, 185, 190, 191,
    199
Memory loss, with ECT, 188
Menninger Clinic study (Menninger Psy-
    chotherapy Research Project), 144–
    145, 170, 223, 348
Meta-analysis method, 90–91, 143–144,
    172, 204–205, 235, 268–269
Millon Multiaxial Clinical Inventory
    (MMCI), 346
Minnesota Multi-Phasic Personality In-
    ventory (MMPI), 327, 329, 333,
    336–337 (Table 10-1), 343–346
Monoamine Oxidase (MAO) inhibitors,
    179, 185–187, 194
Motivation, patient
  lack of, 72–73, 79, 234–235
  and outcome, 256, 257
  treatment duration and, 172

National Institute of Mental Health, xx
Negative therapeutic outcome, 218
Negative therapeutic reaction, 218–220
Negotiation, in treatment, 168–169, 292–
    295, 317–318
"No treatment" recommendation, 213–
    248

Operant conditioning, 122–123
Orientation, treatment. *See also* Thera-
    peutic technique
  directive, 96, 104, 117–131
  experiential, 96, 104, 132–139
  exploratory, 96, 104, 105–117
Outcome research, xix, 170–175, 249–
    276, 353–354
  analysis of data variables in, 276
  bias in, 252, 254, 259
  contamination of, 261
  control groups in, 252, 259, 260
  designs of, 253–265, 270–271
  "ideal study," 270–276
  interpreting, 265–269
  limitations of, 250–253
  meta-analysis method, 90–91, 143–144,
    172, 204–205, 235, 268–269
  outcome measures in, 275–276
  patient variables in, 271–272
  "placebo" in, 252–253, 260, 271
  process measures in, 274–275
  on therapeutic technique, 139–145

  therapist/treatment variables in, 273–
    274
Outpatient care, 2, 17, 47. *See also* Day
    treatment programs
  for maintenance, 42, 43
  for rehabilitation, 26, 28

Paradoxical techniques, 128, 218
Pathology, patient, and outcome, 256,
    257
Patient(s)
  analog, 272
  borderline (*see* Borderline patients)
  as "customer," 293, 294–295
  depressed (*see* Depression)
  education of, in consultation process,
    290–292, 312–317
  and environment, 329, 330
  healthy, in crisis, 236–238
  iatrogenically infantilized, 232–233
  identified, 296
  intelligence of, 342–343
  with minor, chronic problems, 238–239
  motivation of, 72–73, 79, 172, 234–235,
    256, 257
  oppositional, 240
  role induction of, 295, 318–319, 325
  schizophrenic (*see* Schizophrenia)
  spontaneous improvement in, 217
    (Table 7-1), 236–240
Patient role, 61, 68, 134. *See also* Thera-
    pist-patient relationship
Payne Whitney Clinic (New York Hos-
    pital), x, xvi, 353
  evaluation form, 283, 320–323
Peer review manuals, xxii, xxiv
Penn Psychotherapy Project, 350
Pharmacotherapy. *See* Medication
Phenothiazines, 179, 183, 189, 210
Phobias, 110–111, 131, 203. *See also*
    Agoraphobia
Placebo effect, 178–179, 201, 252–253
Polypharmacy, 181, 197, 200
Positive reinforcement, 121–124, 131
Presenting problems, 281–282, 301–303
Primary gain, 223, 224
Privacy, in therapy, 73, 78. *See also* Con-
    fidentiality
Problem-solving techniques, 126–129,
    131
Process, treatment, 258–259, 274–275
Promethazine, 179
Psychoanalysis, 66, 105–112, 115, 156–
    157, 161–162, 295
  analyst role in, 108–109
  contraindications for, 110, 115